SECOND EDITION

SITE-SPECIFIC CANCER SERIES

Head and Neck Cancer

Edited by

Raymond Scarpa, DNP, APNC, AOCN®, and Margaret Hickey, RN, MSN, MS

Oncology Nursing Society
Pittsburgh, Pennsylvania

ONS Publications Department
Publisher and Director of Publications: William A. Tony, BA, CQIA
Managing Editor: Lisa M. George, BA
Assistant Managing Editor: Amy Nicoletti, BA, JD
Acquisitions Editor: John Zaphyr, BA, MEd
Copy Editors: Vanessa Kattouf, BA, Andrew Petyak, BA
Graphic Designer: Dany Sjoen
Editorial Assistant: Judy Holmes

Library of Congress Cataloging-in-Publication Data

Names: Scarpa, Raymond J., editor. | Hickey, Margaret (Margaret M.), editor.
  | Oncology Nursing Society, issuing body.
Title: Head and neck cancer / edited by Raymond Scarpa and Margaret Hickey.
Other titles: Head and neck cancer (Oncology Nursing Society) | Site-specific
  cancer series.
Description: 2nd edition. | Pittsburgh, Pennsylvania : Oncology Nursing
  Society, [2015] | Series: Site-specific cancer series | Includes
  bibliographical references and index.
Identifiers: LCCN 2015026345 | ISBN 9781935864639
Subjects: | MESH: Head and Neck Neoplasms--nursing.
Classification: LCC RC280.H4 | NLM WY 156 | DDC 616.99/491--dc23 LC record available at http://lccn.loc.gov/2015026345

Publisher's Note

This book is published by the Oncology Nursing Society (ONS). ONS neither represents nor guarantees that the practices described herein will, if followed, ensure safe and effective patient care. The recommendations contained in this book reflect ONS's judgment regarding the state of general knowledge and practice in the field as of the date of publication. The recommendations may not be appropriate for use in all circumstances. Those who use this book should make their own determinations regarding specific safe and appropriate patient care practices, taking into account the personnel, equipment, and practices available at the hospital or other facility at which they are located. The editors and publisher cannot be held responsible for any liability incurred as a consequence from the use or application of any of the contents of this book. Figures and tables are used as examples only. They are not meant to be all-inclusive, nor do they represent endorsement of any particular institution by ONS. Mention of specific products and opinions related to those products do not indicate or imply endorsement by ONS. Websites mentioned are provided for information only; the hosts are responsible for their own content and availability. Unless otherwise indicated, dollar amounts reflect U.S. dollars.

ONS publications are originally published in English. Publishers wishing to translate ONS publications must contact ONS about licensing arrangements. ONS publications cannot be translated without obtaining written permission from ONS. (Individual tables and figures that are reprinted or adapted require additional permission from the original source.) Because translations from English may not always be accurate or precise, ONS disclaims any responsibility for inaccuracies in words or meaning that may occur as a result of the translation. Readers relying on precise information should check the original English version.

Printed in the United States of America

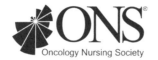

Innovation • Excellence • Advocacy

Contributors

Editors

Raymond Scarpa, DNP, APNC, AOCN®
Advanced Practice Nurse
Department of Otolaryngology/Head and Neck Surgery
University Hospital
Newark, New Jersey
Chapter 1. Overview; Chapter 6. Surgical Management;
Chapter 11. Nursing Research

Margaret Hickey, RN, MSN, MS
Senior Director, Global Patient Advocacy
Novartis Oncology
East Hanover, New Jersey
Chapter 1. Overview; Chapter 3. Pathophysiology

Authors

Cheryl A. Brandt, RN, ACNS-BC, CORLN
Clinical Nurse Specialist
Certified Otorhinolaryngology Nurse
Ear, Nose and Throat Institute
University Hospitals Case Medical Center
Cleveland, Ohio
Chapter 9. Postoperative Management

Cindy J. Dawson, RN, MSN, CORLN
Director, Clinical Functions, Ambulatory Nursing
Department of Nursing and Patient Care Services
University of Iowa Hospitals and Clinics
Iowa City, Iowa
Chapter 5. Patient Assessment

Tara DiFabio, RN, CNP, CORLN
Head and Neck Oncology Nurse Practitioner
Department of Otolaryngology—Head and Neck Surgery
Thomas Jefferson University
Philadelphia, Pennsylvania
Chapter 9. Postoperative Management

Michele Farrington, BSN, RN, CPHON®
Clinical Healthcare Research Associate
Nursing Research, Evidence-Based Practice, and Quality
 and Ambulatory Nursing
University of Iowa Hospitals and Clinics
Iowa City, Iowa
Chapter 4. Prevention and Early Detection

Penelope Stevens Fisher, MS, RN, CORLN
Clinical Instructor of Otolaryngology
Advanced Practice Nurse
Department of Otolaryngology
Division of Head and Neck Surgery
University of Miami
Miami, Florida
Chapter 10. Survivorship

David Anthony (Tony) Forrester, PhD, RN, ANEF, FAAN
Professor, Division of Nursing Science
Rutgers University School of Nursing
Newark, New Jersey
Clinical Professor, Department of Environmental and Occupational Medicine
Rutgers Robert Wood Johnson Medical School
New Brunswick, New Jersey
Chapter 11. Nursing Research

Catherine Jansen, PhD, RN, CNS, AOCNS®
Oncology Clinical Nurse Specialist
Kaiser Permanente Medical Center
San Francisco, California
Chapter 8. Chemotherapy

Joanne Lester, PhD, CNP, AOCN®
Clinical Research Nurse Practitioner
Division of Surgical Oncology
The Ohio State University
Columbus, Ohio
Chapter 6. Surgical Management

Joan Such Lockhart, PhD, RN, CORLN, AOCN®, CNE, ANEF, FAAN
Clinical Professor and MSN Nursing Education Specialty Coordinator
Duquesne University School of Nursing
Pittsburgh, Pennsylvania
Chapter 2. Anatomy and Physiology

Dorothy N. Pierce, DNP, APN-C
Advanced Practice Nurse
Rutgers Cancer Institute of New Jersey
New Brunswick, New Jersey
Chapter 7. Radiation Therapy

Lenore K. Resick, PhD, CRNP, FNP-BC, FAANP, FAAN
Professor Emerita
Duquesne University School of Nursing
Pittsburgh, Pennsylvania
Chapter 2. Anatomy and Physiology

Nancy Roehnelt, PhD, ARNP
Nurse Practitioner
Department of Head, Neck and Endocrine Oncology
Moffitt Cancer Center
Tampa, Florida
Chapter 3. Pathophysiology

Helen Lazio Stegall, BSN, RN, CORLN
Nurse Manager
Department of Otolaryngology—Head and Neck Surgery
University of Iowa Hospitals and Clinics
Iowa City, Iowa
Chapter 4. Prevention and Early Detection

Disclosure

Editors and authors of books and guidelines provided by the Oncology Nursing Society are expected to disclose to the readers any significant financial interest or other relationships with the manufacturer(s) of any commercial products.

A vested interest may be considered to exist if a contributor is affiliated with or has a financial interest in commercial organizations that may have a direct or indirect interest in the subject matter. A "financial interest" may include, but is not limited to, being a shareholder in the organization; being an employee of the commercial organization; serving on an organization's speakers bureau; or receiving research funding from the organization. An "affiliation" may be holding a position on an advisory board or some other role of benefit to the commercial organization. Vested interest statements appear in the front matter for each publication.

Contributors are expected to disclose any unlabeled or investigational use of products discussed in their content. This information is acknowledged solely for the information of the readers.

The contributors provided the following disclosure and vested interest information:

David Anthony (Tony) Forrester, PhD, RN, ANEF, FAAN: Sigma Theta Tau International, Nurse Faculty Leadership Academy, honoraria

Joanne Lester, PhD, CNP, AOCN®: National Comprehensive Cancer Network, research funding; Oncology Nursing Society, other remuneration

Lenore K. Resick, PhD, CRNP, FNP-BC, FAANP, FAAN: National Nursing Centers Consortium, leadership position; Duquesne University, research funding

Contents

Preface

Patients with head and neck cancer are faced with unique and challenging lifestyle changes when confronted with this devastating diagnosis. They will also experience psychological, physiologic, and societal challenges. No other type of malignancy exists that is so visible to the public eye. Patients need to consider complex and sometimes disfiguring treatment options that include surgery, radiation, and/or chemotherapy, and facial and body disfigurements often cannot be concealed. The disease process, along with treatment sequelae, can cause profound dysfunctions in the ability to swallow, breathe, eat, sleep, and communicate, thus affecting basic survival needs. Therefore, a multidisciplinary approach to the care and management of individuals diagnosed with head and neck cancer is necessary for successful outcomes.

Healthcare providers need to be aware of the specific challenges that this patient population experiences. The text in this publication has been updated from the first edition of *Site-Specific Cancer Series: Head and Neck Cancer* with the intent to offer the most current information needed to advocate and care for people with this diagnosis, as well as recommend treatment options and side effect management. This edition has also been updated to include the implications for prevention and detection along with the genetic drivers of head and neck cancer as the carcinogenic process is explored. Patient assessment skills and tools will assist nurses with patient interactions. The advances in surgical interventions are addressed with a discussion on minimally invasive techniques, the use of robotics, and a personalized approach to surgical intervention, with special considerations specific to the geriatric population. New chemotherapeutic agents and the ongoing research with epidermal growth factor receptors and monoclonal antibodies are also examined in this edition. Advances in radiation therapy are discussed with special attention to radiogenomics and the continued development of proton and neutron therapy. Living and surviving with head and neck cancer presents individuals with many challenges and key components of survivorship, and these topics have been addressed. Current nursing research findings in head and neck cancer are summarized, and future directions for nursing research are identified as well.

We thank and acknowledge the passion and commitment of nurses who work with patients with head and neck cancer and their families. It is our hope that this book will serve as a valuable resource. We hope that empowering nurses with knowledge and awareness of the burden of this disease on patients and families, prevention and detection measures, and treatment options and their sequelae will help to achieve the optimal outcomes that patients with head and neck cancer deserve.

CHAPTER 1

Overview

Raymond Scarpa, DNP, APNC, AOCN®, and
Margaret Hickey, RN, MSN, MS

Introduction

Head and neck cancer is often a devastating and debilitating cancer. Although other populations of patients with cancer sustain similar morbidity with treatment, the unique physiologic and psychosocial needs of patients with head and neck cancer often are magnified by the facial disfigurement and multiple sensorimotor functional impairments.

Head and neck carcinoma denotes a malignant process that originates in the upper aerodigestive tract. This area includes the lips, oral and nasal cavities, paranasal sinuses, pharynx, and larynx. It also comprises malignancies found in the salivary, thyroid, and parathyroid glands (Scarpa, 2014). About 90% of tumors found in the upper aerodigestive tract are pathologic squamous cell carcinomas (Rousseau & Badoual, 2011). Other pathologic findings more common in salivary tissue include mucoepidermoid carcinomas, adenocarcinomas, and adenoid cystic carcinomas. Common thyroid carcinomas include papillary, medullary, and anaplastic cell types (American Cancer Society [ACS], 2014c).

According to ACS (2014b), head and neck cancers account for about 3% of all cancers in the United States, with rates twice as high for men than for women. ACS estimates approximately 39,500 new cases of cancer of the oral cavity and pharyngeal carcinomas in 2015 (ACS, 2014b). This is a decrease of approximately 27,000 new cases compared to data recorded in 2005. Incidence rates from 2006 to 2010 were unchanged in men and had decreased by 0.9% annually in women (ACS, 2014a). It is important to note, however, that incidence rates are increasing for cancers in the oral cavity including the oropharynx. This is related to human papillomavirus (HPV) infection. From 2006 to 2010, death rates from oral cancer decreased annually by 1.2% in men and 2.1% in women (ACS, 2014a).

Head and neck cancer is considered to be one of the most debilitating cancers. These malignancies affect basic survival needs (e.g., breathing, eating, communicating) and result in considerable cosmetic and functional deficiencies associated with treatment modalities such as surgery, radiation therapy, and chemotherapy.

Risk Factors

Risk factors for head and neck cancers that originate in the oral cavity and larynx are associated with the combined use of tobacco in any form (e.g., cigarettes, cigars, pipes, chewing tobacco) and alcohol (Turati et al., 2013). The carcinogens found in tobacco products are prone to have a synergistic effect when combined with alcohol, increasing the risk of developing this type of malignancy (Allam, Zhang, Zheng, Gregory, & Windsor, 2011). Other risk factors may include exposure to wood dust, nickel, nitrogen mustard, and asbestos.

Current research has shown a strong link between HPV and oral cancer (Chaturvedi et al., 2011; Jayaprakash, 2011). HPV is a very common sexually transmitted infection in both men and women. About 79 million people are currently infected with this virus, and 14 million are newly infected each year in the United States (Satterwhite et al., 2013). Of more than 150 different HPV strains, about 40 are transmitted through sexual contact. The most common of these HPV strains are types 16 and 18 (Dunne et al., 2014).

Malignant tumors can arise in salivary and endocrine glands in the head and neck region as a result of radiation exposure. This exposure can come from diagnostic procedures or from previous radiation therapy. Inhalation of wood or nickel dust increases the risk of malignancies developing in the nasal cavity and paranasal sinuses. Infection from the Epstein-Barr virus, exposure to wood dust, and ingestion of certain preservatives or dried, salted foods are associated with an increased risk of nasopharyngeal carcinomas (MedicineNet.com, 2014).

The U.S. Surgeon General recently reported that "very large disparities in tobacco use remain across groups defined by race, ethnicity, educational level, and socioeconomic status and across regions of the country" (U.S. Department of Health and Human Services, 2014). This may account for disparities in the risk of head and neck cancers as well. Few studies address the issue of race and the incidence of head and neck cancers. A Surveillance, Epidemiology, and End Results (SEER) database analysis from 1973 to 2001 found an increased incidence of oral and pharyngeal carcinoma among young Caucasians compared with young African Americans. However, conflicting yet smaller studies report higher incidences for African Americans (Blair, 2014). Cancers of the larynx and hypopharynx seem to be more frequent among African Americans and Caucasians than among Asians and Latinos (ACS, 2014a).

Cancer Staging

Patients with head and neck cancer most often present with complaints of a lump or mass, otalgia, dysphagia, voice change, or oral pain. Cervical adenopathy may be present. A workup will include a biopsy or needle aspiration of any suspicious area. Once a malignant diagnosis has been established, additional workup may include a computed tomography scan, positron-emission tomography scan, magnetic resonance imaging scan, or ultrasound. These radiographic studies are done to determine the extent of disease and if any distant metastatic disease is present. The tumor is staged, specific to the primary site, using the data obtained from the biopsy or needle aspiration and radiographic data according to the American Joint Committee on Cancer tumor-node-metastasis staging system. This system gives healthcare professionals a common language to use when describing a malignant process (American Joint Committee on Cancer, 2015). The healthcare provider recommends a treatment plan once the stage is determined (Scarpa, 2009).

Treatment Modalities

Surgery remains the oldest and most successful treatment for malignancies in the head and neck region. Outcomes are determined by disease stage, functional and cosmetic impairments, and the experience of a multidisciplinary team. Advances in surgical techniques, such as robotic-assisted surgery and endoscopic approaches, have led to improved functional outcomes. Radiation and chemotherapy play an important role in adjuvant treatment. Recent advances in radiation therapy, along with the development of new biologic agents and targeted therapies, have improved survival and functional results. In some early-stage carcinomas, radiation therapy may be used alone or in combination with chemo-

therapy. The combination of two or more treatment modalities may be necessary for advanced-stage tumors (Scarpa, 2014).

Summary

For patients with head and neck malignancies, advanced surgical techniques combined with conservative treatment approaches are leading to more favorable outcomes with improved function, cosmetic outcomes, and symptom management. However, caring for these patients continues to present tremendous nursing challenges in all practice settings. Oncology nurses play a critical role in coordinating patient care and providing appropriate interventions and patient education.

The authors would like to acknowledge Mary Jo Dropkin, PhD, RN, and Linda K. Clarke, MS, RN, CORLN, for their contributions to this chapter that remain unchanged from the first edition of this book.

References

Allam, E., Zhang, W., Zheng, C., Gregory, R.L., & Windsor, J.L. (2011). Smoking and oral health. In D. Bernhard (Ed.), *Cigarette smoke toxicity: Linking individual chemicals to human diseases* (pp. 257–280). Hoboken, NJ: John Wiley & Sons.

American Cancer Society. (2014a). Laryngeal and hypopharyngeal cancers. Retrieved from http://www.cancer.org/acs/groups/cid/documents/webcontent/003108-pdf.pdf

American Cancer Society. (2014b). Oral cavity and oropharyngeal cancer. Retrieved from http://www.cancer.org/acs/groups/cid/documents/webcontent/003128-pdf.pdf

American Cancer Society. (2014c). Salivary gland cancer. Retrieved from http://www.cancer.org/acs/groups/cid/documents/webcontent/003137-pdf.pdf

American Joint Committee on Cancer. (2015). What is cancer staging? Retrieved from http://cancerstaging.org/references-tools/Pages/What-is-Cancer-Staging.aspx

Blair, E.A. (2014). Head and neck carcinoma in the young patient. Retrieved from http://emedicine.medscape.com/article/855871-overview

Chaturvedi, A.K., Engels, E.A., Pfeiffer, R.M., Hernandez, B.Y., Xiao, W., Kim, E., … Gillison, M.L. (2011). Human papillomavirus and rising oropharyngeal cancer incidence in the United States. *Journal of Clinical Oncology, 29*, 4294–4301. doi:10.1200/JCO.2011.36.4596

Dunne, E.F., Markowitz, L.E., Saraiya, M., Stokley, S., Middleman, A., Unger, E.R., … Iskander, J. (2014). CDC grand rounds: Reducing the burden of HPV-associated cancer and disease. Retrieved from http://www.cdc.gov/mmwr/preview/mmwrhtml/mm6304a1.htm?s_cid

Jayaprakash, V., Reid, M., Hatton, E., Merzianu, M., Rigual, N., Marshall, J., … Sullivan, M. (2011). Human papillomavirus types 16 and 18 in epithelial dysplasia of oral cavity and oropharynx: A meta-analysis, 1985–2010. *Oral Oncology, 47*, 1048–1054. doi:10.1016/j.oraloncology.2011.07.009

MedicineNet.com. (2014). How common are head and neck cancers? Retrieved from http://www.medicinenet.com/head_and_neck_cancer/page3.htm

Rousseau, A., & Badoual, C. (2011). Head and neck: Squamous cell carcinoma: An overview. *Atlas of Genetics and Cytogenetics in Oncology and Haematology.* Retrieved from http://atlasgeneticsoncology.org//Tumors/Head NeckSCCID5090.html

Satterwhite, C.L., Torrone, E., Meites, E., Dunne, E.F., Mahajan, R., Ocfemia, M.C., ... Weinstock, H. (2013). Sexually transmitted infections among U.S. women and men: Prevalence and incidence estimates, 2008. *Sexually Transmitted Diseases, 40,* 187–193. doi:10.1097/OLQ.0b013e318286bb53

Scarpa, R. (2009). Surgical management of head and neck carcinoma. *Seminars in Oncology Nursing, 25,* 172–182. doi:10.1016/j.soncn.2009.05.007

Scarpa, R. (2014). Surgical care of head and neck cancers. In G.W. Davidson, J.L. Lester, & M. Routt (Eds.), *Surgical oncology nursing* (pp. 65–78). Pittsburgh, PA: Oncology Nursing Society.

Turati, F., Garavello, W., Tramacere, I., Pelucchi, C., Galeone, C., Bagnardi, V., ... Negri, E. (2013). A meta-analysis of alcohol drinking and oral and pharyngeal cancers: Results from subgroup analyses. *Alcohol and Alcoholism, 48,* 107–118. doi:10.1093/alcalc/ags100

U.S. Department of Health and Human Services. (2014). *The health consequences of smoking—50 years of progress: A report of the Surgeon General, 2014.* Retrieved from http://www.surgeongeneral.gov/library/reports/50-years-of-progress

CHAPTER 2

Anatomy and Physiology

Joan Such Lockhart, PhD, RN, CORLN, AOCN®, CNE, ANEF, FAAN, and
Lenore K. Resick, PhD, CRNP, FNP-BC, FAANP, FAAN

Introduction

This chapter provides an overview of head and neck anatomy and physiology. It will focus on the ear, sinonasal area, oral cavity, pharynx, larynx, and structures in the neck, ear, and throat. Head and neck cancer and its medical and surgical treatments often alter the structure of these anatomic features and impact their associated functions: hearing, balance, smelling, tasting, breathing, mastication, swallowing, and speaking. Assessing these changes is essential in developing an appropriate care plan and optimal patient outcomes.

Ear

The ear consists of three anatomic regions: the external ear, the middle ear, and the inner ear (see Figure 2-1). The external ear is the visible portion and extends inward to the lateral surface of the tympanic membrane. It consists of two major structures, the auricle (pinna) and the external auditory canal, which also is known as the acoustic meatus. The auricle houses several landmark structures: the helix, tragus, antitragus, and lobule. The external auditory canal is located near the temporomandibular joint anteriorly and the parotid gland inferiorly.

The auricle and external auditory canal direct sound waves toward the tympanic membrane. The length and shape of the canal and the direction of hair follicles lining the canal protect the tympanic membrane and middle ear from trauma and foreign bodies (VanPutte et al., 2014). The external ear canal of children curves upward and is shorter than that of adults (Isaacson, 2014).

The cartilaginous outer lateral region of the ear canal is covered with thick skin. The bony two-thirds of the inner medial region is lined with thin skin and is very sensitive to pain. The outer lateral aspect of the ear canal contains hair follicles and glands that contribute to the formation of cerumen. Lymph drainage from the external auditory canal flows anteriorly to the preauricular lymph nodes, interiorly to the deep upper cervical nodes, and posteriorly to the lymph nodes in the mastoid region.

The middle ear is an air-filled space located in the temporal bone of the head. The tympanic membrane, a translucent, pearly gray membrane, marks the end of the external auditory canal and the beginning of the middle ear. When sound waves from the environment reach the tympanic membrane, the membrane vibrates, transmitting these vibrations to the three small bones of the middle ear: the malleus, incus, and stapes (Bickley, 2013). These vibrations cause the stapes to move at the oval window of the inner ear, resulting in vibration of the oval window that causes movement of fluids in the inner ear.

For the tympanic membrane to vibrate, the atmospheric pressure both inside and outside the ear must be equal. The eustachian tube, which extends from the middle ear into the nasopharynx, equalizes the atmospheric pressure. It permits air to flow to or from the middle ear, allowing the air pressure of the environment to equal that of the middle ear.

The inner ear contains the facial nerve (cranial nerve VII) and the neuroreceptor organs responsible for balance and hearing. Both balance and hearing are transmitted to the brain by the acoustic (vestibulocochlear) nerve (cranial nerve VIII), which has vestibular and cochlear divisions. *Vestibular* refers to the inner ear, and the vestibule of the ear is responsible for equilibrium. *Cochlear* refers to the cochlea of the inner ear and is responsible for hearing. The structures of the inner ear lie within the protective cavity of the temporal bone.

Nose and Paranasal Sinuses

The nose consists of an outer portion and an inner portion (see Figure 2-2). The framework of the nose consists of nasal bones and portions of the superior maxillary bone. Cartilage comprises the upper and lateral portions of the nose and

Figure 2-1. External, Middle, and Inner Ear

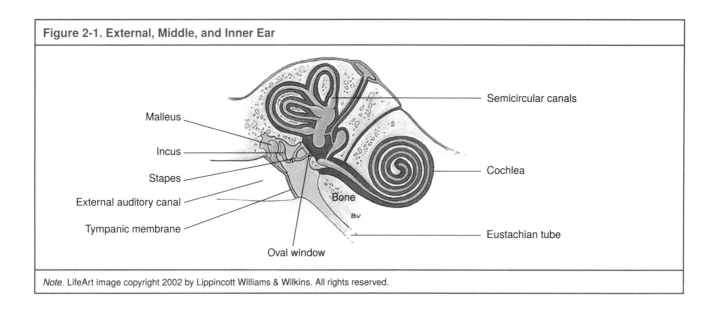

Malleus

Incus

Stapes

External auditory canal

Tympanic membrane

Oval window

Semicircular canals

Cochlea

Bone

Eustachian tube

Figure 2-2. Anatomic Structures of the External Nose

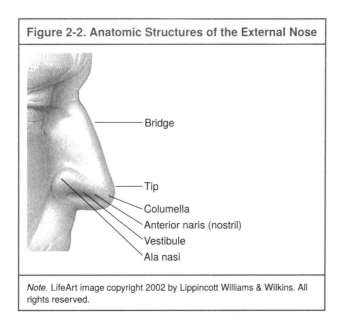

Bridge

Tip

Columella

Anterior naris (nostril)

Vestibule

Ala nasi

the nasal septum. This bony and cartilaginous structure makes up the nasal cavities. The nasal cavities open anteriorly by two pear-shaped nares (nostrils) and posteriorly through openings into the nasopharynx. Soft tissue and skin cover the outside of the nose. The region that is slightly dilated and lies just inside the nose is the nasal vestibule. The vestibule extends into the tip of the nose.

Olfactory and respiratory regions comprise the areas above and behind the nasal vestibule. The frontal sinus, sphenoid sinus, and cribriform plate make up the supralateral boundary of the nose. Inside the nose, the nasal cavity is divided by the nasal septum into two chambers and consists of the vestibule, septum, roof, floor, cribriform, and turbinates (lateral walls) (see Figure 2-3).

The nose receives an extensive blood supply from several branches of the internal and external carotid arteries: the posterior ethmoid arteries, posterior septal nasal arteries, major palatine artery, anterior ethmoid artery, and septal branch of the superior labial artery. Several smaller arteries join together to form a network of vessels on the nasal septum in the anterior portion of the nose called the Kiesselbach plexus or Little area (Marieb, 2015).

The nose protects the lungs by filtering, warming, and moisturizing the air that is inhaled. As air passes through the nasal cavities, it is warmed and moistened by the surfaces of the nasal turbinates and nasal septum. The inhaled air is filtered by coarse hairs (vibrissae) in the nasal mucosa and by precipitation of particles on the turbinates (Marieb, 2015; Zhao & Dalton, 2007).

The nose contains the olfactory nerve (cranial nerve I) endings and serves as the peripheral organ involved in the sense of smell, which also augments the sense of taste. The olfactory receptors lie within the olfactory membrane located high in the nose and originate from the central nervous system.

The paranasal sinuses are named after the skull bones in which they are located: the frontal, ethmoid, maxillary, and sphenoid sinuses (see Figure 2-4). Each sinus is paired. These four sets of air-filled sinuses are lined with ciliated respiratory mucosa, which contain mucus-producing cells. The mucosal lining of all the paranasal sinuses is continuous with that of the mucosa of the nasal cavity.

The paranasal sinuses serve several functions. They protect the brain against frontal trauma by absorbing shock and providing insulation. They help to humidify and warm inhaled air by adding to the surface area of the olfactory membrane. The sinuses also play a role with voice resonance and are thought to aid in the growth of the face without

Figure 2-3. Cross-Sectional View of the Anatomic Structures of the Nose and Nasopharynx

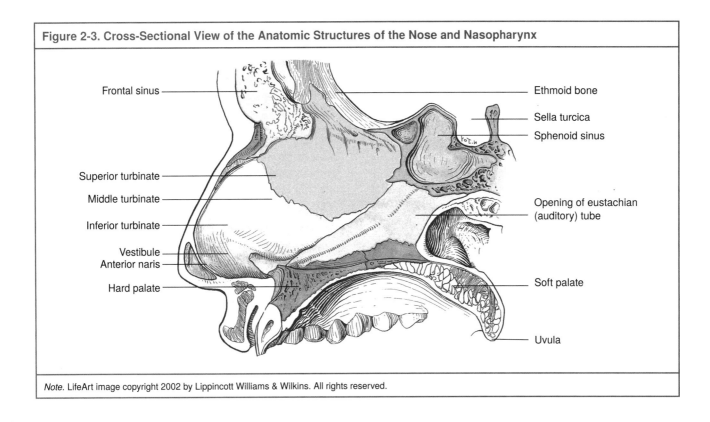

Figure 2-4. Paranasal Sinuses, Anterior View of the Skull and Right Lateral View of the Skull

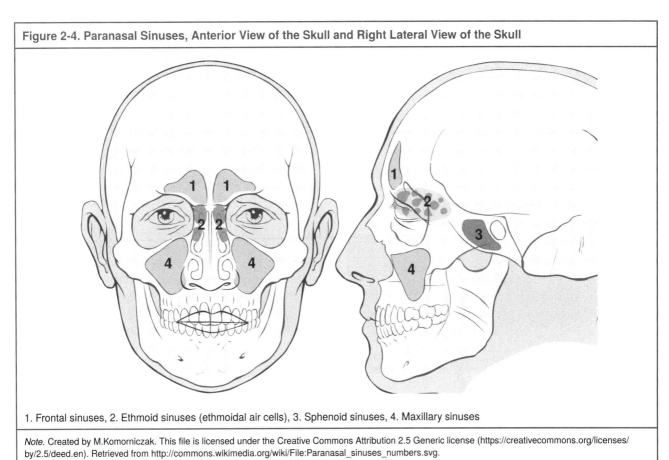

1. Frontal sinuses, 2. Ethmoid sinuses (ethmoidal air cells), 3. Sphenoid sinuses, 4. Maxillary sinuses

adding to the weight of the skull bones (Dalgorf & Harvey, 2013).

Oral Cavity and Salivary Glands

The mouth consists of two parts: the vestibule and the oral cavity (see Figure 2-5). The vestibule is the narrow space that is bordered on the outside by the lips and cheeks and on the inside by the gingivae (gums) and teeth. The oral cavity is surrounded at its anterior and lateral sides by the alveolar arches, teeth, and gingivae and on its posterior side by the oropharynx. The palate borders the oral cavity superiorly, and most of the tongue's base forms the oral cavity's inferior border, or the floor of the mouth. The oral cavity is lined with simple, moist columnar epithelium that is continuous with the lining of the oropharynx. The floor of the mouth is extremely vascular.

The oral cavity contains several structures that play a key role in respiration, mastication, swallowing, and speech production. Structures in the mouth that are key to these functions include the lips, cheeks, buccal mucosa, teeth, gingivae, tongue, hard palate, and soft palate. The mouth also houses the openings of ducts that connect with the salivary glands.

The anatomy housed in the upper portion of the digestive and respiratory tracts discussed throughout this chapter is referred to as the aerodigestive tract (National Cancer Institute, n.d.). This tract is lined with mucous membranes composed of epithelial cells, basement membranes that help these cells attach to their underlying tissue, connective tissue, and occasionally smooth muscle cells (VanPutte et al., 2014). Through mitosis (cell division), epithelial cells are able to replace themselves and regenerate.

Epithelial cells are generally classified according to their number of layers and shape (VanPutte et al., 2014). Many epithelial cells in the aerodigestive tract have more than one layer (stratified) but differ in shape. For example, nonkeratinized (moist) stratified squamous epithelial cells line the mouth, throat, larynx, and esophagus and protect their underlying structures from injury that may occur through abrasion or friction (VanPutte et al., 2014). The larynx is protected by its ciliated stratified columnar epithelium, while pseudostratified columnar epithelial cells that secrete mucus are housed in the pharynx and trachea.

Lips, Cheeks, and Buccal Mucosa

Both the lips and cheeks are constructed of skeletal muscle covered with skin. The orbicularis oris muscle encircles the mouth and forms the bulk of the superior and inferior lips. The buccinator muscles form the bulk of the cheeks and insert into the maxilla and mandible. Externally, the lips appear as dark or reddened areas that are distinctly different in color from the facial skin that surrounds them. This coloring results from capillary blood that shows through the translucent epithelium covering of the lips. A visible margin called the vermilion cutaneous line separates this dark region of the lips from the face. Receptors help the lips to sense both the texture and temperature of food or objects with which they come into contact.

Inside the oral cavity, stratified squamous nonkeratinized epithelium lines the oral surface of the lips, cheeks, and floor of the mouth. A small extension of mucous membrane lining, the labial frenulum, joins the inside of each lip with the mouth lining. The inside portion of the cheeks is referred to as the buccal mucosa. In addition to the buccinator muscles, these lateral walls contain adipose tissue, areolar tissue, blood vessels, and glands that secrete mucus. The space that forms a trough between the lips, cheeks, and teeth is called the vestibule.

The lips close to keep food and fluid in the oral cavity during mastication. The cheeks and buccal mucosa help to control the location of food while it is between the teeth and in the oral cavity and secure the food as the teeth break and grind it into smaller pieces. During speech, the lips help with articulation. Both the lips and cheeks contribute to the animation of the face as it changes expressions for different actions (e.g., kissing, smiling, frowning) through the facial nerve (cranial nerve VII). The trigeminal nerve (cranial nerve V) allows for the jaw to clench as it provides the motor supply to the temporal and masseter muscles. The trigeminal nerve also permits the jaw to move laterally (Marieb, 2015).

Teeth and Gingiva

The teeth are positioned in alveoli, or sockets, located within the processes of the maxilla and mandible. These alve-

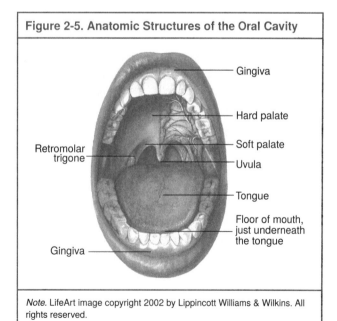

Figure 2-5. Anatomic Structures of the Oral Cavity

Gingiva

Hard palate

Soft palate

Uvula

Retromolar trigone

Tongue

Floor of mouth, just underneath the tongue

Gingiva

olar ridges are covered by gingivae, dense fibrous connective tissue layered with stratified squamous epithelium. The teeth are held firmly in place by periodontal ligaments and cementum, a bone-like substance produced by the periodontal membrane that lines the alveoli. The teeth are innervated by branches of the trigeminal nerve (cranial nerve V), specifically the superior and inferior alveolar nerves. Branches of the maxillary artery, the superior and inferior alveolar arteries, supply blood to the teeth.

The cutting, tearing, grinding, and crushing abilities of the teeth make them instrumental during mastication. This mechanical action of the teeth turns large bites of food into small pieces that can be mixed readily with saliva, broken down by digestive enzymes, and easily swallowed. The teeth also play an important role in the articulation of various sounds during speech.

The trigeminal nerve (cranial nerve V) comprises three branches that together supply somatic motor or proprioceptive and cutaneous sensory innervation to and from the face and jaw: ophthalmic (V1), maxillary (V2), and mandibular (V3) (VanPutte et al., 2014). The ophthalmic and maxillary nerves are only sensory in nature. The ophthalmic branch innervates the scalp, forehead, nose, upper eyelid, and cornea. The maxillary nerve supplies the maxillary teeth, palate, and gingiva. Conversely, the mandibular nerve has both sensory and motor functions that innervate the lowest region of the face and jaw. It supplies sensation to the mandibular teeth, tongue, and gingiva and supplies movement and proprioception to the muscles involved in chewing (mastication), as well as to the soft palate, throat, and middle ear (VanPutte et al., 2014).

Tongue

The tongue extends from its anterior tip, or apex, which is visible through the opening of the oral cavity, to its posterior attachment, or base, in the oropharynx. The tongue occupies most of the oral cavity. The anterior two-thirds of the tongue is attached by its undersurface to the floor of the mouth by a fold of mucous membrane called the lingual frenulum. The posterior one-third of the tongue continues toward the oropharynx, where it is attached by mucous membranes (see Figure 2-6).

The tongue itself is a large muscular structure constructed of interlocking skeletal fibers. The dorsal surface of the tongue is covered with three types of papillae that are small extensions of the tongue's mucosa: fungiform, filiform, and circumvallate. Fungiform papillae contain the receptors for taste, called taste buds. Filiform papillae lack taste buds but provide the tongue with a rough surface that assists with eating and chewing. A third type of papillae, circumvallate papillae, is positioned directly in front of the sulcus terminalis near the back of the tongue and contains taste buds. The remaining dorsal surface of the posterior tongue lacks papillae but contains a few taste buds as well as a mass of lymph

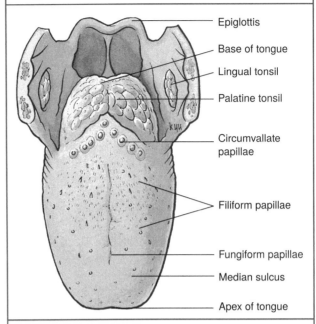

Figure 2-6. Surface View of the Dorsal Surface of the Tongue

- Epiglottis
- Base of tongue
- Lingual tonsil
- Palatine tonsil
- Circumvallate papillae
- Filiform papillae
- Fungiform papillae
- Median sulcus
- Apex of tongue

tissue called the lingual tonsil. The ventral side, or undersurface, of the tongue has a relatively smooth appearance. Wharton ducts of the submandibular glands bring saliva into the oral cavity in this area, near the lingual frenulum.

The tongue also plays a significant role in communication. The mobility of the tongue provides articulation and facilitates pronunciation of words, specifically consonants such as *D*, *K*, and *T*.

An overview of the swallowing process illustrates the important role that the tongue plays in mastication and the initial voluntary phase of swallowing. Swallowing (deglutition) involves three phases: voluntary, pharyngeal, and esophageal (VanPutte et al., 2014). As food enters the mouth in the voluntary phase, the tongue positions the food and allows it to be chewed and broken down into smaller particles by the teeth. The tongue moves its position within the mouth and changes its shape to allow food particles to mix with saliva. The taste buds provide the many sensations associated with eating. The facial nerve (cranial nerve VII) provides taste sensation to the anterior two-thirds of the tongue (salty, sweet, sour, and bitter), whereas the glossopharyngeal nerve (cranial nerve IX) provides these taste sensations to the posterior tongue (Bickley, 2013). The tongue actively moves the chewed bolus of food toward the oropharynx to be swallowed. To do this, the tongue elevates within the mouth and contracts against the hard palate, pushing the food toward the back of the pharynx.

The second pharyngeal phase of swallowing involves the soft palate elevating and closing off the nasopharynx (Van-Putte et al., 2014). Both the pharynx and the larynx elevate as the pharyngeal muscles constrict, pushing the bolus of food through the pharynx downward toward the esophagus. The opening of the larynx is protected as the vestibular and vocal folds expand medially, and the epiglottis shields the larynx from the food entering it. The pharyngeal constrictor muscles contract, while the upper esophageal sphincter relaxes and allows the bolus to reach the esophagus. In the last esophageal phase of swallowing, peristaltic contractions of the esophagus move the food bolus from the pharynx toward the stomach, where the digestion process continues (VanPutte et al., 2014).

Hard and Soft Palates

The palate forms the roof of the mouth (see Figure 2-5). The entire palate consists of two continuous portions, the anterior hard palate and the posterior soft palate. The uvula, a small piece of tissue hanging inferiorly from the midline edge of the soft palate, easily can locate the soft palate.

A thick layer of rough mucosa covers the hard palate, which is marked by a midline ridge (palatine raphe). The soft palate connects to the tongue and oropharyngeal wall by two vertical pairs of folds, the anterior and posterior pillars. These folds, the soft palate, and the uvula together form an arch above and posterior to the tongue. The opening of this arch is referred to as the fauces. The palatine tonsils lie in the fossae between the anterior and posterior pillars.

Like the tongue, the hard and soft palates play an important role in mastication, swallowing, and speech production. The hard palate provides a firm, rough surface against which the tongue can move food particles as they gradually mix with saliva. The soft palate moves upward and closes the entrance to the nasopharynx. This action prevents food and fluids from entering the nasopharynx during swallowing. The movement of the soft palate is considered an involuntary reflex action rather than a voluntary conscious movement, as with the tongue. As food moves into the oropharynx, the soft palate returns to its resting position, allowing normal respiration to resume.

Salivary Glands

Three major pairs of salivary glands exist: parotid, submandibular (submaxillary), and sublingual. The main purpose of these glands is to produce saliva, with the submandibular glands secreting the majority (i.e., more than two-thirds). Each set of glands has its specific lymphatic network that drains into lymph nodes in the head and neck region. The salivary glands produce an average of 1–1.5 liters of saliva each day (VanPutte et al., 2014).

The parotid glands are the largest pair of salivary glands, located superficially behind the mandible and directly below and anterior to the ears. Branches of the facial nerve (cranial nerve VII) divide the parotid gland into a superficial lobe and a deep lobe, connected by tissue referred to as the isthmus. The superficial lobe is larger than the deep lobe. Stensen ducts drain saliva from the parotid glands and open into the oral mucosa in the vestibule, next to the second upper molars.

The submandibular (submaxillary) glands are the second largest salivary glands, located near the inner surface of the mandible. Wharton ducts carry saliva to the mouth and open on the floor of the mouth on either side of the frenulum.

The sublingual glands are the smallest pair of salivary glands. They are located under the mucosa of the floor of the mouth under the tongue and anterior to the submandibular glands. The sublingual glands contain approximately 10–12 ducts that drain saliva into the floor of the mouth (Seeley, Stephens, & Tate, 2002).

The parotid and submandibular glands produce the majority (90%) of the body's saliva (Seeley et al., 2002). Saliva consists of several substances, including electrolytes, amylase, proteins such as mucin, lysozyme, immunoglobulin A, and waste products from the body's metabolism (Marieb, 2015). These substances not only aid with digestion and prevent tooth decay but also protect the body against invading microorganisms.

Saliva helps individuals accomplish several key processes, such as digestion, taste, swallowing, and speech. In addition to these functions, saliva also protects the oral structures against invasion by microorganisms. Saliva assists with digestion through the enzyme amylase, which breaks down ingested carbohydrates into maltose. As a person chews food, chemicals in the food become dissolved in the saliva. This process enables the taste buds in the fungiform papillae of the tongue to sense various tastes. Saliva moistens the food particles and allows them to adhere together to form a bolus. This bolus then moves toward the pharynx to be swallowed. Because saliva acts as a lubricant in the mouth, it also facilitates the production of speech. Moistened with saliva, the tongue, lips, and teeth can move freely within the oral cavity so that words can be pronounced (Andresen et al., 2008).

Pharynx

The pharynx is a funnel-shaped passageway that connects the nasal cavity with the larynx and the mouth with the esophagus (see Figure 2-7). The superior end of the pharynx begins at the base of the skull and extends downward for approximately 12 cm (4.7 in.) to the level of the larynx near the sixth cervical vertebra (Logan, Reynolds, & Hutchings, 2010).

The pharynx consists anatomically of three primary regions: the nasopharynx, oropharynx, and laryngopharynx (hypopharynx). Each of these regions contains vital structures that play an important role in breathing, swallowing, and speaking.

Figure 2-7. Midsagittal Section of the Head and Neck, Showing the Structures of the Upper Respiratory Tract

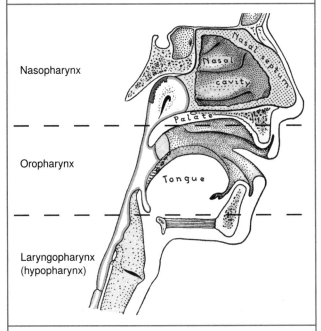

Nasopharynx

Oropharynx

Laryngopharynx (hypopharynx)

The pharynx serves several purposes related to breathing and swallowing. Except for its most superior region, the nasopharynx (which transports air), the pharynx is a common pathway for air, food, and fluids. As a person inspires air through the nose or mouth, it travels downward through the pharynx. As air travels to the lungs, it passes through the larynx, trachea, and right and left bronchi. When a person ingests food or fluids through the mouth, the pharynx channels the food bolus downward through the esophagus toward the stomach. Unlike in the mouth, no digestion takes place in the pharynx. The muscles of the pharynx assist with sound production and speech by changing the shape of the pharynx.

Nasopharynx

The most superior portion of the pharynx, the nasopharynx, is located behind the nose and nasal cavity and in front of the sphenoid bone. The nasopharynx starts at the base of the skull inferior to the sphenoid bone and extends downward to the lower border of the soft palate. The lining of the nasopharynx is continuous with that of the nose and nasal cavity. The pseudostratified columnar epithelium lining of the nasopharynx contains cilia that assist with removal of mucus and secretions.

Because the nasopharynx is located above the mouth, it serves as a passageway for the transport of air but not food.

During the swallowing process, the inferior opening of the nasopharynx is sealed off by the upward movement of the soft palate and uvula. This protective mechanism prevents food from entering the nasopharynx during swallowing.

The nasopharynx houses two important structures: the pharyngeal tonsils and the openings of the auditory (pharyngotympanic, or eustachian) tubes. Each of these structures is paired. The pharyngeal tonsils, commonly referred to as adenoids when enlarged, are clumps of lymphoid tissue positioned high on the posterior wall of the nasopharynx behind the nasal cavity.

Oropharynx

The oropharynx, the middle segment of the pharynx, starts at the inferior end of the nasopharynx. The oropharynx lies behind the oral cavity and is continuous with it. The oropharynx extends superiorly from the soft palate and extends downward to the upper border of the epiglottis. Unlike the nasopharynx, the oropharynx serves as a passageway for both air and food.

The lining of the oropharynx differs from that of the nasopharynx. Its stratified squamous epithelial lining helps to protect the oropharynx from mechanical and chemical irritation caused by food and fluids that come into contact with it during swallowing.

The oropharynx houses two additional tonsils: the palatine and lingual tonsils. The pair of palatine tonsils is embedded in the lateral mucosal walls between the two sets of arches in the oral cavity and is larger in size than the adenoids. The lingual tonsil is not paired and covers the base of the tongue. Combined, these tonsils in the oropharynx and the pharyngeal tonsils of the nasopharynx form a circle of lymphatic tissue called the Waldeyer ring that serves as an initial line of defense against pathogens that enter the pharynx (Andresen et al., 2008).

Laryngopharynx (Hypopharynx)

The third segment of the pharynx is the laryngopharynx, or hypopharynx, located behind the epiglottis and extending from the level of the hyoid bone to the lower edge of the cricoid cartilage of the larynx, level with the sixth cervical vertebra. The laryngopharynx is located behind the larynx and partially encircles it on either side. Like the oropharynx, the laryngopharynx is a common passageway for both food and air. These two pathways separate at the level of the larynx. Food and fluids travel from the laryngopharynx through the esophagus to the stomach. Air passes through the structures of the larynx downward through the trachea, bronchi, and lungs. This movement of air is delayed to permit swallowing to occur.

The laryngopharynx consists of pharyngeal walls, the pyriform sinuses, and the postcricoid area. The pyriform sinus is a space located on each side of the thyroid cartilage in the larynx. The laryngopharynx is continuous with the oropharynx superiorly and esophagus inferiorly. The stratified squamous epithelium lining of the laryngopharynx is similar to that of the oropharynx. The laryngopharynx also has a rich supply of lymphatics.

The larynx connects the pharynx with the trachea. The larynx lies between the fourth and sixth cervical vertebrae and is approximately 5 cm (2 in.) long (Marieb, 2015). The larynx is attached from the hyoid bone at the level of the third cervical vertebra superiorly, opens into the laryngopharynx, and is continuous with the trachea inferiorly.

The larynx serves important functions related to breathing, swallowing, and speech production. First, cartilages of the larynx keep the airway open so that air exchange can occur during respiration. Second, the larynx prevents aspiration of food, fluids, and saliva during swallowing through the protective actions of the epiglottis and vocal cords. The larynx enables the cough reflex and Valsalva maneuver (bearing down against a closed glottis) to occur. Third, the larynx aids with phonation by creating sounds through vibrations of the vocal cords.

The hyoid bone lies just above the larynx at the level of the third cervical vertebra but is not considered part of the larynx. It is attached to the larynx by muscles and membranes and supports the base of the tongue (see Figure 2-8).

The larynx is composed of a framework of nine cartilages, three that are single (unpaired) and six that are paired. The single cartilages of the larynx are the thyroid cartilage, the cricoid cartilage, and the epiglottis. The thyroid cartilage lies at the level of the fourth and fifth cervical vertebrae and is shaped like a shield. The thyroid cartilage is commonly referred to as the Adam's apple because of its midline laryngeal prominence that often is evident on a person's neck. The angle of this prominence is more obvious in males than in females because of sex hormones secreted in males during adolescence.

The cricoid cartilage lies directly beneath the thyroid cartilage at the level of the sixth cervical vertebra and is shaped like a signet ring, with the band (arch) at the front and the stone (lamina) at the back of the larynx. The cricoid is the only cartilage that entirely encircles the larynx. This thick cartilage is one of the most important of all laryngeal cartilages and provides the base for many laryngeal functions. The cricoid cartilage marks the beginning of the trachea.

The leaf-shaped epiglottis is attached to the anterior edge of the thyroid cartilage and extends superiorly to the back portion of the tongue. During swallowing, the larynx moves upward and the epiglottis tips over the larynx to shield the opening. This action of the epiglottis prevents food, fluids, and saliva from entering the larynx. If food or fluids enter the larynx, the cough reflex initiates to help the body expel the substance. During quiet respiration, the superior flap of the

Figure 2-8. Anterior View of the Larynx

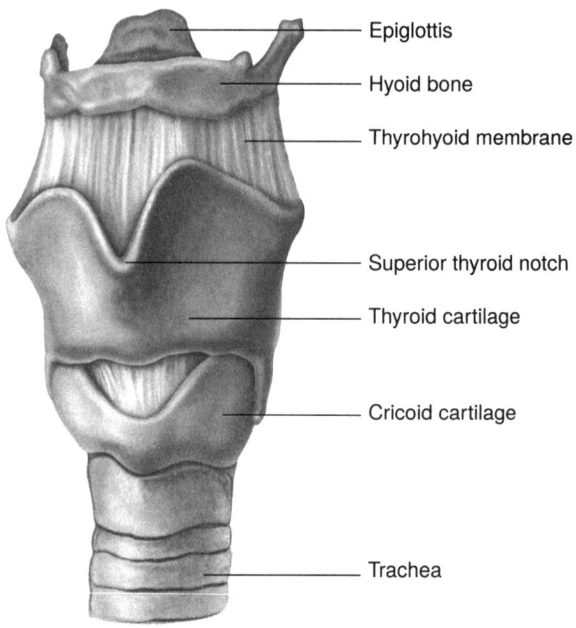

- Epiglottis
- Hyoid bone
- Thyrohyoid membrane
- Superior thyroid notch
- Thyroid cartilage
- Cricoid cartilage
- Trachea

epiglottis extends upward, allowing air to pass freely through the larynx.

Three smaller sets of paired cartilages—the arytenoid, cuneiform, and corniculate cartilages—comprise a portion of the lateral and posterior laryngeal walls. Two pairs of ligaments stretch from the anterior side of the arytenoid cartilage to the posterior surface of the thyroid cartilage. The most superior pair of ligaments are the false vocal cords, or the vestibular folds. The false vocal cords do not play a direct role in sound production but help to protect the airway.

The inferior pair of ligaments, two V-shaped bands of elastic tissue, form the true vocal cords. These vocal cords lie directly beneath the thyroid cartilage and above the cricoid cartilage. The space between the vocal cords is referred to as the glottis. During quiet breathing, the vocal cords remain apart to permit the flow of air to and from the lungs through the glottis. The vocal cords are the primary structures responsible for protecting the airway. They act as a sphincter muscle and close during the pharyngeal phase of swallowing. When air passes this area, they vibrate, producing a sound. Recognizable speech is produced when this sound is formed into words by the lips and tongue.

The true vocal cords come together to allow a person to perform a Valsalva maneuver, in which expired air is forced against a closed glottis, mouth, or nose. This maneuver is useful in a variety of everyday activities, such as lifting heavy objects or having a bowel movement. The vagus nerve (cranial nerve X) provides the motor supply to the palate, pharynx, and larynx, as well as sensation to the pharynx and larynx.

The larynx anatomically consists of three regions that are referred to in the classification and clinical treatment plan of laryngeal tumors; superior to inferior, they are the supraglottis, glottis, and subglottis. The most superior segment of the larynx, the supraglottic region, extends from the epiglottis superiorly downward to the level of the true vocal cords. This area has a rich blood and lymphatic supply. The second segment of the larynx is the glottic region, which consists mainly of the true vocal cords. This region has a sparse blood and lymphatic supply. The third segment of the larynx, the subglottic region, starts just below the true vocal cords and extends inferiorly to the lower border of the cricoid cartilage. This region contains a rich lymphatic supply.

The lining of the larynx is continuous with that of the pharynx. The larynx is lined with pseudostratified ciliated columnar epithelium that helps to remove both mucus and debris. Stratified squamous epithelium covers both the false and true vocal cords.

The larynx receives its blood supply from the laryngeal and cricothyroid arteries, branches of the external carotid, and common carotid arteries. The laryngeal and thyroid veins drain blood from the head and neck and return it to the heart via the internal jugular vein. The larynx receives most of its motor and sensory supply from the recurrent laryngeal nerve and the superior laryngeal nerves.

Trachea

The trachea is a 10–12 cm (4–4.8 in.) tube approximately 2.5 cm (1 in.) in diameter (Marieb, 2015) that lies anterior to the esophagus and connects the larynx at the cricoid cartilage with both mainstem bronchi and lungs. The walls of the trachea are supported with C-shaped hyaline cartilages.

Esophagus

The esophagus is a 25 cm (10 in.) tube that lies behind the trachea and connects the pharynx with the stomach (Marieb, 2015). The muscular walls of the esophagus remain collapsed unless peristalsis moves food toward the stomach. Unlike in the oral cavity, no digestion of food occurs in the esophagus.

General Head and Neck Anatomy and Physiology

Skull and Facial Bones

The human skull consists of 22 bones—8 cranial bones and 14 facial bones (Marieb, 2015). The uppermost portion

of the skull is called the roof or skull cap (cranial vault); the floor of the cranial vault is referred to as the skull base. Three cavities exist within the skull: the cranial cavity, nasal cavity, and orbital cavities. The cranial cavity is formed by cranial bones, which house and protect the brain, eyeballs, and ears. The nasal septum divides the nasal cavity lengthwise into two halves. The two orbital cavities contain the eyeballs.

Eight bones, two paired and four unpaired, form the cranial cavity itself: frontal (1), parietal (2), temporal (2), occipital (1), sphenoid (1), and ethmoid (1). The frontal, parietal, temporal, and occipital bones form the top and sides of the cranium, and the sphenoid and ethmoid bones comprise the orbits and the floor of the skull base. The junctions between the bones of the cranium are immovable joints, commonly referred to as sutures.

The facial skeleton comprises the anterior portion of the skull. Fourteen facial bones, six paired and two unpaired, exist: the mandible (1), condyloid joint (2), maxilla (2), zygomatic (2), nasal (2), lacrimal (2), palatine (2), and vomer (1).

The mandible is a horseshoe-shaped bone that houses the sockets for the roots of the lower teeth. The mandible is movable and connects with the temporal bone at the condyloid joints. The maxillae contain the sockets for the roots of the upper teeth and form the anterior part of the hard palate. The zygomatic bones form the cheekbones and connect with the maxillae and the temporal and frontal bones. The nasal bones create the bridge of the nose. The lacrimal bones contain the opening in which the nasolacrimal duct transports tears from the lacrimal duct to the nasal cavity. The palatine bones form the posterior portion of the hard palate. The vomer bone lies behind the palatine bone and forms the inferior portion of the nasal cavity. The maxillae, frontal, sphenoid, and ethmoid bones house the air-filled paranasal sinuses and connect with the nose.

Major Neck Regions

For descriptive purposes, the neck consists of two sections: an anterior triangle and a posterior triangle. Figure 2-9 illustrates these anatomic landmarks. The sternocleidomastoid muscle divides both triangles and borders them as it extends obliquely from the mastoid area downward to the clavicle and the manubrium of the sternum.

Major Blood Supply

Two pairs of major veins, the external and internal jugular veins, drain blood in the head and neck (see Figure 2-10). The external jugular vein runs diagonally over the surface of the sternocleidomastoid muscle and drains blood from the superficial region of the posterior portions of the head and neck into the subclavian veins. The internal jugular veins lie deeper than the external veins and drain blood from the

Figure 2-9. Anterior and Posterior Triangles of the Neck

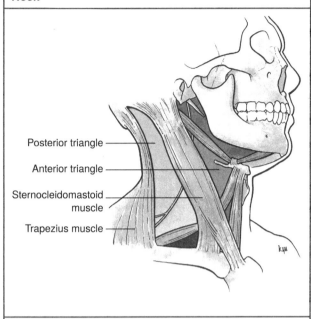

Posterior triangle

Anterior triangle

Sternocleidomastoid muscle

Trapezius muscle

Note. LifeArt image copyright 2002 by Lippincott Williams & Wilkins. All rights reserved.

anterior portion of the face, head, neck, and venous sinuses of the cranial vault. The internal jugular veins connect with the subclavian veins to create the brachiocephalic veins.

Three vessels also drain into the brachiocephalic veins: the lingual veins, the superior thyroid veins, and the facial veins. The lingual veins drain the mouth and tongue, whereas the superior thyroid veins drain the thyroid and deep posterior face. The facial veins drain blood from the superior and anterior facial structures.

Blood that reaches the head and neck originates from three vessels that branch from the aortic arch: the brachiocephalic artery, the left common carotid artery, and the left subclavian artery. Each of these three arteries further separates into one or more smaller arteries as it approaches the structures of the face, head, and neck.

The first vessel, the brachiocephalic artery, separates at the level of the right clavicle into two vessels: the right subclavian artery and the right common carotid artery. The right subclavian artery provides blood to the upper part of the right arm but branches into the right vertebral artery that carries blood to the right brain. The right common carotid artery further divides into two vessels: the right external carotid artery and the right internal carotid artery. Branches of the right external carotid artery nourish the

Figure 2-10. Underlying Structures of the Neck, Anterior View

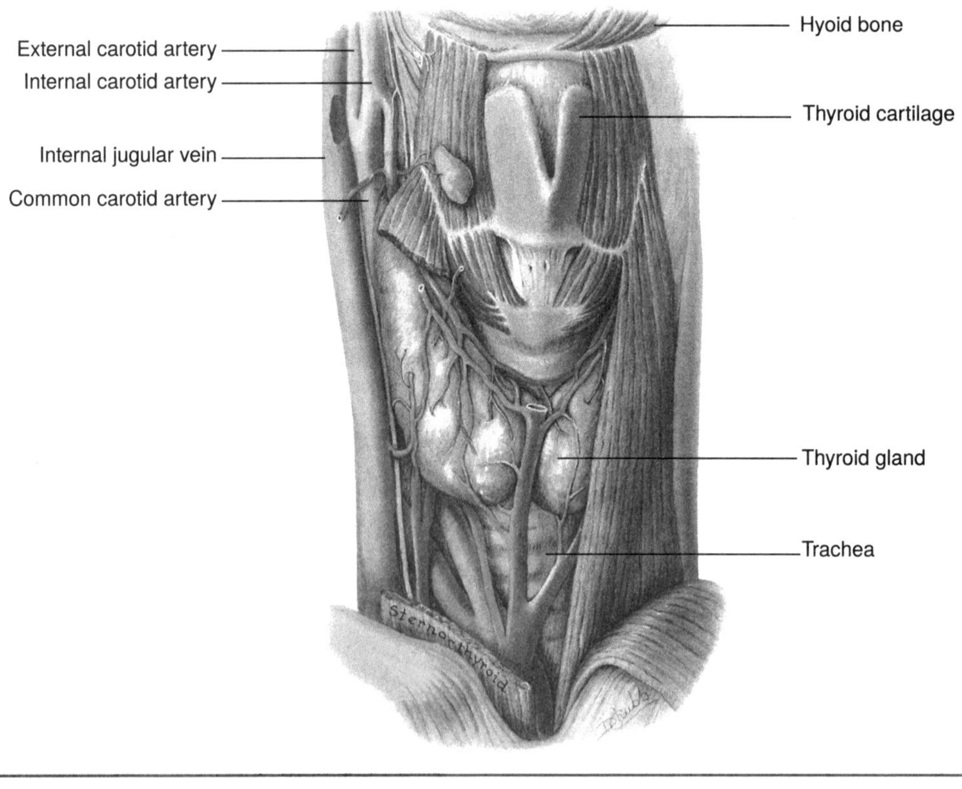

External carotid artery

Internal carotid artery

Internal jugular vein

Common carotid artery

Hyoid bone

Thyroid cartilage

Thyroid gland

Trachea

Note. LifeArt image copyright 2002 by Lippincott Williams & Wilkins. All rights reserved.

right side of the face, head, and neck region. Branches of the right internal carotid artery carry blood toward vessels that supply the right brain.

The second vessel, the left common carotid artery, extends from the aortic arch into two vessels: the left internal carotid artery and the left external carotid artery. The left internal carotid artery joins vessels that nourish the left brain. The left external carotid artery supplies blood to vessels that feed the left side of the face, head, and neck.

The third vessel, the left subclavian artery, branches from the aortic arch to supply the upper portion of the left arm and divides into the left vertebral artery. Branches of the left vertebral artery supply blood to the left brain.

Major Muscle Groups

The head and neck region contains several major muscle groups that enable movement of the face, head, tongue, neck, and shoulders. The sternocleidomastoid muscle (SCM) of the anterior and lateral neck and the trapezius muscle of the scapular region are two muscles that can be affected by diseases of and treatments to the head and neck region.

The SCM extends from the upper sternum (manubrium) medially and the clavicle to the mastoid process behind the ear (see Figure 2-11). Contraction of the SCM on one side enables the head to rotate to the opposite side and extends the head. For example, contraction of the right SCM enables the head to turn toward the left side. The neck flexes when both SCM muscles contract. The trapezius muscle extends from the scapula, clavicle, and thoracic vertebrae to the occipital protuberance. The trapezius muscle allows the shoulders to rise, lower, and adduct/abduct and extends the head and neck. It also elevates, depresses, retracts, rotates, and fixes the scapula. The accessory nerve

---

Figure 2-11. Muscles of the Neck, Anterior Superficial and Posterior Superficial

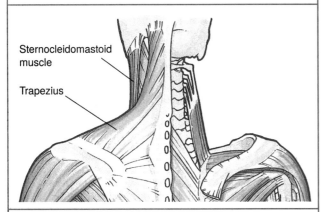

Sternocleidomastoid muscle

Trapezius

(cranial nerve XI) provides the SCM and trapezius muscles with their motor supply.

Lymphatic Supply and Cervical Lymph Nodes

The head and neck region contains a comprehensive lymphatic network that drains lymph, a protein-rich fluid, from the tissues of the body and returns it to the heart by way of the bloodstream. This connection between the lymphatic and circulatory systems is a closed one-way path, but a permeable one. Figure 2-12 illustrates the extensive lymphatic drainage system of the head and neck region.

Fluid drained from the interstitial spaces in the head and neck enters the microscopic and permeable lymph capillaries located near blood capillaries and travels through deep and superficial lymphatic collecting vessels. Lymph enters the cervical lymph nodes via afferent lymphatic vessels and exits using the efferent lymphatic vessels.

Cervical lymph nodes are superficial groups of nodes located along the lymphatic vessels on either side of the neck and are one of the three sets of lymph nodes (along with inguinal and axillary nodes) in the body. Lymph nodes are small, measuring less than 1 cm. Some nodes are round, whereas others are oval or bean-shaped. A capsule made of thick fibrous tissue encases each node.

Lymph nodes defend the body through two mechanisms. First, cervical lymph nodes filter fluid drained from the head and neck region before returning it to the bloodstream, where it travels throughout the body. Macrophages in the nodes act as phagocytes, removing and destroying bacteria, viruses, and other harmful particles that enter the lymph fluid. Second, lymphocytes located in the nodes search the lymph fluid for antigens, such as bacteria, viruses, cancer cells, and other foreign bodies, and destroy them before they have an opportunity to harm the body. Because the flow of lymph fluid exiting the lymph node is slower than that entering the node, the lymph nodes have time to cleanse the lymph that passes through it. In addition to defending the body, the lymphatic system also helps the body to maintain its fluid balance and assists with the absorption of fats.

After being filtered by one or more lymph nodes, lymph passes through large collecting vessels, called trunks, into two lymphatic ducts on each side of the thoracic region: the right lymphatic duct and the left thoracic duct. The right lymphatic duct drains fluid from the right upper body. This includes the right side of the head and neck, the right portion of the upper arm, and the right side of the chest. The thoracic duct drains lymph from the left side of the head and neck and the remaining portions of the body.

Cervical lymph nodes undergo various changes as they encounter infections and cancer. For example, superficial lymph nodes become swollen and painful if they are obstructed, as they destroy the many microscopic organisms that enter the lymph fluid. These nodes also swell without pain, as cancer cells

Figure 2-12. Lymphatic Drainage System of the Head and Neck

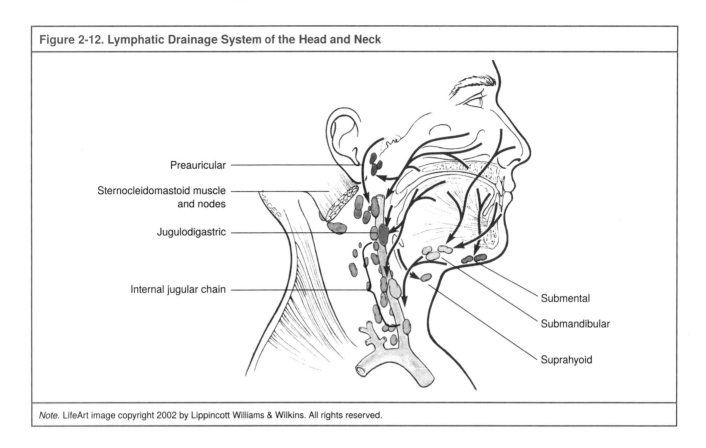

Preauricular

Sternocleidomastoid muscle and nodes

Jugulodigastric

Internal jugular chain

Submental

Submandibular

Suprahyoid

separate from a malignant tumor in the body, enter the lymphatic system, and become trapped in the nodes. In this situation, lymph nodes basically provide a route for cancer cells to spread to other sites in the body. Finally, diseases or surgery can cause the lymphatic ducts of regional lymph nodes to become obstructed or infected. This condition can result in lymphedema, a severe localized swelling of the area drained by the affected nodes. Enlarged cervical lymph nodes or neck masses, known as lymphadenopathy, frequently result from reactive hyperplasia, infection, metastatic tumors, or lymphoma.

The appearance of lymph fluid varies in color, including clear, opaque, or yellow-tinged. Lymph fluid that is drained from the digestive viscera is referred to as chyle and appears milky white because it contains digested fats. Lymph also contains other substances extracted from the plasma and cells of the body, including water, proteins, nutrients, hormones, enzymes, and wastes. Lymph contains many lymphocytes, other white blood cells, and some red blood cells. Lymph fluid moves slowly through the lymphatic network, with approximately three liters returning to the body's bloodstream every 24 hours (Marieb, 2015).

Summary

Understanding alterations in ear, nose, throat, head, and neck anatomy and physiology is essential in determining the impact of head and neck cancer and its treatment. This knowledge aids in planning appropriate nursing interventions and evaluating patient outcomes.

References

Andresen, H.G., Hickey, M.M., Higgens, T.S., Huntoon, M.B., LeGrand, M.S., McGuire, M.A., ... Sievers, A.E.F. (2008). Normal anatomy and physiology. In L.L. Harris & M.B. Huntoon (Eds.), *Core curriculum for otorhinolaryngology and head/neck nursing* (2nd ed., pp. 39–78). New Smyrna Beach, FL: Society of Otorhinolaryngology and Head-Neck Nurses.

Bickley, L.S. (2013). *Bates' guide to physical examination and history taking* (11th ed.). Philadelphia, PA: Lippincott Williams & Wilkins.

Dalgorf, D.M., & Harvey, R.J. (2013). Chapter 1: Sinonasal anatomy and function. *American Journal of Rhinology and Allergy, 1*(Suppl. 1), S3–S6. doi:10.2500/ajra.2013.27.3888

Isaacson, G. (2014). Endoscopic anatomy of the pediatric middle ear. *Otolaryngology—Head and Neck Surgery, 150*, 6–15. doi:10.1177/0194599813509589

Logan, B.M., Reynolds, P., & Hutchings, R.T. (2010). *McMinn's color atlas of head and neck anatomy* (4th ed.). Philadelphia, PA: Mosby.

Marieb, E.N. (2015). *Essentials of human anatomy and physiology* (11th ed.). Boston, MA: Pearson Education.

National Cancer Institute. (n.d.). NCI dictionary of cancer terms. Retrieved from http://www.cancer.gov/dictionary?cdrid=44811

VanPutte, C., Regan, J., Russo, A., Seeley, R., Stephens, T.D., & Tate, P. (2014). *Seeley's anatomy and physiology* (10th ed.). New York, NY: McGraw-Hill.

Zhao, K., & Dalton, P. (2007). The way the wind blows: Implications of modeling nasal airflow. *Current Allergy and Asthma Reports, 7*, 117–125. doi:10.1007/s11882-007-0009-z

CHAPTER 3

Pathophysiology

Nancy Roehnelt, PhD, ARNP, and Margaret Hickey, RN, MSN, MS

Introduction

Pathophysiology is the study of the biologic and physical manifestations of diseases as they correlate with underlying abnormalities and physiologic disturbances. It is not about the treatment of disease, but rather the processes within the body that result in the signs and symptoms of a disease. Pathophysiology is often referred to as *carcinogenesis* when pertaining to cancer, and it represents the disease process when normal cells are transformed into cancer cells by a progression at the cellular level.

Carcinogenesis

Carcinogenesis is the result of genetic and epigenetic mutations that occur in a normal cell, causing that cell to become a cancer cell. Cancer results after a progressive series of events that incrementally increase the extent of deregulation within a cell line. These events include a failure of DNA repair, activation of oncogenes, and loss of tumor suppressor function. Known DNA genetic mutations associated with head and neck cancer that are involved in the deregulation of the cell's programming for apoptosis and proliferation include p53, CDKN2A, PIK3CA, NOTCH1, and Nrf2 (Riaz, Morris, Lee, & Chan, 2014). Head and neck cancer is also driven by epigenetic changes. Epigenetic changes modify the activation of certain genes, but the epigenetic influence does not change the sequence of the cell's DNA. An example of epigenetic change is the silencing of DNA repair enzymes. These DNA repair enzymes function to mend DNA damage once it is recognized by the cell and to prevent mutation that could result in unregulated cell division and cancer (Bakhtiar, Ali, & Barh, 2015).

Carcinogenesis is the result of not one insult to the DNA, but from multiple insults to the integrity of the cell's DNA and the DNA's protective mechanisms. Chronic or significant exposure to carcinogens is the most obvious explanation. Carcinogens can be chemical, such as tobacco smoke or asbestos; physical, such as ionizing radiation; or biologic, such as viruses. The DNA repair mechanism usually repairs the cell's damaged DNA or eliminates the cell, thus halting its progression into a cancer cell. The abnormal cell that escapes the repair process and the immune system undergoes a second series of events that allow it to grow and continue to manifest changes. It may be years before cancer manifests; this stage between exposure and diagnosis is called the *latency period*. Nadler and Zurbenko (2014) applied mathematical modeling to estimate latency periods for 44 types of cancer. They reported that the majority of cancers have a latency period of at least 10 years. They estimated a wide range of latency periods for head and neck cancer diagnoses. For example, hypopharyngeal cancer was found to have the shortest latency period, estimated at 9.6 years, and laryngeal cancer was the longest, at 35.4 years. The latency period for oropharyngeal cancer was 12.3 years, and for pharyngeal and other oral cavity cancers, it was estimated at 16.9 years.

Initiation

Cancer initiates with one or more irreversible genetic mutations, and any daughter cell produced by the division of a mutated cell will carry that mutation (CancerQuest, 2012a). Classes of genes involved in initiation are (a) oncogenes that accelerate cell growth, (b) mutated DNA mismatch-repair genes that fail to repair mistakes during cell division, and (c) mutated tumor suppressor genes that fail to stop cellular proliferation (Lea, Calzone, Masny, & Bush, 2002).

Proto-oncogenes are present and function normally to stimulate cellular growth and include genes that inhibit cellular apoptosis, or programmed cell death. When a proto-oncogene is defective or mutated, it is known as an *oncogene*. Oncogenes are dominant; one defective allele can predispose the cell to unchecked cellular growth. If the cell has one normal gene (proto-oncogene) at a site and one mutated gene (oncogene), the abnormal product takes control. Numerous oncogenes have been identified in head and neck cancer, including *ras, myc, abl,* and *HER2* (Singh, 2008). No single oncogene can cause cancer by itself. It can, however, increase the rate of mitosis of the cell and put the cells at increased risk for acquiring additional mutations. A clone of an actively dividing cell is at risk for developing subclones with second, third, or multiple oncogenes.

Promotion

Once carcinogenesis has been initiated and a cell has undergone mutation, it is susceptible to the actions of promoting factors that facilitate proliferation. Promoting factors, unlike initiating factors, do not bind to DNA or other macromolecules within the cell. Rather, many bind to cell surface receptors, impacting downstream intracellular pathways and stimulating proliferation (CancerQuest, 2010a). Promoting factors may also influence the microenvironment, creating favorable conditions for proliferation. Unlike the irreversible mutations of the initiation phase, promotion requires repeated and prolonged exposure and may be reversible. Promoting factors stimulate the initiated cells to continue to propagate abnormally, resulting in hyperplasia. Hyperplasia is the earliest stage in which the altered cell divides in an uncontrolled manner, resulting in an excess of cells in a certain region. These cells continue to have a normal appearance but are atypical because of the overpopulation (CancerQuest, 2010b). An example of a hyperplastic head and neck lesion is leukoplakia. Leukoplakia is identified as a white patch in the mouth that cannot be scraped or wiped away and cannot be diagnosed as another condition. Leukoplakia lesions are associated with exposure to irritants, such as tobacco or alcohol. Hyperplasia of keratinocytes can be seen during microscopic assessment of leukoplakia, and genetic changes have also been demonstrated (Oral Cancer Foundation, 2014). Patients with oral leukoplakia must be followed over time, as it has been demonstrated that 8%–15% of these cases can later become cancerous lesions (Brigham and Women's Hospital, n.d.).

Progression

Progression, the third stage of neoplastic development, is separate from initiation and promotion. Like initiation, progression involves molecular genetic changes; however, these changes are very different from the genetic changes of initiation. Karyotype changes result during the progression stage. All tumors that advance to malignancies have an altered number of chromosomes. An increase in tumor growth rate, invasiveness, and the potential for metastasis as well as alterations in the cell morphology and chemistry occur during the progression stage (CancerQuest, 2010a). Cellular progression occurs in four steps: benign hyperplasia, dysplasia, neoplasia, and carcinoma. Hyperplasia is increased cellular proliferation that can lead to increased organ tissue. Dysplasia is abnormal-

ity of growth and differentiation, often a precursor to neoplasia. Neoplasia is cell overgrowth that can form a tumor. The World Health Organization (WHO) classifies neoplasia as four categories: benign, in situ, malignant, and neoplasia of uncertain origins or behavior (WHO, 2013). Malignant neoplasms are known as carcinoma. Carcinoma represents cells that have undergone DNA damage or alterations that cause uncontrollable growth and potential to spread outside of the tumor and organ tissue. In patients with head and neck cancer, leukoplakia and erythroplakia are clinically identifiable lesions of the oral cavity that may undergo malignant transformation. As cells continue to multiply uncontrolled, the risk of additional genetic alterations increases, and if this process continues, dysplasia is the next stage. *Dysplasia* describes the transformation from normal to abnormal cells. An increase in immature cells also occurs, often appearing disordered and with greater variability between the cells. The cells cannot yet be described as cancerous, but they no longer look or behave normally (Open University, 2013). Based on the degree of nuclear abnormality, dysplasia is graded as either mild, moderate, or severe. In the transition from mild to severe dysplasia, nuclear abnormalities become more marked and mitoses become more apparent; these changes involve increasing depth of the epithelium. In severe dysplasia, 25% will develop into carcinoma. *Carcinoma* describes dysplastic cells that have invaded into surrounding tissue and have the ability to travel to other sites. *Neoplasia* is the abnormal rate of proliferation of the dysplastic cell.

Carcinoma in situ is severe dysplasia where the group of abnormal cells stays in one place and does not invade surrounding tissue. Carcinoma in situ of the head and neck is characterized by the presence of dysplastic changes throughout the entire thickness of the epithelium, with loss of normal maturation. These cells have an abnormally fast mitotic rate and bear little or no resemblance to normal cells. They may regress or become more primitive in their capabilities, often unable to complete normal functions. An example would be a liver cell that no longer makes liver-specific proteins. Cells of this type are referred to as *dedifferentiated* or *anaplastic*. Carcinoma in situ lesions often are described as preinvasive because they are limited to one area. Carcinoma in situ is irreversible and is expected to become an invasive carcinoma if left untreated. These growths are considered to have the potential to become invasive and are treated as malignant growths. Tumors of this type often are curable by surgery because the abnormal cells are limited to one area.

Once the dysplastic squamous cells move beyond the borders of the basement membrane, or basal lamina, the lesion is referred to as *invasive squamous cell carcinoma* (Saunders & Wakely, n.d.). As the tumor continues to grow, it can invade surrounding tissues or metastasize outside of the local area. Benign tumors do not spread to tissues around them or to other parts of the body and are not cancerous. However, benign tumors still can cause serious health problems because they may put pressure on other organs and impair function. For example, meningioma, a common, usually benign brain tumor, is slow growing but, given the limited space within the skull, can have serious consequences, causing considerable morbidity or even death.

Characteristics of Cancer Cells

Cancer cells are different from normal cells in that they are able to form a tumor and eventually metastasize to other parts of the body. Normal cells require growth signals before they can move from a resting state into an active proliferative state. Cancer cells will proliferate in the absence of these growth signals. Noticeable changes also occur in the physical properties of the cell. Alterations in the cytoskeleton of the cell affect cellular adhesion and motility. Cancer cells do not exhibit contact inhibition, one of the cellular growth inhibitory signals. Normal cellular growth is checked as cells respond to contact inhibition and cease to divide when they sense they are being "crowded" by other cells. The reduction of cell-to-cell and cell-to-extracellular matrix adhesion allows large masses of cells to form. Without contact inhibition, tumor cells continue to divide, even when surrounded by other cells, and the cells continue to "pile up," eventually forming a tumor. Normal cellular adhesion prevents normal cells from moving. The cytoskeletal alterations affecting cellular adhesion allow the cancer cells to move about. Cancer cells must be able to move and migrate in order to spread, so they often secrete enzymes that digest the barriers to migration and enable invasion into neighboring tissues, aiding in the spread of the tumor (CancerQuest, 2012b). The shape and organization of the nuclei of cancer cells may be markedly different from the nuclei of normal cells of the same origin. These changes are useful in diagnosing and staging tumors.

The changes seen in individual cells are mirrored by the behavior of the tumors. For a tumor to grow and invade neighboring tissues, several major changes must occur. Hanahan and Weinberg (2011) have detailed a model of cancer growth and metastasis. Cancer cells and tumors must acquire a specific set of abilities. These include (a) sustained growth signaling, (b) insensitivity to growth suppressors, (c) resistance to apoptosis, (d) limitless replicative potential, (e) induction of angiogenesis, and (f) tissue invasion and metastasis.

Sustained Growth Signaling

Normal cells will not reproduce unless they receive external signals that cause the cells to enter the cell cycle. A cell that divides without proper growth signals results in a population of daughter cells that also divide autonomously of growth signals. Cancer cells are able to proliferate by entering the cell cycle independent of external signaling. They acquire growth signal autonomy through three processes.

- Many cancer cells acquire the ability to synthesize growth factors to which they are responsive, eliminating dependence on other cells within the tissue.
- Cell surface receptors transmit growth signals into the cell interior. Receptor overexpression may cause the cancer cell to become hyperresponsive to low levels of growth factor that would not normally trigger proliferation.
- Cancer cells can switch the types of extracellular matrix receptors they express to favor ones that transmit pro-growth signals.

Insensitivity to Growth Suppressors

Normal cell division is restricted through multiple antigrowth signals. These signals include both soluble growth inhibitors and inhibitors fixed in the extracellular matrix and on the surfaces of nearby cells. Two distinct mechanisms exist to block cells from entering the cell cycle and dividing. One forces cells out of active proliferation into the resting (G_0) phase until some future extracellular growth signal permits it to reenter the cell cycle. A second mechanism occurs in which cells permanently relinquish their ability to divide by entering a postmitotic state. This state usually is associated with cellular differentiation when a precursor cell continues to differentiate, acquiring its final functional capabilities. Cancer cells must evade these antigrowth signals specifically through disruptions of the pathways that govern the transit of the cell through the cell cycle. At the molecular level, many, if not all, of the antiproliferative signals are channeled through the retinoblastoma protein (pRb) and its two relatives, p17 and p130. Disruption of the pRb pathway releases E2F transcription factors, allowing cell proliferation. This makes cells insensitive to antigrowth factors that normally operate along this pathway. Human tumors have been found to disrupt the pRb pathway in a variety of ways, therefore creating insensitivity to antigrowth signals (Hanahan & Weinberg, 2011).

Normal cells will stop dividing when they are in contact with neighboring cells. The cell-to-cell contact immobilizes cells and sends signals to the dividing cells to stop them from dividing. Cancer cells undergo cytoskeletal changes, rendering them nonresponsive to this normal cellular growth brake.

Resistance to Apoptosis

In normal tissue, a balance between new cells is created through cell division and the loss of cells through cell death. Apoptosis eliminates cells that become damaged and is a precisely choreographed series of steps during which (a) the cellular membranes are disrupted, (b) the cytoplasmic and nuclear skeletons are broken down, (c) the cytosol is extruded, (d) the chromosomes are degraded, (e) the cell is fragmented, and (f) the debris is consumed by nearby phagocytic cells. This process is a normal and necessary safeguard that allows for the identification and elimination of mutated or damaged cells.

The ability of tumor cell populations to grow is a result of not only the rate of cell proliferation, but also the rate of cell death. Increasing evidence suggests that the resistance to apoptosis is a hallmark of most, if not all, types of cancer. Apoptotic machinery can be divided into two components—sensors and effectors. Sensors monitor the extracellular and intracellular environment for conditions of normality or abnormality that indicate whether a cell will live or die. Extracellular sensors are maintained for most cells by the cellular matrix and cell-to-cell adherence-based survival signals. Intracellular sensors monitor the cell and activate the "death pathway" in response to detection of abnormalities, including DNA damage, signaling imbalance provoked by oncogenes, or hypoxia.

When activated, the intracellular and extracellular sensors send signals to regulate the effectors of apoptotic death. The signals that prompt apoptosis converge on the mitochondrion, which responds by releasing cytochrome c, a potent catalyst of apoptosis. The ultimate effectors of apoptosis include an array of intracellular proteases called *capsases*. The capsases trigger activation of a dozen or more effector capsases that execute the death program. Cancer cells can acquire resistance to apoptosis through a variety of strategies. The most common is the loss of a proapoptotic regulator, involving mutation of the *p53* tumor suppressor gene (Hanahan & Weinberg, 2011).

Limitless Replicative Potential and Immortality

In theory, deregulation of cellular proliferation through growth signal autonomy, insensitivity to antigrowth signals, and resistance to apoptosis should suffice in leading to the vast cell populations that create tumors. However, this disruption of cell-to-cell signaling alone does not guarantee expansive tumor growth. Many, if not all, mammalian cells carry an intrinsic cell autonomous program that limits cell multiplication. This appears to operate independently of the pathways previously described. It, too, must be disrupted for cancer cells to expand to an overt and potentially life-threatening tumor. Although normal cells can divide only a finite number of times before stopping cell division and dying, cancer cells have the ability to divide endlessly without appearing to "age." In many cancers, this is because of the activation of the enzyme telomerase. Telomerase functions to maintain the integrity of the chromosomes during cell division (Hanahan & Weinberg, 2011).

Induction of Angiogenesis

Oxygen and nutrients supplied by the vasculature are crucial for cell function and survival. During organ formation, blood supply is ensured through coordinated growth of new blood vessels. In normal cellular growth, once a tissue is formed, the growth of new blood vessels, or angiogenesis, is transitory and carefully regulated.

The development of blood vessels is an essential step in the growth and metastasis of a tumor. Tumors can grow up to 1–2 mm without neovascularization, but they cannot metastasize and grow above this size without new blood vessel growth (National Cancer Institute [NCI], 2011). For a tumor to progress in size, it must develop angiogenic ability. Tumor cells or adjacent cells produce angiogenic growth factors to stimulate the formation of new blood vessels. Angiogenic activators include vascular endothelial growth factor (VEGF), basic fibroblast growth factor, and transforming growth factors. Without angiogenesis, tumor cell proliferation is inhibited because it is matched or exceeded by apoptosis. The ability to induce or sustain angiogenesis seems to be acquired in a discrete step during tumor development when tumor cell proliferation exceeds apoptosis (Hanahan & Weinberg, 2011).

Tissue Invasion and Metastasis

During the development of most cancers, primary cancer cells can move through the blood or lymphatic systems or through direct contact to another location. When a cancer cell moves, it may divide and form a tumor at the new site. Metastatic tumors often interfere with organ function and lead to the morbidity and mortality seen with cancer. The majority of cancer deaths are a result of metastasis of the cancer to sites distant from the primary site (CancerQuest, 2014).

Invasion and metastasis are closely allied processes. For cells to move through the body, they must first "climb" over and around neighboring cells. They do this by rearranging their cytoskeleton and attaching to other cells and the extracellular matrix via proteins on the outside of their plasma membrane. Cells migrate, or move, until stopped by the basal lamina (or basement membrane). To cross this membrane, cancer cells secrete enzymes called *matrix metalloproteases*. These enzymes degrade the proteins in the basal lamina and allow continued migration and invasion into adjacent tissues as well as to distant locations via adjacent blood vessels or lymphatic vessels (CancerQuest, 2014).

Metastasis can occur through invasion of the cancer cells by direct contact with other organs or via cancer cell migration into the lymphatic system or vasculature. The lymphatic system is an extensive network with lymphatic flow throughout the body, much like the circulatory system. Cancer cells move into the lymphatic system and can then deposit nearby or distantly from the primary tumor site. The tumor cells can be found in the lymph nodes. This helps to identify the extent of metastatic disease and tumor staging (CancerQuest, 2014). Hematogenous metastasis, the spread of cancer cells through the circulatory system, results from cells migrating among the blood vessel epithelial cells. Once in the blood, the cancer cell embolism is carried through the circulatory system until it finds a suitable location in which to settle and reenter the tissues. Hematogenous and lymphatic metastases result in the cancer cells settling in a distant location and forming a new tumor. The tumor cells that have metastasized to a distant location retain the characteristics they had when they were in their original location.

How cancers of the head and neck behave is dependent on the site of origin. Each anatomic site predisposes the metastatic pattern and prognosis. Regional invasion usually reaches beyond the anatomic limits of the primary site deep into the neighboring structures and along tissue planes. The perineural route is also an important pathway for metastasis of head and neck cancer. Intracranial spread can occur along the peripheral branches of the cranial nerves.

Regional and distant metastases are most likely caused by invasion of the lymphatic system because the head and neck region is rich in lymphatic drainage. The greater the size and thickness of the primary tumor, the more likely lymph node metastasis will be present. Spread to the cervical lymph nodes affects progression-free survival and overall survival of patients with head and neck squamous cell cancer (Li, Shen, Di, & Song, 2012). If the primary site is near the midline, contralateral or bilateral metastases should be anticipated. Important prognostic factors in head and neck cancer include tumor size, lymph node spread, and distant metastasis. With lymph node spread, the presence of extracapsular nodal involvement of the tumor is an important negative prognostic factor in head and neck cancer (Ridge, Mehra, Lango, & Feigenberg, 2014). The more aggressive and poorly differentiated tumors tend to metastasize early to regional lymph nodes and beyond.

Distant metastasis is not commonly seen in squamous cell carcinoma of the head and neck. The most common sites of distant metastasis secondary to hematogenous spread are the lungs, bones (frequently the vertebrae, ribs, and skull), and liver (Li et al., 2012).

Epidemiology

According to the American Cancer Society (ACS), head and neck cancer, including all sites of origin, will account for 3.9% of new cancer cases in the United States in 2015, with an estimated 64,970 new cases and 13,070 deaths occurring. Approximately 1.1% of men and women will be diagnosed with oral cavity and pharynx cancer at some point during their lifetime (ACS, 2015a). The median age at diagnosis is 62 years, and the median age at death is 67 years. Despite new treatment options, the prognosis has remained unchanged over the past 40 years, with approximately 50% of patients dying from their disease (NCI Surveillance, Epidemiology, and End Results Program, 2012). Recent years have shown a decrease in the incidence of head and neck cancer but an increase in

the incidence of a subtype of oropharyngeal cancer associated with human papillomavirus (HPV) infection (ACS, 2015a).

Head and neck cancer is categorized by the location in which it occurs. The oral cavity, larynx, and pharynx are the three most common categorical sites, and tumors of the nasal, sinus, and salivary glands are relatively uncommon.

Carcinogens

A malignant transformation of epithelial cells as a result of extended exposure to carcinogens and a cascade of genetic and epigenetic changes results in the different subtypes of head and neck cancer. The carcinogens that influence the molecular changes include those related to infection, occupation, and lifestyle.

Alcohol and tobacco, including smokeless tobacco, are the two most important risk factors for head and neck cancer. People who use both tobacco and alcohol are at greater risk compared to people who use either tobacco or alcohol alone. It has been estimated that 75% of head and neck cancers are caused by tobacco and alcohol use. Tobacco and alcohol use are not risk factors for salivary gland cancer (Hashibe et al., 2009; Simard, Torre, & Jemal, 2014). Viruses, such as HPV—especially type 16—are a risk factor for oropharyngeal cancer. Although the presence of HPV in the tumor has been implicated as a positive prognostic factor, alcohol and tobacco use are correlated with the acceleration of invasive carcinoma and a poorer prognosis (Chaturvedi et al., 2011). The Epstein-Barr virus (EBV) is a risk factor for nasopharyngeal cancer and salivary gland cancer (NCI, 2013). Asian ancestry, particularly Chinese ancestry, is a risk factor for nasopharyngeal cancer (NCI, 2014a). Paan, also called *betel quid*, is habitually used among immigrants from Southeast Asia and increases the risk of oral cancer (Crozier & Sumer, 2010). Maté, a tea-like beverage typically consumed by South Americans, has also been associated with an increased risk of cancers of the mouth, throat, esophagus, and larynx (Stefani et al., 2011). Frequent consumption of preserved or salted foods during childhood increases the risk for developing nasopharyngeal cancer (ACS, 2015b). Occupational exposure to wood dust also is a risk factor for nasopharyngeal cancer (ACS, 2015b). Exposures to asbestos and synthetic fibers have been associated with cancer of the larynx, but the increase in risk remains controversial. Industrial exposure to wood or nickel dust or formaldehyde is a risk factor for cancers of the paranasal sinuses and nasal cavity (Luce et al., 2002). Radiation to the head and neck increases risk for cancer of the salivary glands (NCI, 2014b).

Cancer Cell Types

Squamous cell carcinoma accounts for more than 90% of head and neck carcinomas. Historically, it was believed these tumors differed only by anatomic site of origin; however, recent evidence suggests they are more heterogeneous. Distinct subtypes exist, with molecular genetic profiles differing in risk factors such as pathogenesis and clinical behavior (e.g., the unique molecular genetic profile of HPV-related carcinoma) (Pai & Westra, 2009). Fewer than 10% of head and neck cancer cases are represented by mucoepidermoid carcinoma, adenoid cystic carcinoma, and adenocarcinoma, all of which may arise in the salivary glands. Very rare cancers of the head and neck are represented by tumors with neuroendocrine features, including carcinoid, small cell undifferentiated cancer, and esthesioneuroblastoma (also called *olfactory neuroblastoma*) or Hodgkin lymphoma and non-Hodgkin lymphoma (Ridge et al., 2014). Head and neck cancers encompass a diverse group of tumors that may be aggressive in their biologic behavior.

Squamous cell carcinoma is a malignant neoplasm of epithelial origin that develops from the epithelial cells lining the surface of the upper airway and aerodigestive tract. Squamous cell carcinomas are mucosal lesions that are usually visible at the surface; they rarely develop beneath intact-appearing mucosa. *Squamous cell carcinoma* can be used interchangeably with *epidermoid carcinoma*, although the latter is less commonly used.

Morphologic appearance of squamous cell carcinoma is variable, and these tumors may appear as plaques, nodules, or wart-like growths. These lesions may be scaly or ulcerated, white, red, or brown (Rousseau & Badoual, 2011b). Invasive squamous cell carcinoma initially infiltrates the subepithelial fibrous tissue. The tissue invaded in later stages depends on the site of the tumor. Muscle invasion is a common feature, and bone and cartilage invasion is usually a late phenomenon. Perivascular spread or perineural spread along the nerve sheath can be seen at all head and neck sites. Locoregional spread results from invasion of the lymphatic capillaries, with subsequent metastasis to cervical lymph nodes. Hematogenous metastasis is uncommon, but if it occurs, the most common site of metastasis is the lung (Li et al., 2012).

Squamous cell carcinoma may arise from dysplastic epithelium or may arise without dysplastic changes being noted. The hallmark of invasive squamous cell carcinoma (especially in low-grade lesions) is the presence of keratin, or keratin pearls, on histologic evaluation. Keratin is the end product of squamous cell degeneration and normally is found in skin and squamous mucosa, excluding the larynx. Keratin pearls are eosinophilic and roundish and have a thin membrane. For reasons unknown, keratin pearls are not found in carcinoma in situ (Saunders & Wakely, n.d.).

Microscopically, the nuclei of malignant squamous cells are rich with DNA and will stain dark (i.e., hyperchromatic). The nucleus is likely to be large in proportion to the cytoplasm; the nuclear-cytoplasmic ratio may be 1:1 instead of the normal 1:4 or 1:6. The nuclear shape may be variable. Mitotic figures may be numerous and often are abnormal in appearance, with large spindles in one area and shrunken spindles in others. Giant tumor cells may be present with a single huge polymorphic nucleus and others with two or more nuclei. The orientation of tumor cells to one another is erratic compared to the orderly arrangement seen in normal tissue. Large masses of cells are seen, and "fingers" of tumor cells may invade adjacent normal tissue (Saunders & Wakely, n.d.).

Verrucous Carcinoma

Verrucous carcinoma is a rare variant of low-grade squamous cell carcinoma, first described by Lauren Ackerman in 1948. It is an uncommon variant in the United States, usually occurring in White males in their sixth decade (Alan, Agacayak, Kavak, & Ozcan, 2015). It typically appears at sites of chronic irritation and inflammation. HPV may be a risk factor for development of verrucous carcinoma, as can use of chewing tobacco, snuff, and betel nuts. It most frequently is found in the oral cavity. HPV 16 frequently has been identified in these lesions. Verrucous carcinoma is characterized as an exophytic, gray, bulky lesion with a papillomatous and fungating appearance. Verrucous carcinoma is sometimes described as a well-differentiated papillomatous tumor because of the papillomatous character of the lesion. This well-differentiated squamous carcinoma is much less invasive and rarely metastasizes. In the rare instance that metastasis occurs, it is usually to regional lymph nodes. However, these tumors can become problematic because they may grow to be quite large and potentially may lead to upper airway obstruction (Rousseau & Badoual, 2011b; Saunders & Wakely, n.d.).

Microscopically, the cells show none of the mitoses or dysplastic features usually seen with squamous carcinoma. The surface shows characteristic "church spire" formations because of extensive keratinization (Saunders & Wakely, n.d.). This lesion is composed of highly differentiated squamous cells, is broadly based, and has a large blunt-ended network of ridges with an intact basement membrane. An inflammatory reaction is often present in the underlying tissue (Rousseau & Badoual, 2011b).

Undifferentiated Carcinoma

WHO's histopathologic grading system describes three types of nasopharyngeal cancer: WHO grade 1, keratinizing squamous cell carcinoma and nonkeratinizing squamous cell carcinoma; WHO grade 2, differentiated carcinoma; and WHO grade 3, undifferentiated carcinoma. Undifferentiated nonkeratinizing carcinoma is the classic nasopharyngeal carcinoma (Wei & Sham, 2005). Subtypes of nasopharyngeal carcinoma previously included lymphoepithelioma, which is now classified as WHO grade 3, undifferentiated carcinoma. This is characterized by the presence of lymphocyte infiltration (WHO, 2013). Lymphoepithelioma has also been described as Regaud tumors and represents a well-defined collection of epithelium that is surrounded by lymphocytes and fibrous tissue. This is compared to Schmincke tumors, in which the tumor cells are diffuse and mixed with inflammatory cells. EBV seems to play an important etiologic role in WHO grade 2 nonkeratinizing squamous cell carcinoma and WHO grade 3 undifferentiated carcinoma. Nasopharyngeal carcinoma may present as cervical lymphadenopathy, as it often metastasizes early to cervical lymph nodes (Brennan, 2006).

Spindle Cell Carcinoma

Spindle cell carcinoma is a rare and unusual form of poorly differentiated squamous cell carcinoma with elongated or spindled epithelial cells that resemble sarcoma spindle cell morphology. It may be invasive or in situ and can be well to poorly differentiated. The nuclei of the spindle cell components are hyperchromatic with large reddish nucleoli and many mitoses present. Mononucleated giant cells may also be seen, and necrosis is often present (Saunders & Wakely, n.d.). Spindle cell carcinoma may also be referred to as *sarcomatoid squamous cell carcinoma* and *polypoid squamous cell carcinoma* (Rousseau & Badoual, 2011b).

There seem to be no specific risk factors, such as smoking, associated with spindle cell carcinoma. When lymph node metastases are found, the cell type may represent either the spindle cell or squamous cell component. Surgery is the most effective therapy; however, overall prognosis is poor (Saunders & Wakely, n.d.).

Histologic Grading

Grading is done according to the degree that the cells have departed histologically from their normal appearance. Five grading categories exist for head and neck cancer (with the exception of thyroid cancers): grade (G) X, grade cannot be assessed; G1, well differentiated; G2, moderately differentiated; G3, poorly differentiated; and G4, undifferentiated (Stevenson, 2013). Individual pathologists' experiences and criteria will account for occasional differences in grading of the same specimen (Saunders & Wakely, n.d.).

In general, the more poorly differentiated a lesion, the higher the incidence of regional metastases and the poorer the prognosis. However, tumor grade has not always been directly correlated with clinical behavior. Aggressive behavior can be more accurately predicted by perineural spread, lymphatic invasion, and tumor extension beyond the lymph node capsule. HPV-positive tumors tend to be nonkeratinizing and poorly differentiated; yet, patients often have better outcomes than patients with oropharyngeal cancer who do not have an HPV-positive disease (Ridge et al., 2014).

Salivary Gland Tumors

Salivary gland neoplasms are histologically diverse. These neoplasms include benign and malignant tumors. Salivary gland tumor grading is used mostly for mucoepidermoid carcinoma, adenocarcinoma, adenoid cystic carcinoma, squamous cell carcinoma, and not otherwise specified (NOS). NCI (2014b) lists the categories of salivary gland carcinomas according to histologic grade (see Figure 3-1).

Adenoid Cystic Carcinoma

Adenoid cystic carcinoma (previously known as cylindroma) is a slow-growing but aggressive neoplasm with a remarkable ability to recur. It is a very lethal type of tumor, even when treated early (NCI, 2014b). This neoplasm usually presents as a slow-growing swelling in the preauricular or submandibular region. Perineural invasion can result in pain and facial paralysis and is an unfavorable sign (Saunders & Wakely, n.d.). Regardless of histologic grade, adenoid cystic carcinomas have an unusually slow biologic growth, a protracted course, and, ultimately, a poor outcome. The 10-year survival rate is reported to be less than 50% for all grades (NCI, 2014b). These carcinomas typically recur, and late distant metastasis occurs with patients dying of pulmonary metastasis. Clinical stage may be a better prognostic indicator than histologic grade. In a retrospective review of 92 cases, a tumor size greater than 4 cm was associated with an unfavorable clinical course in all cases (NCI, 2014b).

This malignant tumor is poorly encapsulated, and although it seems to be well defined within the gland, infiltration of the surrounding tissue usually occurs. Morpholog-

---

Figure 3-1. Categories for Salivary Gland Carcinomas by Grade

Low Grade
- Acinic cell carcinoma
- Basal cell adenocarcinoma
- Clear cell carcinoma
- Cystadenocarcinoma
- Epithelial-myoepithelial carcinoma
- Mucinous adenocarcinoma
- Polymorphous low-grade adenocarcinoma

Low Grade, Intermediate Grade, and High Grade
- Adenocarcinoma, not otherwise specified
- Mucoepidermoid carcinoma
- Squamous cell carcinoma

Intermediate Grade and High Grade
- Myoepithelial carcinoma

High Grade
- Anaplastic small cell carcinoma
- Carcinosarcoma
- Large cell undifferentiated carcinoma
- Small cell undifferentiated carcinoma
- Salivary duct carcinoma

Note. Based on information from National Cancer Institute, 2014b.

ically, three growth patterns have been described: cribriform (classic), tubular, and solid (basaloid). The tumors are categorized according to the predominant pattern. The cribriform pattern shows epithelial cell nests forming a cylindrical pattern and giving it a classic "Swiss cheese" appearance. The tubular pattern is defined as such because of the tubular structures that are lined by stratified cuboidal epithelium. The solid pattern shows solid groups of cuboidal cells. The cribriform pattern is the most common, whereas the solid pattern is the least common. Solid adenoid cystic carcinoma is a high-grade lesion with reported recurrence rates of up to 100%, compared with 50%–80% for the tubular and cribriform types (NCI, 2014b; Rajendran, 2009; Saunders & Wakely, n.d.).

Mucoepidermoid Carcinoma

Mucoepidermoid carcinoma is the most common malignant salivary gland neoplasm in both adults and children. Usually, they grow slowly and present as painless masses. They are poorly encapsulated or unencapsulated and easily infiltrate surrounding tissue. A wide range of biologic behavior may be seen. The majority of these tumors do not metastasize; however, if metastasis occurs, it is to the regional nodes, bone, lung, and brain. Patients with well-differentiated tumors have a 90% five-year survival rate, whereas those with poorly differentiated tumors may have only a 20% five-year survival rate (Saunders & Wakely, n.d.). This malignant epithelial tumor is composed of mucoid and epidermoid squamous cells. The mucoid cells are large with distinct borders and have a foamy cytoplasm that stains with mucin. The epidermoid squamous cells may show large nuclei with prominent nucleoli and an eosinophilic cytoplasm. The squamous cells are arranged in nests or solid areas in conjunction with mucoid cells. There may be some keratin deposits, but usually no large pearls as with squamous carcinoma. In addition to mucous and epidermal cells, there are "intermediate" cells, which are round- or oval-shaped and basaloid with scant pink cytoplasm (Saunders & Wakely, n.d.). Microscopic grading of mucoepidermoid carcinoma helps to determine prognosis. Mucous cells and cysts are prominent in low-grade tumors with minimal dysplastic cells. High-grade lesions are more squamous than mucinous and have significant pleomorphism and mitotic activity (Saunders & Wakely, n.d.).

Adenocarcinoma

Adenocarcinoma is a malignant neoplasm with a microscopic glandular growth pattern. These tumors are particularly common in the head and neck, especially in tumors of the salivary glands. Approximately 20 specific types of malignant epithelial salivary gland tumors exist. Clinically, patients typically present with a slowly enlarging mass in the parotid region. Pain related to the tendency for perineural invasion is a symptom in more than one-third of patients (Saunders & Wakely, n.d.).

Adenocarcinoma, Not Otherwise Specified

The term *adenocarcinoma, NOS,* is used for a subset of adenocarcinoma neoplasms that do not easily fit into the defined tumor subtypes. Approximately 40% occur in the major salivary glands and 60% in the minor glands. The mean patient age at diagnosis is 58 years (NCI, 2014b).

Adenocarcinoma, NOS, is a salivary gland carcinoma that presents a glandular growth pattern microscopically. The borders tend to be irregular and there may be extension outside of the gland, as found in other adenocarcinomas. Histologic diagnosis is one of exclusion more than inclusion. This tumor is graded according to the degree of differentiation, a manner similar to other salivary lesions. Tumor grades include low, intermediate, and high. Low-grade tumors may be well circumscribed with focal infiltration and contain well-formed duct-like structures with bland features and few mitoses. High-grade tumors also show glandular differentiation but with more solid areas of tumor growth, more mitoses, and greater nuclear variability. Giant tumor cells also may be present (Saunders & Wakely, n.d.).

Rare Adenocarcinomas

The glandular tissue of the salivary glands, both major and minor, lends itself to a number of rare adenocarcinomas. Because these pathologies are extremely rare, they will not be discussed in detail here, but a list is provided (NCI, 2014b).
• Basal cell adenocarcinoma
• Clear cell carcinoma
• Cystadenocarcinoma
• Sebaceous adenocarcinoma
• Sebaceous lymphadenocarcinoma
• Oncocytic carcinoma
• Salivary duct carcinoma
• Mucinous adenocarcinoma

Acinic Cell Carcinoma

Acinic cell carcinoma (also known as *acinic cell adenocarcinoma*) is a low-grade malignant epithelial neoplasm in which the cells express acinar differentiation. The term *acinic cell carcinoma* is used because of the differentiation between serous acinar cells and mucous acinar cells (NCI, 2014b). The largest series of salivary tumors to date was reported in the Armed Forces Institute of Pathology (AFIP) salivary gland registry. AFIP identified acinic cell carcinoma as the third most common malignancy of salivary glands. Seventeen percent of primary malignant salivary gland tumors and approximately 6% of all salivary gland neoplasms were acinic cell carcinomas. Most of these (more than 80%) occurred in the parotid gland. Women were affected more than men, and the mean age at diagnosis was 44 years (NCI, 2014b). According to Aly (2013), multiple considerations can determine a poor prognosis. The more advanced stage of the disease, pain, tumor fixation, neural invasion, involvement of deep lobe of parotid, increased mitotic rate, necrosis, and multinodularity, desmoplasia, anaplasia, or dedifferentiated components are poor prognostic factors.

Polymorphous Low-Grade Adenocarcinoma

Polymorphous low-grade adenocarcinoma (PLGA) is a malignant epithelial tumor that is limited to the minor salivary glands, most commonly the salivary glands of the palate. A bland, uniform nucleus and diverse architecture that infiltrates, particularly with perineural invasion, characterize these lesions. This neoplasm can be benign or malignant. The average age at diagnosis is 59 years, and it is twice as common in women as in men (NCI, 2014b).

PLGA typically presents as a firm, nontender swelling and usually runs a moderately indolent course. Cervical metastasis is rare, and wide excision often leads to cure. Microscopic perineural invasion does not seem to negatively affect prognosis. Death from this tumor is uncommon (Saunders & Wakely, n.d.).

Malignant Mixed Tumors

Malignant mixed tumors include three distinct entities: carcinoma ex pleomorphic adenoma, carcinosarcoma, and metastasizing mixed tumor. Most salivary neoplasms are carcinoma ex pleomorphic adenoma. Carcinosarcoma and metastasizing mixed tumor are rare.

Carcinoma Ex Pleomorphic Adenoma

Carcinoma ex pleomorphic adenoma (also known as *carcinoma ex mixed tumor*) is a carcinoma arising from or within a benign pleomorphic adenoma. Diagnosis requires the identification of benign tumor in the tissue sample. The AFIP database reports that carcinoma ex pleomorphic adenoma comprises 6% of all malignant salivary gland tumors. The tumor occurs most commonly in the parotid gland (Rousseau & Badoual, 2011a). Presentation is commonly a painless mass, and facial paralysis occurs in approximately one-third of patients. Tumor stage, histologic grade, and the extent of invasion are important prognostic factors (NCI, 2014b). Prognosis can be excellent when the malignant tumor is confined in the benign nodule and poor when the malignancy infiltrates into nearby soft tissues. Depending on the series cited, survival rates vary: 25%–65% at 5 years, 18%–50% at 10 years, 10%–35% at 15 years, and 0%–38% at 20 years (Rousseau & Badoual, 2011a).

Carcinosarcoma

Carcinosarcoma (also known as *true malignant mixed tumor*) is an extremely rare salivary gland malignancy that contains both carcinoma and sarcoma components. Most of these tumors occur in the major salivary glands and present with swelling, pain, nerve palsy, and ulceration. Carcinosarcoma is an aggressive high-grade malignancy (NCI, 2014b).

Metastasizing Mixed Tumor

Metastasizing mixed tumor is a very rare histologically benign salivary gland neoplasm that unexplainably metastasizes. It often occurs in the major salivary glands following a single well-defined primary mass. Often, a long interval occurs between the diagnosis of the primary tumor and the metastases. The histologic features are those seen in pleomorphic adenoma (NCI, 2014b).

Rare Carcinomas

The remaining salivary gland carcinomas are extremely rare and will not be discussed but are included in the following list (NCI, 2014b).
• Primary squamous cell carcinoma
• Epithelial-myoepithelial carcinoma
• Anaplastic small cell carcinoma
• Undifferentiated carcinoma
• Small cell undifferentiated carcinoma
• Large cell undifferentiated carcinoma
• Myoepithelial carcinoma
• Adenosquamous carcinoma
• Carcinoid neuroendocrine carcinoma

Molecular Genetics

Critically altered pathways in head and neck cancer include p53, epidermal growth factor receptor (EGFR), VEGF receptor, and other molecules that may serve as therapeutic targets (Chen, Sturgis, Etzel, Wei, & Li, 2008; Ragin, Modugno, & Gollin, 2007; Singh, 2008).

p53

The *p53* gene is a tumor suppressor gene. When *p53* is mutated and no longer able to act as a stop signal for cell division, the cells divide uncontrollably and can form tumors. Mutation of *p53* has been identified in 50% of head and neck malignances. Endogenous genetic alterations are not the only disrupters of *p53* function; HPV, specifically HPV 16, is a risk factor for oropharyngeal head and neck squamous cell carcinoma. E6 is a viral oncoprotein of HPV 16 and inactivates *p53* (Klein & Grandis, 2010).

Epidermal Growth Factor Receptor

EGFR is a tyrosine kinase receptor that is highly expressed on epithelial cells. EGFR is overexpressed in the majority of head and neck squamous cell carcinoma malignancies. EGFR is upstream of phosphoinositol 3-kinase (PI3K) and protein kinase B (Akt). EGFR is also upstream of mitogen-activated protein kinase (MAPK), which is stimulated through the Ras/Raf pathway. The downstream signaling along these pathways modulates cell migration, adhesion, and proliferation. Activation of the receptor is important for the innate immune response in human skin (Klein & Grandis, 2010).

Hepatocyte Growth Factor and c-Met

The hepatocyte growth factor (HGF) and its receptor c-Met promote cell proliferation, survival, motility, and invasion. High levels of HGF or c-Met correlate with poor prognosis in head and neck cancer. HGF has been shown to be a regulator of both MAPK and PI3K pathways. Activation of these pathways contributes to the expression of the proangiogenic factors, VEGF, and interleukin-8, and the promotion of tumor progression and angiogenesis (Dong et al., 2004; Knowles et al., 2009).

Insulin-Like Growth Factor-1 Receptor

The insulin-like growth factor-1 receptor (IGF-1R) is a protein found on the surface of human cells. The receptor is activated by insulin-like growth factor-1 (IGF-1). IGF-1 binds to IGF-1R and initiates intracellular signaling; IGF-1 is one of the most potent natural activators of the Akt signaling pathway. IGF-1R signaling is required for survival and growth of the cancer cell. IGF-1R has been implicated in the progression and survival of head and neck squamous cell carcinoma. Similar to c-Met, IGF-1R signals via Akt and MAPK, contributing to rapid tumor progression through apoptosis evasion, increased motility, changes in cell adhesion, and enhancement of proliferation. IGF-1R controls focal-adhesion kinase expression, contributing to increased motility and metastatic potential with IGF-1R overexpression. IGF-1R inhibition leads to decreased MAPK and PI3K signaling and is associated with a decrease in growth and motility (Limesand, Chibly, & Fribley, 2013).

Mammalian Target of Rapamycin

Mammalian target of rapamycin (mTOR) regulates cell growth, proliferation, motility, and survival and is a signaling molecule downstream of the PI3K/Akt pathway. Activation of the mTOR pathway is prevalent in head and neck squamous cell carcinoma independent of EGFR or *p53* status. *Akt* is an oncogene and involved in the transmitting of growth signals and interacts with mTOR. Expression of phosphorylated Akt contributes to mTOR activation and consequential cell proliferation. Unopposed activation of mTOR, as a result of silencing of the tumor suppressor gene phosphatase and tensin homolog (*PTEN*), contributes to malignant progression (Iglesias-Bartolome, Martin, & Gutkind, 2013).

Vascular Endothelial Growth Factor and Receptors

VEGF and its receptors are involved in head and neck squamous cell carcinoma. VEGF is an important signaling protein involved in angiogenesis. All members of the VEGF family stimulate cellular responses by binding to tyrosine kinase receptors on the cell surface, causing them to become activated. This response can lead to tumor expression of proangiogenic factors that allow for unregulated or less regulated blood vessel growth and formation. An "angiogenic switch" stimulates the growth of new vessels. Oxygen deprivation, inflammation, oncogenic mutations, and mechanical stress activate the angiogenic switch. This process results in increased tumor vascularization (Holmes, Roberts, Thomas, & Cross, 2007).

p16

The *p16* gene is a regulator of the cell cycle. It slows cell progression from G_1 phase to S phase and therefore acts as a tumor suppressor that is implicated in the prevention of cancers. The protein product is a tumor suppressor protein (Ai et al., 2003). It is frequently mutated or deleted in a wide variety of tumors, including oropharyngeal squamous cell carcinoma. Tissue samples of primary oral squamous cell carcinoma display hypermethylation in the promoter regions of *p16*. Cancer cells show a significant increase in the accumulation of methylation in CpG islands in the promoter region of *p16*. This epigenetic change leads to the loss of tumor suppressor gene function through methylation, thus causing the downregulation of gene expression and the decrease in the levels of the *p16* protein (Demokan et al., 2012; Khor et al., 2013). Immunohistochemistry is used to detect the presence of *p16* and is now being explored as a prognostic biomarker for patients with oropharyngeal squamous cell carcinoma. The presence of *p16* biomarker has been shown to be the strongest indicator of disease course, and it is associated with a more favorable prognosis as measured by cancer-specific survival, recurrence-free survival, and locoregional control (Oguejiofor et al., 2013).

Summary

Cancer is a general term for a group of diseases that result from genetic cellular changes, causing abnormal and uncontrolled cellular division, interfering with apoptosis, and altering the normal function and appearance of cells. As more is learned about the genetic code and cellular processes, a greater understanding of carcinogenesis is unfolding.

Head and neck cancer represents the sixth most common cancer worldwide and accounts for 3.9% of new cancer cases in the United States. Despite new treatment options, the prognosis has remained unchanged over the past 40 years, with approximately 50% of patients ultimately dying from their disease. The incidence of head and neck cancers is decreasing, but an increase has been seen in the incidence of oropharyngeal head and neck cancer associated with HPV.

The epidemiology, natural history, and treatment approach are dependent on the tumor anatomic site. Squamous cell carcinoma is the most common pathology and accounts for more than 90% of head and neck tumors. Head and neck cancers frequently are aggressive, and, unfortunately, most patients with head and neck cancer have metastatic disease at the time of diagnosis (43% nodal involvement and 10% distant metastasis). Patients with head and neck cancer often develop a second primary lesion, usually of the upper aerodigestive tract or lung, at an annual rate of 3%–7% (Ridge et al., 2014). If patients with a single cancer continue to smoke and use alcohol, the cure rate for the initial cancer, regardless of treatment modality, is diminished, and the risk of a second cancer increases (NCI, 2013). Lifestyle modification plays a major role in patients' response to therapy, as well as reducing the chance of recurrence and the development of a second primary malignancy.

References

Ackerman, L.V. (1948). Verrucous carcinoma of the oral cavity. *Surgery, 23,* 670–678.

Ai, L., Stephenson, K.K., Ling, W., Zuo, C., Mukunyadzi, P., Suen, J.Y., … Fan, C.Y. (2003). The p16 (CDKN2a/INK4a) tumor-suppressor gene in head and neck squamous cell carcinoma: A promoter methylation and protein expression study in 100 cases. *Modern Pathology, 16,* 944–950.

Alan, H., Agacayak, S., Kavak, G., & Ozcan, A. (2015). Verrucous carcinoma and squamous cell papilloma of the oral cavity: Report of two cases and review of literature. *European Journal of Dentistry, 9,* 453–456. doi:10.4103/1305-7456.163224

Aly, F. (2013). Salivary glands: Epithelial/myoepithelial tumors: Acinic cell carcinoma. Retrieved from http://www.pathologyoutlines.com/topic/salivaryglandsaciniccell.html

American Cancer Society. (2015a). *Cancer facts and figures 2015.* Retrieved from http://www.cancer.org/acs/groups/content/@editorial/documents/document/acspc-044552.pdf

American Cancer Society. (2015b). Oral cavity and oropharyngeal cancer. Retrieved from http://www.cancer.org/cancer/oralcavityandorophary ngealcancer/detailedguide/oral-cavity-and-oropharyngeal-cancer-key -statistics

Bakhtiar, S.M., Ali, A., & Barh, D. (2015). Epigenetics in head and neck cancer. In M. Verma (Ed.), *Cancer epigenetics: Risk assessment, diagnosis, treatment, and prognosis* (pp. 751–769). New York, NY: Springer Press.

Brennan, B. (2006). Nasopharyngeal carcinoma. *Orphanet Journal of Rare Diseases, 1,* 23. doi:10.1186/1750-1172-1-23

Brigham and Women's Hospital. (n.d.). Oral leukoplakia. Retrieved from http://www.brighamandwomens.org/departments_and_services/surgery/services/oralmedicine/imported%20files/leukoplakia.pdf

CancerQuest. (2010a). Cancer initiation, promotion, and progression. Retrieved from http://www.cancerquest.org/cancer-initiation -promotion-progression.html

CancerQuest. (2010b). Stages of tumor development. Retrieved from http://www.cancerquest.org/stages-tumor-progression.html

CancerQuest. (2012a). Cancer genes. Retrieved from http://www.cancer quest.org/cancer-genes-overview.html

CancerQuest. (2012b). Changes in physical properties of cancer cells. Retrieved from http://www.cancerquest.org/cancer-cell-physical -properties.html

CancerQuest. (2014). Overview of metastasis. Retrieved from http://www .cancerquest.org/metastasis-overview.html

Chaturvedi, A.K., Engels, E.A., Pfeiffer, R.M., Hernandez, B.Y., Xiao, W., Kim, E., … Gillison, M.L. (2011). Human papillomavirus and rising oropharyngeal cancer incidence in the United States. *Journal of Clinical Oncology, 29,* 4294–4301. doi:10.1200/JCO.2011.36.4596

Chen, X., Sturgis, E.M., Etzel, C.J., Wei, Q., & Li, G. (2008). *p73* G4C14-to-A4T14 polymorphism and risk of human papillomavirus-associated squamous cell carcinoma of the oropharynx in never smokers and never drinkers. *Cancer, 113,* 3307–3314. doi:10.1002/cncr.23976

Crozier, E., & Sumer, B.D. (2010). Head and neck cancer. *Medical Clinics of North America, 94,* 1031–1046. doi:10.1016/j.mcna.2010.05.014

Demokan, S., Chuang, A., Suoğlu, Y., Ulusan, M., Yalnız, Z., Califano, J.A., & Dalay, N. (2012). Promoter methylation and loss of $p16^{INK4a}$ gene expression in head and neck cancer. *Head and Neck, 34,* 1470–1475. doi:10.1002/hed.21949

Dong, G., Lee, T.L., Yeh, N.T., Geoghegan, J., Van Waes, C., & Chen, Z. (2004). Metastatic squamous cell carcinoma cells that overexpress c-Met exhibit enhanced angiogenesis factor expression, scattering and metastasis in response to hepatocyte growth factor. *Oncogene, 23,* 6199–6208. doi:10.1038/sj.onc.1207851

Hanahan, D., & Weinberg, R.A. (2011). The hallmarks of cancer: The next generation. *Cell, 144,* 646–674. doi:10.1016/j.cell.2011.02.013

Hashibe, M., Brennan, P., Chuang, S.C., Boccia, S., Castellsague, X., Chen, C., … Boffetta, P. (2009). Interaction between tobacco and alcohol use and the risk of head and neck cancer: Pooled analysis in the International Head and Neck Cancer Epidemiology Consortium. *Cancer Epidemiology, Biomarkers and Prevention, 18,* 541–550. doi:10.1158/1055-9965.EPI-08-0347

Holmes, K., Roberts, O.L., Thomas, A.M., & Cross, M.J. (2007). Vascular endothelial growth factor receptor-2: Structure, function, intracellular signalling and therapeutic inhibition. *Cell Signaling, 19,* 2003–2012. doi:10.1016/j.cellsig.2007.05.013

Iglesias-Bartolome, R., Martin, D., & Gutkind, J.S. (2013). Exploiting the head and neck cancer oncogenome: Widespread PI3K-mTOR pathway alterations and novel molecular targets. *Cancer Discovery, 3,* 722–725. doi:10.1158/2159-8290.CD-13-0239

Khor, G.H., Froemming, G.R., Zain, R.B., Abraham, M.T., Omar, E., Tan, S.K., … Thong, K.L. (2013). DNA methylation profiling revealed promoter hypermethylation-induced silencing of p16, DDAH2 and DUSP1 in primary oral squamous cell carcinoma. *International Journal of Medical Sciences, 10,* 1727–1739. doi:10.7150/ijms.6884

Klein, J.D., & Grandis, J.R. (2010). The molecular pathogenesis of head and neck cancer. *Cancer Biology and Therapy, 9,* 1–7. doi:10.4161/cbt.9.1.10905

Knowles, L.M., Stabile, L.P., Egloff, A.M., Rothstein, M.E., Thomas, S.M., Gubish, C.T., … Siegfried, J.M. (2009). HGF and c-Met participate in paracrine tumorigenic pathways in head and neck squamous cell cancer. *Clinical Cancer Research, 15,* 3740–3750. doi:10.1158/1078-0432.CCR-08-3252

Lea, D.H., Calzone, K.A., Masny, A., & Bush, A.M. (2002). *Genetics and cancer care: A guide for oncology nurses.* Pittsburgh, PA: Oncology Nursing Society.

Li, X., Shen, Y., Di, B., & Song, Q. (2012). Metastasis of head and neck squamous cell carcinoma. In X. Li (Ed.), *Squamous cell carcinoma* (pp. 3–32). Retrieved from http://cdn.intechopen.com/pdfs-wm/27527.pdf

Limesand, K.H., Chibly, A.M., & Fribley, A. (2013). Impact of targeting insulin-like growth factor signaling in head and neck cancers. *Growth Hormone and IGF Research, 23*(5), 135–140. doi:10.1016/j.ghir.2013.06.001

Luce, D., Leclerc, A., Bégin, D., Demers, P.A., Gérin, M., Orlowski, E., … Bofetta, P. (2002). Sinonasal cancer and occupational exposures: A pooled analysis of 12 case-control studies. *Cancer Causes and Control, 13,* 147–157. doi:10.1023/A:1014350004255

Nadler, D.L., & Zurbenko, I.G. (2014). Estimating cancer latency times using a Weibull model. *Advances in Epidemiology, 2014,* Article ID 746769. doi:10.1155/2014/746769

National Cancer Institute. (2011). Angiogenesis inhibitors. Retrieved from http://www.cancer.gov/cancertopics/factsheet/Therapy/angiogenesis-inhibitors

National Cancer Institute. (2013). Head and neck cancers. Retrieved from http://www.cancer.gov/cancertopics/factsheet/Sites-Types/head-and-neck

National Cancer Institute. (2014a). Nasopharyngeal cancer treatment (PDQ®). Retrieved from http://www.cancer.gov/cancertopics/pdq/treatment/nasopharyngeal/HealthProfessional#section_1.1

National Cancer Institute. (2014b). Salivary gland cancer treatment (PDQ®). Retrieved from http://www.cancer.gov/cancertopics/pdq/treatment/salivarygland/HealthProfessional#_408_toc

National Cancer Institute Surveillance, Epidemiology, and End Results Program. (2012). SEER Stat Fact Sheets: Oral cavity and pharynx cancer. Retrieved from http://seer.cancer.gov/statfacts/html/oralcav.html

Oguejiofor, K.K., Hall, J.S., Mani, N., Douglas, C., Slevin, N.J., Homer, J., … West, C.M. (2013). The prognostic significance of the biomarker p16 in oropharyngeal squamous cell carcinoma. *Clinical Oncology, 25,* 630–638. doi:10.1016/j.clon.2013.07.003

Open University. (2013). Introduction to histopathology. Retrieved from http://www.open.edu/openlearn/science-maths-technology/science/biology/introduction-histopathology/content-section-2.1

Oral Cancer Foundation. (2014). Histopathology, biology and markers. Retrieved from http://www.oralcancerfoundation.org/cdc/cdc_chapter2.php

Pai, S.I., & Westra, W.H. (2009). Molecular pathology of head and neck cancer: Implications for diagnosis, prognosis, and treatment. *Annual Review of Pathology, 4,* 49–70. doi:10.1146/annurev.pathol.4.110807.092158

Ragin, C.C., Modugno, F., & Gollin, S.M. (2007). The epidemiology and risk factors of head and neck cancer: A focus on human papillomavirus. *Journal of Dental Research, 86,* 104–114. doi:10.1177/154405910708600202

Rajendran, R. (2009). Malignant tumors of the salivary glands. In R. Rajendran & B. Sivapathasundharam (Eds.), *Shafer's textbook of oral pathology* (6th ed., pp. 230–242). New Delhi, India: Elsevier.

Riaz, N., Morris, L.G., Lee, W., & Chan, T.A. (2014). Unraveling the molecular genetics of head and neck cancer through genome-wide approaches. *Genes and Diseases, 1,* 75–86. doi:10.1016/j.gendis.2014.07.002

Ridge, J.A., Mehra, R., Lango, M.N., & Feigenberg, S. (2014). Head and neck tumors. In D.G. Haller, L.D. Wagman, K.A. Camphausen, & W.J. Hoskins (Eds.), *Cancer management: A multidisciplinary approach: Medical, surgical, and radiation oncology.* Retrieved from http://www.cancernetwork.com/head-and-neck-tumors

Rousseau, A., & Badoual, C. (2011a). Head and neck: Salivary gland tumors: An overview. *Atlas of Genetics and Cytogenetics in Oncology and Haematology, 15,* 533–541. doi:10.4267/2042/45043

Rousseau, A., & Badoual, C. (2011b). Head and neck: Squamous cell carcinoma: An overview. *Atlas of Genetics and Cytogenetics in Oncology and Haematology, 16,* 145–155. Retrieved from http://atlasgeneticsoncology.org/Tumors/HeadNeckSCCID5090.html

Saunders, W.H., & Wakely, P. (n.d.). Atlas of head and neck pathology. Retrieved from http://ent.osu.edu/atlas-head-and-neck-pathology

Simard, E.P., Torre, L.A., & Jemal, A. (2014). International trends in head and neck cancer incidence rates: Differences by country, sex and anatomic site. *Oral Oncology, 50,* 387–403. doi:10.1016/j.oraloncology.2014.01.016

Singh, B. (2008). Molecular pathogenesis of head and neck cancers. *Journal of Surgical Oncology, 97,* 634–639. doi:10.1002/jso.21024

Stefani, E.D., Moore, M., Aune, D., Deneo-Pellegrini, H., Ronco, A.L., Boffetta, P., … Landó, G. (2011). Maté consumption and risk of cancer: A multi-site case-control study in Uruguay. *Asian Pacific Journal of Cancer Prevention, 12,* 1089–1093.

Stevenson, M.M. (2013). Head and neck cancer staging: TNM classification for head and neck cancer. Retrieved from http://emedicine.medscape.com/article/2007181-overview

Wei, W.I., & Sham, J.S.T. (2005). Nasopharyngeal carcinoma. *Lancet, 365,* 2041–2054. doi:10.1016/S0140-6736(05)66698-6

World Health Organization. (2013). *International classification of diseases for oncology* (3rd ed.). Retrieved from http://apps.who.int/iris/bitstream/10665/96612/1/9789241548496_eng.pdf?ua=1

CHAPTER 4

Prevention and Early Detection

Helen Lazio Stegall, BSN, RN, CORLN, and
Michele Farrington, BSN, RN, CPHON®

Introduction

Cancer prevention and early detection are strategies aimed at decreasing the incidence and increasing the survival of patients with head and neck cancer. These strategies involve several common themes. One is an understanding of the risk factors associated with head and neck carcinoma. Understanding the risk factors allows for appropriate lifestyle choices and more effective cancer screening of at-risk populations, subsequently providing an opportunity for early detection. This may lead to earlier initiation of treatment, which may increase the chance of survival. Chemoprevention prevents or delays the development of cancer through the use of medications, vitamins, or other agents. Research in this area may prove useful in preventing or suppressing some types of cancers, such as with human papillomavirus (HPV) and its relationship to oral cavity malignancies and the current trend toward vaccination.

Risk Factors

The World Health Organization (WHO) defines a risk factor as "any attribute, characteristic, or exposure of an individual that increases the likelihood of developing a disease or injury" (WHO, 2015, para. 1). Humans are exposed continually and simultaneously to a broad spectrum of biologic, chemical, and physical forces. To complicate matters even more, each individual reacts differently to these forces, which are conditioned by heredity, age, sex, and a multitude of other factors (National Cancer Institute [NCI], 2015). Current evidence suggests cancer is multifactorial; no single cause for any type of cancer has been identified (Cancer Research UK, 2014).

Because of the location of head and neck tumors and the functions of the vital structures involved, patients with head and neck cancer often are faced with challenging and potentially life-altering conditions. An understanding of risk fac-

tors could lead to earlier detection and treatment, thereby decreasing morbidity and mortality in this patient population.

Upper Aerodigestive Tract Cancers

Cancers found in the oral cavity, oropharynx, hypopharynx, larynx, or esophagus are collectively known as upper aerodigestive tract cancers (Anantharaman et al., 2011). Tobacco (Gandini et al., 2008; Wyss et al., 2013) and alcohol use (Boffetta & Hashibe, 2006) contribute to an increased risk of cancer development in the upper aerodigestive tract (Anantharaman et al., 2011; Bakri, Hussaini, Holmes, Cannon, & Rich, 2010; IARC Working Group on the Evaluation of Carcinogenic Risks to Humans, 2010; Pfister et al., 2011; Shin & Saba, 2014). Combined use of tobacco and alcohol is associated with 44% of upper aerodigestive tract cancers, whereas 29% of these cancers are associated with only tobacco use and 1% of these cancers are associated with only alcohol use (Anantharaman et al., 2011).

Multiple chemicals are found in both tobacco and tobacco smoke and are known to be carcinogenetic. Some of these chemicals include cyanide, benzene, formaldehyde, methanol, acetylene, and ammonia. All tissues and vital organs that come in contact with these chemicals will experience harmful effects (American Cancer Society [ACS], 2014b). ACS (2014b) reports that the smoke from tobacco is composed of more than 7,000 chemicals, including more than 70 chemicals that are known carcinogens (e.g., tar, carbon monoxide, nitrogen oxide). The carcinogenic effects of tobacco initiate both genetic mutations and the proliferation of cell clones in the mucosa. In turn, the entire epithelial field of the upper aerodigestive tract is at increased risk for development of cancer because of these widespread genetic abnormalities (Boyle et al., 2010).

Smokeless tobacco (snuff), commonly used worldwide, is dry or moist tobacco that is finely ground and comes packaged in cans or pouches. Smokeless tobacco often contains sweeteners and flavorings (e.g., vanilla, mint, fruit) designed to increase its appeal with younger people. Many harmful effects may result from use of smokeless tobacco, some of which include mouth, tongue, cheek, gum, throat, and esophageal cancer; leukoplakia (white patches in the mouth); receding gums; and gingivitis (gum disease) (ACS, 2013; Boffetta, Hecht, Gray, Gupta, & Straif, 2008).

Cigar smoking continues to be popular among teenagers and young adults, and evidence suggests it poses an increased risk for development of head and neck cancer (ACS, 2014a; Wyss et al., 2013). Most full-size cigars contain the same amount of nicotine found in several cigarettes. Larger cigars typically contain 100–200 mg of nicotine but can contain as much as 444 mg. Increased risk of lip, oral cavity, esophageal, or laryngeal cancer exists for people who regularly smoke cigars, but actual health risks are dependent on the number of cigars smoked and how the cigar is smoked. An ACS (2014a) study comparing cigar smokers who inhale deeply to nonsmokers found that cigar smokers were seven times more likely to die from an oral cancer and 39 times more likely to die from laryngeal cancer than nonsmokers.

New products on the market (e.g., electronic cigarettes [e-cigarettes], electronic cigars [e-cigars]) are sold over the counter and are not currently held to the same regulations as conventional cigarettes and cigars. These electronic nicotine delivery devices generate nicotine aerosol or vapor along with flavorings and other chemicals via an inhaled aerosol without the combustion of tobacco. More research is needed on these products to determine what associated risks exist for both the user and the public (Chatham-Stephens et al., 2014; Czogala et al., 2014; Goniewicz et al., 2014; McGill, 2013).

As previously mentioned, alcohol consumption is a major risk factor for head and neck cancer, specifically cancers arising from the oral cavity (excluding the lips), larynx, oropharynx, and hypopharynx (Baan et al., 2007). An increased risk of head and neck cancer development is associated with the consumption of more than three alcoholic beverages per day in both men and women (Freedman, Schatzkin, Leitzmann, Hollenbeck, & Abnet, 2007). In addition to causing cell damage, alcohol consumption depletes the body of selenium and vitamin A, which compromises the immune system (Clugston & Blaner, 2012; Rametta et al., 2013; Rua et al., 2014) and decreases the body's ability to protect itself from cancer (NCI, 2014a).

A third common risk factor for development of an upper aerodigestive tract cancer is betel nut quid, which is chewed as a popular custom in South Asia. Various ingredients, including tobacco, lime, spices, and betel nut, are placed in a betel leaf that is folded and held in the mouth for hours or days (Crozier & Sumer, 2010). Prolonged exposure or repeated use of betel nut quid can lead to inflammation and fibro-

sis of the oral cavity tissue, resulting in potentially malignant lesions (Auluck, Rosin, Zhang, & Sumanth, 2008).

The healthcare team is in an ideal position to address ways to prevent morbidity and mortality related to tobacco, alcohol, and betel nut quid use through provision of patient education and access to available resources. Patient education should be approached using multiple interactive and reinforcing strategies. To address tobacco use, members of the healthcare team need to ask all patients about use of any form of tobacco on every visit. If patients report using tobacco, the healthcare team must assess their readiness to quit; no matter the level of readiness, the importance of quitting must be discussed. Additional assistance should be provided through referrals to support groups, self-help resources, and community services. Finally, appropriate follow-up should be arranged. Alcohol and betel nut quid use must also be routinely and consistently assessed and addressed in a similar manner to ensure that patients understand the consequences and risks associated with these behaviors.

Unlike other tumors of the upper aerodigestive tract, tobacco and alcohol use are not as strongly linked with nasopharyngeal carcinoma (NPC). The risk of developing NPC is often associated with gender (men are affected twice as often as women), race/ethnicity, diet, Epstein-Barr virus (EBV), genetic factors, and family history. Workplace exposure to formaldehyde or wood dust may also increase the risk of NPC (ACS, 2015c). Although NPC is uncommon in the United States, with incidence rates of less than one case per 100,000 people, it is one of the most common cancers in southern China and southeastern Asia (ACS, 2015c; Wang, Zhang, & Ma, 2013). NPC is strongly associated with a diet rich in salt-cured fish and meat commonly eaten in China and other regions where NPC is common. As diets change and become more "Westernized," the incidence of NPC is decreasing (ACS, 2015c; Tsao et al., 2014). Despite the strong association between EBV infection and NPC, the exact etiology remains unclear. A study published in 2013 demonstrated that plasma EBV DNA analysis is sensitive for the detection of early and clinically silent NPC and proposed serology testing for EBV as an efficient and cost-effective screening test for high-risk populations (Chan et al., 2013).

Potentially Malignant Disorders

Oral squamous cell carcinomas (SCCs) may develop from a number of potentially malignant disorders (PMDs). Increasing awareness about oral PMDs may lead to improved diagnosis and treatment of these lesions and subsequently help to prevent malignant transformation (Mortazavi, Baharvand, & Mehdipour, 2014). A published report in 2011 noted that the transformation rate for patients with leukoplakia, the most common of the oral PMDs, ranges from 0.13% to 17.5%, illustrating the importance of screening, identification, and treatment of oral PMDs (Amagasa, Yamashiro, & Uzawa, 2011). PMDs of the oral mucosa can easily be detected visually on clinical examination, often presenting as leukoplakia, erythroplakia, or together in the same lesion as erythroleukoplakia (Carnelio, Rodrigues, Shenoy, & Fernandes, 2011).

Leukoplakia

Oral leukoplakia is a white plaque or patch that cannot be rubbed off and cannot be diagnosed as any other condition or disease. The original WHO definition for leukoplakia was established in 1978 and most recently updated in 2005, describing it as "white plaques of questionable risk having excluded (other) known diseases or disorders that carry no increased risk for cancer" (Warnakulasuriya, Johnson, & van der Waal, 2007, p. 577). These lesions vary in size and shape and are not associated with any physical or chemical causative agent except tobacco (Abidullah, Kiran, Gaddikeri, Raghoji, & Ravishankar, 2014). Leukoplakia with candidal infection leads to a higher rate of malignant transformation than uninfected leukoplakia (Bartie, Williams, Wilson, Potts, & Lewis, 2004). Specifically, *Candida albicans* has been associated with oral and esophageal cancer development for many years. Typical presentation of oral candidiasis is a chronic white patch that accumulates on the lining of the mouth, but other sites of the oral mucosa may be affected (Bakri et al., 2010).

Erythroplakia

Erythroplakia is defined as "a chronic red mucosal macule which cannot be given another specific diagnostic name and cannot be attributed to traumatic, vascular, or inflammatory causes" (Bouquot, 1994, p. 11). Erythroplakia occurs less frequently than leukoplakia and is seen more commonly in middle-aged and older adult men and presents on the floor of the mouth, soft palate, or buccal mucosa (Reichart & Philipsen, 2005). The actual annual malignant transformation rate for erythroplakia is unknown but is much higher than leukoplakia (Syrjänen et al., 2011; van der Waal, 2014).

Oral Lichen Planus

Oral lichen planus, a chronic inflammatory disease that affects the mucous membrane of the oral cavity (Lavanya, Jayanthi, Rao, & Ranganathan, 2011), is another condition sometimes placed in the "potentially malignant" category (Mattila, Rautava, & Syrjänen, 2012; Syrjänen et al., 2011). Although the exact etiology is unknown, oral lichen planus is thought to be a mucocutaneous autoimmune disease (Lavanya et al., 2011). The oral lesions appear in different forms and are not usually thought to have malignant potential (van der Waal, 2014).

Screening of the easily accessible oral cavity and oropharynx to identify PMDs should routinely be done by dentists, dental hygienists, and primary care providers (PCPs) (Brocklehurst et al., 2013). Education and training for dental professionals and PCPs must be an area of focus, with time and attention dedicated to the importance of comprehensive examinations performed competently by members of the healthcare team (Maybury, Horowitz, & Goodman, 2012).

Sinonasal Tumors

Tumors of the nasal cavity and paranasal sinuses are rare (Turner & Reh, 2012), accounting for less than 3% of cancers of the upper aerodigestive tract and less than 1% of all cancers (Baier, Völter, Steigerwald, Müller, & Schwager, 2005). However, these tumors are usually advanced at diagnosis and associated with a poor prognosis (Jensen, Nikoghosyan, Windemuth-Kieselbach, Debus, & Münter, 2011; Khademi, Moradi, Hoseini, & Mohammadianpanah, 2009; Turner & Reh, 2012). Sinonasal tumors may develop in the maxillary, ethmoid, frontal, or sphenoid sinuses or the nasal cavity but are more commonly found in the maxillary sinuses or nasal cavity (ACS, 2015b). Occupational exposures have often been linked and documented with these types of cancers, one example being wood dust and sinonasal adenocarcinoma (Mensi et al., 2013). Exposure to the following have been confirmed or suspected to cause an increased risk of sinonasal tumor development: wood dust, leather dust, nickel compounds, hexavalent chromium compounds, welding fumes, arsenic, mineral oils, organic solvents, and textile dust (d'Errico et al., 2009; Samant & Kruger, 2007; Straif et al., 2009). In addition, viruses (e.g., EBV, HPV type 16 or 18) and other microorganisms may play a role in the development of these tumors (Irigaray et al., 2007).

Individuals who work in industries where potential occupational exposures occur should talk with their healthcare team about ways to reduce their risk of cancer development. The discussion must also address how often checkups are needed to facilitate early detection in individuals at increased risk of sinonasal tumor development.

Salivary Gland Tumors

Little evidence is available regarding the etiology of malignant salivary gland tumors, and, in most instances, no known risk factors can be identified (Mendenhall, Werning, & Pfister, 2011). However, a few risk factors may be associated with development of these tumors, including older age, male gender, radiation exposure, and family history. The following potential risk factors must also be considered, although none have a large body of supporting evidence for a direct linkage with development of a salivary gland tumor: occupational exposures (e.g., nickel alloy dust, silica dust, asbestos mining, plumbing, rubber products manufacturing, woodworking), tobacco use, alcohol use, and a diet low in vegetables and high in animal fat (ACS, 2015e; American Society of Clinical Oncology, 2014; NCI, 2014b).

As with many cancers of the head and neck region, individuals must create and maintain healthy lifestyles to reduce the risk of salivary gland tumor development. A healthy lifestyle is contingent on daily choices and habits, such as good nutrition, exercise, adequate sleep, limited alcohol consumption, and absence of tobacco use.

Skin Carcinomas and Melanoma

Skin cancers, such as basal cell carcinoma (BCC), SCC, and melanoma, can be found in the area of the head and neck. Sun exposure is the primary risk factor for skin cancers (Ouyang, 2010), but genetic makeup, family history, immune system suppression, age, and xeroderma pigmentosum also play a role (Daya-Grosjean & Sarasin, 2005; Markovic et al., 2007). Multiple additional factors influence the development of these cancers, including outdoor occupations, amount of sun exposure, natural versus artificial light, and increased exposure to ultraviolet (UV) radiation caused by changes in the ozone (Dessinioti, Antoniou, Katsambas, & Stratigos, 2010; Eggermont, Spatz, & Robert, 2014; Markovic et al., 2007). The time between UV damage and the clinical onset of BCC may be as long as 20–50 years (Dessinioti et al., 2010).

The presence of a dysplastic nevus, an atypical mole, increases an individual's risk for development of skin melanoma (Silva, Sá, Avila, Landman, & Duprat Neto, 2011; Stratigos & Katsambas, 2009). The amount of risk is determined by the number of dysplastic nevi; if an individual has 10 or more dysplastic nevi, then the risk of developing melanoma is 12 times greater than for the general population (Skin Cancer Foundation, 2015).

Individuals with particular skin types and coloring are more sensitive to the effects of UV radiation and are at an increased risk for developing skin melanoma. This includes those with red or blond hair, freckles, and fair skin that burns easily and tans with difficulty (Dessinioti et al., 2010; Ouyang, 2010; Raimondi et al., 2008; Stratigos & Katsambas, 2009). As opposed to cumulative sun exposure, which influences nonmelanoma skin cancer, skin melanoma risk is associated with intermittent, intense sun exposure (Dessinioti et al., 2010; Eggermont et al., 2014).

One of the most important risk factors for development of skin melanoma is a family history (Gandini et al., 2005; Stratigos & Katsambas, 2009), as 5%–10% of individuals who develop melanoma have a family history (Bataille & de Vries, 2008). If a first-degree relative has a history of skin melanoma, the individual is twice as likely to develop melanoma as someone without a family history (Markovic et al., 2007).

Lip cancer is a type of oral cancer that may result from sun exposure. Most cases of lip cancer are found on the lower lip and are SCCs. Avoiding excessive sun exposure and wearing sunscreen on the lips may decrease one's risk of developing this type of cancer (HealthGrades, 2015). Actinic cheilitis, a form of actinic keratosis, is a potentially malignant change seen in the lip after an individual has sustained sun damage that must be monitored for malignant transformation into SCC (Dessinioti et al., 2010; Skin Cancer Foundation, 2014).

Thyroid Carcinomas

External radiation exposure to the head and neck region is one cause of thyroid cancer. Historical evidence links thyroid cancer with contamination caused by radioactive fallout from atomic bomb explosions and nuclear reactor meltdowns. Thyroid cancers have developed in individuals given external beam radiation treatments as children for medical diagnostics or as part of treatment plans (Schneider & Chen, 2013).

The latent period between radiation exposure and the diagnosis of thyroid carcinomas is usually 10–20 years (Schneider & Chen, 2013). Thyroid cancer occurs in approximately 5%–15% of thyroid nodules depending on age, sex, radiation exposure history, family history, and other factors related to dietary intake (e.g., iodine, selenium, goitrogen, carcinogen) and thyroid-stimulating hormone levels (Cooper et al., 2009; Schneider & Chen, 2013).

Human Papillomavirus

HPV is the most common sexually transmitted infection in the United States and has been linked to the development of cervical cancer. There have been more than 100 types of HPV identified; 40 of these types infect the mucosal epithelium. High-risk HPV type 16 is the cause of approximately 50% of cervical cancers throughout the world. Since 2006, a vaccine has been available to prevent infection with four types of HPV (Centers for Disease Control and Prevention, 2014).

Head and neck SCCs can occur in nonsmokers and nondrinkers (Deschler, Richmon, Khariwala, Ferris, & Wang, 2014), which suggests the presence of other risk factors. Since the 1970s, HPV has been linked with a subset of these cancers (Kreimer, Clifford, Boyle, & Franceschi, 2005; Woods et al., 2014). Approximately 26% of all patients with head and neck cancer and 36% of the oropharyngeal SCC subgroup of patients harbor HPV (Gillison et al., 2008; Hardefeldt, Cox, & Eslick, 2014). In addition, the probability of an oropharyngeal cancer attributed to HPV is five times more likely than other cancers of the oral cavity, larynx, or hypopharynx (Combes & Franceschi, 2014). Specifically, HPV type 16 has been associated with oropharyngeal cancer (Ang et al., 2010; Pfister et al., 2011; Shin & Saba, 2014; Syrjänen et al., 2011). HPV is most strongly linked with head and neck cancer of the tonsils or base of the tongue (Pfister et al., 2011; Woods et al., 2014). The current risk factors associated with HPV-related SCC include younger age at presentation, sexual behaviors, oral HPV infection, immunodeficiency, male gender, and higher socioeconomic status (Woods et al., 2014).

The link between prophylactic HPV vaccination and prevention of oropharyngeal SCC is unclear at this time (Pfister et al., 2011; Woods et al., 2014). No studies have looked at the efficacy of HPV vaccination in preventing oral HPV infection (Chaturvedi, 2012; Kreimer & Chaturvedi, 2011; Shin & Saba, 2014). Once efficacy of the HPV vaccination in preventing oral HPV infection has been established, recommendations should include vaccination for both genders because oropharyngeal cancers occur in both men and women (D'Souza et al., 2007). The full effects of HPV vaccination on cancer incidence will not be detected for several decades (Ramqvist & Dalianis, 2010).

Diet

A diet rich in fruits and vegetables is critical for preventing cancer (Freedman et al., 2014; Liu, Wang, Leng, & Lv, 2013). Diets lacking in fruits and vegetables deplete the body of the protection provided by their primary nutrients, antioxidants (Rahal et al., 2014). Antioxidants protect cells from the damaging effects of unstable molecules known as free radicals. Additional studies are needed regarding the efficacy and safety of antioxidants in helping to slow or prevent the free radical cell damage associated with cancer development (Ratnam, Ankola, Bhardwaj, Sahana, & Kumar, 2006).

Patients with head and neck cancer have a frequent incidence of poor-fitting dentures, loss of teeth or bone, frequent oral infections, and sores resulting from poor oral hygiene (Mahmood, Butterworth, Lowe, & Rogers, 2014). These factors, coupled with heavy alcohol consumption and tobacco use, can lead to compromised nutrition in this patient population. Maintaining a healthy diet along with head and neck cancer screening and prevention are important topics for continued research in this patient population. However, this does not preclude the healthcare team's need for patient education focused on the importance of routine and systematic evidence-based oral care.

Cancer Screening

Significant controversy exists in the literature regarding cancer screening recommendations. The debate centers on the benefits of generalized screening for head and neck cancers in asymptomatic individuals versus individuals previously identified as being at increased risk (Moyer, 2014). Easy accessibility and ability for inspection has led to increased focus on screening of the oral cavity and orophar-

ynx (Brocklehurst et al., 2013; Radoï & Luce, 2013; Shin & Saba, 2014). Although there may be insufficient evidence to establish that screening results in decreased morbidity and mortality from oral and oropharyngeal cancers (Epstein, Güneri, Boyacioglu, & Abt, 2012), ACS recommends an oral cavity examination as part of all cancer-related checkups and recommends that regular dental checkups include an examination of the entire mouth (ACS, 2015d). Regular dental checkups, at least annually, may facilitate earlier detection of oral and pharyngeal cancer, thereby reducing the public health burden caused by these diseases (Langevin et al., 2012; Walsh et al., 2013). Time and attention must be focused on ensuring that education and training are provided to dental professionals regarding why routine performance of comprehensive cancer screening examinations is warranted and how to competently perform these examinations (Maybury et al., 2012).

Similar controversy exists regarding skin cancer screening and early detection programs, which have the potential to decrease morbidity and mortality from skin melanoma (Stratigos & Katsambas, 2009). This controversy focuses on the benefits of population-based screening versus screening subgroups that are at increased risk for developing skin melanoma (Stratigos & Katsambas, 2009). In light of these inconsistent recommendations, the focus must shift to education of the healthcare team and general public regarding risk factor awareness for certain types of cancer (Stratigos & Katsambas, 2009), as well as risk reduction strategies (e.g., tobacco cessation, alcohol cessation) (Shin & Saba, 2014).

Chemoprevention

Many cancers develop as a result of exposure to carcinogens and cancer-promoting agents. This exposure creates a stepwise accumulation of cellular and genetic changes that may eventually develop into a malignant tumor. An increased understanding of the biology of this carcinogenesis, as well as the high mortality rates associated with recurrent disease and second primary tumors, have led researchers to focus on chemoprevention (Kim, Amin, & Shin, 2010; Kozyreva, D'Silva, & Vaughan, 2013).

Chemoprevention is the use of natural, synthetic, or biologic chemical agents to suppress, reverse, or prevent the multistep process that leads to cancer formation (Tsao, Kim, & Hong, 2004). Primary chemoprevention includes the use of chemopreventive agents to reverse the progression of PMDs, and secondary chemoprevention focuses on preventing the development of subsequent cancers in patients who have already received cancer-directed therapy (Kozyreva et al., 2013; Shin & Saba, 2014).

The principle of chemoprevention for epithelial carcinomas of the head and neck is built on the concept of multistep carcinogenesis and field cancerization (Shin & Saba, 2014;

Smith & Saba, 2005). Field cancerization describes the diffuse epithelial damage caused by exposure to inhaled carcinogens. The entire epithelial surface of the upper aerodigestive tract is at increased risk for the development of potentially malignant and, in turn, malignant lesions (Sheth, 2006).

Development of a second primary tumor is associated with a worse prognosis for patients with head and neck cancer (Priante, Castilho, & Kowalski, 2011). Second primary tumors may develop from influences related to treatment effects, lifestyle factors, environmental exposures, or host factors but most likely develop as a result of a combination of influences, including gene-environment and gene-gene interactions (Travis et al., 2006).

As research and knowledge has expanded around the epithelial field changes often observed in patients with head and neck cancer, second primary cancers have been found to be genetically related to the primary cancer (Sheth, 2006). Studies of PMDs of the head and neck have been a particular focus for chemoprevention research, as PMDs (e.g., leukoplakia, erythroplakia) associated with carcinogen exposure are precursors of malignant tumors (Brocklehurst et al., 2013; Radoï & Luce, 2013). Although advances in multidisciplinary cancer treatment have slightly improved the mortality rate from epithelial malignancies, the development of locally recurrent diseases and second primary tumors continues to affect the morbidity and mortality of this patient population (Lee et al., 2011; Sheth, 2006).

Numerous agents, such as retinoids and vitamin A (beta-carotene), alpha-tocopherol (vitamin E), biochemoprevention, selenium, cyclooxygenase-2 (COX-2) inhibitors, tyrosine kinase inhibitors, ONYX-015 (attenuated adenovirus), and protease inhibitors, are being investigated as potential systemic agents that may interrupt or inhibit the development of head and neck cancers (Kozyreva et al., 2013; Shin & Saba, 2014; Smith & Saba, 2005). Retinoids have been the main focus of chemoprevention research because of their inhibiting effect on tumor cell proliferation and their ability to normalize cell differentiation of malignant and potentially malignant lesions (Kozyreva et al., 2013; Shin & Saba, 2014), but a major limitation is retinoid-related toxicity (Shin & Saba, 2014; Smith & Saba, 2005).

Vitamin A (retinol) functions in the body to regulate normal growth and differentiation of a wide variety of cell types: epithelial cells of the respiratory and digestive tracts, nervous and immune systems, skin, and bone (National Institutes of Health [NIH], 2013; Smith & Saba, 2005). Vitamin A can be obtained by individuals in their diet, both from animal sources as preformed retinoids (retinyl esters) or from plant sources such as provitamin carotenoids (e.g., beta-carotene). These sources of vitamin A are converted to retinol and stored in the liver (NIH, 2013). Current research involves the use of various natural and synthetic vitamin A derivatives, alone or combined, to prevent cancer development (Sheth, 2006; Shin & Saba, 2014).

Retinoids might be effective in suppressing the formation of head and neck cancers with primary prevention studies demonstrating variable regression of leukoplakia resulting from the use of retinol and/or beta-carotene (Sheth, 2006; Shin & Saba, 2014). Secondary prevention studies using beta-carotene and other retinol derivatives have also shown decreased incidence of second primary head and neck cancers (Sheth, 2006). Although the retinoid compounds have been associated with relatively good overall response rates, the most notable issue from these studies was the serious dose-related toxicity of vitamin A. Symptoms of toxicity include increased intracranial pressure, dizziness, nausea, headaches, skin irritation, joint pain, bone pain, coma, and even death (NIH, 2013).

To date, great strides have been made in demonstrating the role retinoids may have in the chemoprevention of head and neck carcinomas. However, research gaps remain concerning the degree to which retinoid compounds reduce the rate of primary and secondary tumors and the most effective treatment regimen (e.g., dose and prescribed treatment course) that balances the chemopreventive effects with the toxic side effects. Future research must address the development of additional less toxic, more effective chemopreventive compounds with a more standardized approach to chemoprevention in head and neck cancers (Shin & Saba, 2014).

Summary

An estimated 45,780 new cases of oral cavity and pharyngeal cancer are expected in 2015 (ACS, 2015a). Current evidence suggests that cancer prevention strategies, coupled with early diagnosis (Harris, Phillips, Sayer, & Moore, 2013) and new developments in chemotherapy treatment, play an important role in the diagnosis, staging, treatment, and overall outcome for individuals experiencing these types of cancers.

The authors would like to acknowledge Margaret L. Colwill, RN, BSN, CORLN, for her contribution to this chapter that remains unchanged from the first edition of this book.

References

Abidullah, M., Kiran, G., Gaddikeri, K., Raghoji, S., & Ravishankar, T.S. (2014). Leuloplakia—Review of a potentially malignant disorder. *Journal of Clinical and Diagnostic Research, 8*(8), ZE01–ZE04. doi:10.7860/JCDR/2014/10214.4677

Amagasa, T., Yamashiro, M., & Uzawa, N. (2011). Oral premalignant lesions: From a clinical perspective. *International Journal of Clinical Oncology, 16*, 5–14. doi:10.1007/s10147-010-0157-3

American Cancer Society. (2013). Smokeless tobacco. Retrieved from http://www.cancer.org/cancer/cancercauses/tobaccocancer/smokeless-tobacco

American Cancer Society. (2014a). Cigar smoking. Retrieved from http://www.cancer.org/acs/groups/cid/documents/webcontent/002965-pdf.pdf

American Cancer Society. (2014b). Questions about smoking, tobacco, and health. Retrieved from http://www.cancer.org/cancer/cancercauses/tobaccocancer/questionsaboutsmokingtobaccoandhealth/questions-about-smoking-tobacco-and-health-cancer-and-health

American Cancer Society. (2015a). *Cancer facts and figures 2015.* Retrieved from http://www.cancer.org/acs/groups/content/@editorial/documents/document/acspc-044552.pdf

American Cancer Society. (2015b). Nasal cavity and paranasal sinus cancers. Retrieved from http://www.cancer.org/acs/groups/cid/documents/webcontent/003123-pdf.pdf

American Cancer Society. (2015c). Nasopharyngeal cancer. Retrieved from http://www.cancer.org/acs/groups/cid/documents/webcontent/003124-pdf.pdf

American Cancer Society. (2015d). Oral cavity and oropharyngeal cancer. Retrieved from http://www.cancer.org/acs/groups/cid/documents/webcontent/003128-pdf.pdf

American Cancer Society. (2015e). Salivary gland cancer. Retrieved from http://www.cancer.org/acs/groups/cid/documents/webcontent/003137-pdf.pdf

American Society of Clinical Oncology. (2014). Salivary gland cancer: Risk factors. Retrieved from http://www.cancer.net/cancer-types/salivary-gland-cancer/risk-factors

Anantharaman, D., Marron, M., Lagiou, P., Samoli, E., Ahrens, W., Pohlabeln, H., … Macfarlane, G.J. (2011). Population attributable risk of tobacco and alcohol for upper aerodigestive tract cancer. *Oral Oncology, 47,* 725–731. doi:10.1016/j.oraloncology.2011.05.004

Ang, K.K., Harris, J., Wheeler, R., Weber, R., Rosenthal, D.I., Nguyen-Tân, P.F., … Gillison, M.L. (2010). Human papillomavirus and survival of patients with oropharyngeal cancer. *New England Journal of Medicine, 363,* 24–35. doi:10.1056/NEJMoa0912217

Auluck, A., Rosin, M.P., Zhang, L., & Sumanth, K.N. (2008). Oral submucous fibrosis, a clinically benign but potentially malignant disease: Report of 3 cases and review of the literature. *Journal of the Canadian Dental Association, 74,* 735–740.

Baan, R., Straif, K., Grosse, Y., Secretan, B., El Ghissassi, F., Bouvard, V., … Cogliano, V. (2007). Carcinogenicity of alcoholic beverages. *Lancet Oncology, 8,* 292–293. doi:10.1016/S1470-2045(07)70099-2

Baier, G., Völter, C., Steigerwald, I., Müller, J., & Schwager, K. (2005). Malignant paranasal sinus tumors. Diagnosis, therapy, and results. *HNO, 53,* 957–965. doi:10.1007/s00106-005-1251-0

Bakri, M.M., Hussaini, M.H., Holmes, R.A., Cannon, D.R., & Rich, M.A. (2010). Revisiting the association between candidal infection and carcinoma, particularly oral squamous cell carcinoma. *Journal of Oral Microbiology, 2.* doi:10.3402/jom.v2i0.5780

Bartie, K.L., Williams, D.W., Wilson, M.J., Potts, A.J., & Lewis, M.A. (2004). Differential invasion of *Candida albicans* isolates in an in vitro model of oral candidosis. *Oral Microbiology and Immunology, 19,* 293–296. doi:10.1111/j.1399-302X.2004.00155.x

Bataille, V., & de Vries, E. (2008). Melanoma—Part 1: Epidemiology, risk factors, and prevention. *BMJ, 337,* a2249. doi:10.1136/bmj.a2249

Boffetta, P., & Hashibe, M. (2006). Alcohol and cancer. *Lancet Oncology, 7,* 149–156. doi:10.1016/S1470-2045(06)70577-0

Boffetta, P., Hecht, S., Gray, N., Gupta, P., & Straif, K. (2008). Smokeless tobacco and cancer. *Lancet Oncology, 9,* 667–675. doi:10.1016/S1470-2045(08)70173-6

Bouquot, J.E. (1994). Oral leukoplakia and erythroplakia: A review and update. *Practical Periodontics and Aesthetic Dentistry, 6,* 9–17.

Boyle, J.O., Gümüs, Z.H., Kacker, A., Choksi, V.L., Bocker, J.M., Zhou, X.K., … Dannenberg, A.J. (2010). Effects of cigarette smoke on the human oral mucosal transcriptome. *Cancer Prevention Research, 3,* 266–278. doi:10.1158/1940-6207.CAPR-09-0192

Brocklehurst, P., Kujan, O., O'Malley, L.A., Ogden, G., Shepherd, S., & Glenny, A.M. (2013). Screening programmes for the early detection and prevention of oral cancer. *Cochrane Database of Systematic Reviews, 2013*(11). doi:10.1002/14651858.CD004150.pub4

Cancer Research UK. (2014). What causes cancer? Retrieved from http://www.cancerresearchuk.org/cancer-help/about-cancer/causes-symptoms/causes/what-causes-cancer

Carnelio, S., Rodrigues, G.S., Shenoy, R., & Fernandes, D. (2011). A brief review of common oral premalignant lesions with emphasis on their management and cancer prevention. *Indian Journal of Surgery, 73,* 256–261. doi:10.1007/s12262-011-0286-6

Centers for Disease Control and Prevention. (2014). Human papillomavirus. Retrieved from http://www.cdc.gov/vaccines/pubs/pinkbook/hpv.html

Chan, K.C., Hung, E.C., Woo, J.K., Chan, P.K., Leung, S.F., Lai, F.P., … Lo, Y.M. (2013). Early detection of nasopharyngeal carcinoma by plasma Epstein-Barr virus DNA analysis in a surveillance program. *Cancer, 119,* 1838–1844. doi:10.1002/cncr.28001

Chatham-Stephens, K., Law, R., Taylor, E., Melstrom, P., Bunnell, R., Wang, B., … Centers for Disease Control and Prevention. (2014). Notes from the field: Calls to poison centers for exposures to electronic cigarettes—United States, September 2010–February 2014. *Morbidity and Mortality Weekly Report, 63,* 292–293. Retrieved from http://www.cdc.gov/mmwr/preview/mmwrhtml/mm6313a4.htm

Chaturvedi, A.K. (2012). Epidemiology and clinical aspects of HPV in head and neck cancers. *Head and Neck Pathology, 6*(Suppl. 1), S16–S24. doi:10.1007/s12105-012-0377-0

Clugston, R.D., & Blaner, W.S. (2012). The adverse effects of alcohol on vitamin A metabolism. *Nutrients, 4,* 356–371. doi:10.3390/nu4050356

Combes, J.D., & Franceschi, S. (2014). Role of human papillomavirus in non-oropharyngeal head and neck cancers. *Oral Oncology, 50,* 370–379. doi:10.1016/j.oraloncology.2013.11.004

Cooper, D.S., Doherty, G.M., Haugen, B.R., Kloos, R.T., Lee, S.L., Mandel, S.J., … Tuttle, R.M. (2009). Revised American Thyroid Association management guidelines for patients with thyroid nodules and differentiated thyroid cancer. *Thyroid, 19,* 1167–1214. doi:10.1089/thy.2009.0110

Crozier, E., & Sumer, B.D. (2010). Head and neck cancer. *Medical Clinics of North America, 94,* 1031–1046. doi:10.1016/j.mcna.2010.05.014

Czogala, J., Goniewicz, M.L., Fidelus, B., Zielinska-Danch, W., Travers, M.J., & Sobczak, A. (2014). Secondhand exposure to vapors from electronic cigarettes. *Nicotine and Tobacco Research, 16,* 655–662. doi:10.1093/ntr/ntt203

Daya-Grosjean, L., & Sarasin, A. (2005). The role of UV induced lesions in skin carcinogenesis: An overview of oncogene and tumor suppressor gene modifications in xeroderma pigmentosum skin tumors. *Mutation Research, 571,* 43–56. doi:10.1016/j.mrfmmm.2004.11.013

d'Errico, A., Pasian, S., Baratti, A., Zanelli, R., Alfonzo, S., Gilardi, L., … Costa, G. (2009). A case-control study on occupational risk factors for sino-nasal cancer. *Occupational and Environmental Medicine, 66,* 448–455. doi:10.1136/oem.2008.041277

Deschler, D.G., Richmon, J.D., Khariwala, S.S., Ferris, R.L., & Wang, M.B. (2014). The "new" head and neck cancer patient—Young, nonsmoker, nondrinker, and HPV positive: Evaluation. *Otolaryngology—Head and Neck Surgery, 151,* 375–380. doi:10.1177/0194599814538605

Dessinioti, C., Antoniou, C., Katsambas, A., & Stratigos, A.J. (2010). Basal cell carcinoma: What's new under the sun. *Photochemistry and Photobiology, 86,* 481–491. doi:10.1111/j.1751-1097.2010.00735.x

D'Souza, G., Kreimer, A.R., Viscidi, R., Pawlita, M., Fakhry, C., Koch, W.M., … Gillison, M.L. (2007). Case-control study of human papillomavirus and oropharyngeal cancer. *New England Journal of Medicine, 356,* 1944–1956. doi:10.1056/NEJMoa065497

Eggermont, A.M., Spatz, A., & Robert, C. (2014). Cutaneous melanoma. *Lancet, 383,* 816–827. doi:10.1016/S0140-6736(13)60802-8

Epstein, J.B., Güneri, P., Boyacioglu, H., & Abt, E. (2012). The limitations of the clinical oral examination in detecting dysplastic oral lesions and oral squamous cell carcinoma. *Journal of the American Dental Association, 143,* 1332–1342. doi:10.14219/jada.archive.2012.0096

Freedman, D.A., Peña-Purcell, N., Friedman, D.B., Ory, M., Flocke, S., Barni, M.T., & Hébert, J.R. (2014). Extending cancer prevention to improve fruit and vegetable consumption. *Journal of Cancer Education, 29*, 790–795. doi:10.1007/s13187-014-0656-4

Freedman, N.D., Schatzkin, A., Leitzmann, M.F., Hollenbeck, A.R., & Abnet, C.C. (2007). Alcohol and head and neck cancer risk in a prospective study. *British Journal of Cancer, 96*, 1469–1474. doi:10.1038/sj.bjc.6603713

Gandini, S., Botteri, E., Iodice, S., Boniol, M., Lowenfels, A.B., Maisonneuve, P., & Boyle, P. (2008). Tobacco smoking and cancer: A meta-analysis. *International Journal of Cancer, 122*, 155–164. doi:10.1002/ijc.23033

Gandini, S., Sera, F., Cattaruzza, M.S., Pasquini, P., Zanetti, R., Masini, C., ... Melchi, C.F. (2005). Meta-analysis of risk factors for cutaneous melanoma: III. Family history, actinic damage and phenotypic factors. *European Journal of Cancer, 41*, 2040–2059. doi:10.1016/j.ejca.2005.03.034

Gillison, M.L., D'Souza, G., Westra, W., Sugar, E., Xiao, W., Begum, S., & Viscidi, R. (2008). Distinct risk factor profiles for human papillomavirus type 16-positive and human papillomavirus type 16-negative head and neck cancers. *Journal of the National Cancer Institute, 100*, 407–420. doi:10.1093/jnci/djn025

Goniewicz, M.L., Knysak, J., Gawron, M., Kosmider, L., Sobczak, A., Kurek, J., ... Benowitz, N. (2014). Levels of selected carcinogens and toxicants in vapour from electronic cigarettes. *Tobacco Control, 23*, 133–139. doi:10.1136/tobaccocontrol-2012-050859

Hardefeldt, H.A., Cox, M.R., & Eslick, G.D. (2014). Association between human papillomavirus (HPV) and oesophageal squamous cell carcinoma: A meta-analysis. *Epidemiology and Infection, 142*, 1119–1137. doi:10.1017/S0950268814000016

Harris, M.S., Phillips, D.R., Sayer, J.L., & Moore, M.G. (2013). A comparison of community-based and hospital-based head and neck cancer screening campaigns: Identifying high-risk individuals and early disease. *JAMA Otolaryngology—Head and Neck Surgery, 139*, 568–573. doi:10.1001/jamaoto.2013.3153

HealthGrades. (2015). Lip cancer. Retrieved from http://www.healthgrades.com/conditions/lip-cancer

IARC Working Group on the Evaluation of Carcinogenic Risks to Humans. (2010). Alcohol consumption and ethyl carbamate. *IARC Monographs on the Evaluation of Carcinogenic Risks to Humans, 96*, 3–1383.

Irigaray, P., Newby, J.A., Clapp, R., Hardell, L., Howard, V., Montagnier, L., ... Belpomme, D. (2007). Lifestyle-related factors and environmental agents causing cancer: An overview. *Biomedicine and Pharmacotherapy, 61*, 640–658. doi:10.1016/j.biopha.2007.10.006

Jensen, A.D., Nikoghosyan, A.V., Windemuth-Kieselbach, C., Debus, J., & Münter, M.W. (2011). Treatment of malignant sinonasal tumours with intensity-modulated radiotherapy (IMRT) and carbon ion boost (C12). *BMC Cancer, 11*, 190. doi:10.1186/1471-2407-11-190

Khademi, B., Moradi, A., Hoseini, S., & Mohammadianpanah, M. (2009). Malignant neoplasms of the sinonasal tract: Report of 71 patients and literature review and analysis. *Oral and Maxillofacial Surgery, 13*, 191–199. doi:10.1007/s10006-009-0170-8

Kim, J.W., Amin, A.R., & Shin, D.M. (2010). Chemoprevention of head and neck cancer with green tea polyphenols. *Cancer Prevention Research, 3*, 900–909. doi:10.1158/1940-6207.CAPR-09-0131

Kozyreva, O., D'Silva, K.J., & Vaughan, C.W. (2013, November 22). Chemoprevention strategies in head and neck cancer. Retrieved from http://emedicine.medscape.com/article/855712-overview#aw2aab6b2

Kreimer, A.R., & Chaturvedi, A.K. (2011). HPV-associated oropharyngeal cancers—Are they preventable? *Cancer Prevention Research, 4*, 1346–1349. doi:10.1158/1940-6207.CAPR-11-0379

Kreimer, A.R., Clifford, G.M., Boyle, P., & Franceschi, S. (2005). Human papillomavirus types in head and neck squamous cell carcinomas worldwide: A systematic review. *Cancer Epidemiology, Biomarkers and Prevention, 14*, 467–475. doi:10.1158/1055-9965.EPI-04-0551

Langevin, S.M., Michaud, D.S., Eliot, M., Peters, E.S., McClean, M.D., & Kelsey, K.T. (2012). Regular dental visits are associated with earlier stage at diagnosis for oral and pharyngeal cancer. *Cancer Causes and Control, 23*, 1821–1829. doi:10.1007/s10552-012-0061-4

Lavanya, N., Jayanthi, P., Rao, U.K., & Ranganathan, K. (2011). Oral lichen planus: An update on pathogenesis and treatment. *Journal of Oral and Maxillofacial Pathology, 15*, 127–132. doi:10.4103/0973-029X.84474

Lee, J.J., Wu, X., Hildebrandt, M.A., Yang, H., Khuri, F.R., Kim, E., ... Hong, W.K. (2011). Global assessment of genetic variation influencing response to retinoid chemoprevention in head and neck cancer patients. *Cancer Prevention Research, 4*, 185–193. doi:10.1158/1940-6207.CAPR-10-0125

Liu, J., Wang, J., Leng, Y., & Lv, C. (2013). Intake of fruit and vegetables and risk of esophageal squamous cell carcinoma: A meta-analysis of observational studies. *International Journal of Cancer, 133*, 473–485. doi:10.1002/ijc.28024

Mahmood, R., Butterworth, C., Lowe, D., & Rogers, S.N. (2014). Characteristics and referral of head and neck cancer patients who report chewing and dental issues on the patient concerns inventory. *British Dental Journal, 216*, E25. doi:10.1038/sj.bdj.2014.453

Markovic, S.N., Erickson, L.A., Rao, R.D., Weenig, R.H., Pockaj, B.A., Bardia, A., ... Melanoma Study Group of the Mayo Clinic Cancer Center. (2007). Malignant melanoma in the 21st century, part 1: Epidemiology, risk factors, screening, prevention, and diagnosis. *Mayo Clinic Proceedings, 82*, 364–380. doi:10.4065/82.3.364

Mattila, R., Rautava, J., & Syrjänen, S. (2012). Human papillomavirus in oral atrophic lichen planus lesions. *Oral Oncology, 48*, 980–984. doi:10.1016/j.oraloncology.2012.04.009

Maybury, C., Horowitz, A.M., & Goodman, H.S. (2012). Outcomes of oral cancer early detection and prevention statewide model in Maryland. *Journal of Public Health Dentistry, 72*(Suppl. 1), S34–S38. doi:10.1111/j.1752-7325.2012.00320.x

McGill, N. (2013). Research on e-cigarettes examining health effects: Regulations due. *The Nation's Health, 43*(5), 1–10. Retrieved from http://thenationshealth.aphapublications.org/content/43/5/1.2.full

Mendenhall, W.M., Werning, J.W., & Pfister, D.G. (2011). Treatment of head and neck cancer. In V.T. DeVita Jr., T.S. Lawrence, & S.A. Rosenberg (Eds.), *Cancer: Principles and practice of oncology* (9th ed., pp. 729–780). Philadelphia, PA: Lippincott Williams & Wilkins.

Mensi, C., Consonni, D., Sieno, C., De Matteis, S., Riboldi, L., & Bertazzi, P.A. (2013). Sinonasal cancer and occupational exposure in a population-based registry. *International Journal of Otolaryngology, 2013*, Article ID 672621. doi:10.1155/2013/672621

Mortazavi, H., Baharvand, M., & Mehdipour, M. (2014). Oral potentially malignant disorders: An overview of more than 20 entities. *Journal of Dental Research, Dental Clinics, Dental Prospects, 8*(1), 6–14. doi:10.5681/joddd.2014.002

Moyer, V.A. (2014). Screening for oral cancer: U.S. Preventive Services Task Force recommendation statement. *Annals of Internal Medicine, 160*, 55–60. doi:10.7326/M13-2568

National Cancer Institute. (2014a). Cancer prevention overview (PDQ®): Risk factors. Retrieved from http://www.cancer.gov/cancertopics/pdq/prevention/overview/patient/page3

National Cancer Institute. (2014b). Salivary gland cancer treatment (PDQ®). Retrieved from http://www.cancer.gov/cancertopics/pdq/treatment/salivarygland/HealthProfessional

National Cancer Institute. (2015). Risk factors for cancer. Retrieved from http://www.cancer.gov/about-cancer/causes-prevention/risk

National Institutes of Health. (2013). Vitamin A. Retrieved from http://ods.od.nih.gov/factsheets/VitaminA-HealthProfessional

Ouyang, Y.H. (2010). Skin cancer of the head and neck. *Seminars in Plastic Surgery, 24*, 117–126. doi:10.1055/s-0030-1255329

Pfister, D.G., Ang, K.K., Brizel, D.M., Burtness, B.A., Cmelak, A.J., Colevas, A.D., ... National Comprehensive Cancer Network. (2011).

Head and neck cancers. *Journal of the National Comprehensive Cancer Network, 9,* 596–650.

Priante, A.V., Castilho, E.C., & Kowalski, L.P. (2011). Second primary tumors in patients with head and neck cancer. *Current Oncology Reports, 13,* 132–137. doi:10.1007/s11912-010-0147-7

Radoï, L., & Luce, D. (2013). A review of risk factors for oral cavity cancer: The importance of a standardized case definition. *Community Dentistry and Oral Epidemiology, 41,* 97–109. doi:10.1111/j.1600-0528.2012.00710.x

Rahal, A., Kumar, A., Singh, V., Yadav, B., Tiwari, R., Chakraborty, S., & Dhama, K. (2014). Oxidative stress, prooxidants, and antioxidants: The interplay. *BioMed Research International, 2014,* Article ID 761264. doi:10.1155/2014/761264

Raimondi, S., Sera, F., Gandini, S., Iodice, S., Caini, S., Maisonneuve, P., & Fargnoli, M.C. (2008). MC1R variants, melanoma and red hair color phenotype: A meta-analysis. *International Journal of Cancer, 122,* 2753–2760. doi:10.1002/ijc.23396

Rametta, S., Grosso, G., Galvano, F., Mistretta, A., Marventano, S., Nolfo, F., ... Biondi, A. (2013). Social disparities, health risk behaviors, and cancer. *BMC Surgery, 13*(Suppl. 2), S17. doi:10.1186/1471-2482-13-S2-S17

Ramqvist, T., & Dalianis, T. (2010). Oropharyngeal cancer epidemic and human papillomavirus. *Emerging Infectious Diseases, 16,* 1671–1677. doi:10.3201/eid1611.100452

Ratnam, D.V., Ankola, D.D., Bhardwaj, V., Sahana, D.K., & Kumar, M.N. (2006). Role of antioxidants in prophylaxis and therapy: A pharmaceutical perspective. *Journal of Controlled Release, 113,* 189–207. doi:10.1016/j.jconrel.2006.04.015

Reichart, P.A., & Philipsen, H.P. (2005). Oral erythroplakia—A review. *Oral Oncology, 41,* 551–561. doi:10.1016/j.oraloncology.2004.12.003

Rua, R.M., Ojeda, M.L., Nogales, F., Rubio, J.M., Romero-Gómez, M., Funuyet, J., ... Carreras, O. (2014). Serum selenium levels and oxidative balance as differential markers in hepatic damage caused by alcohol. *Life Sciences, 94,* 158–163. doi:10.1016/j.lfs.2013.10.008

Samant, S., & Kruger, E. (2007). Cancer of the paranasal sinuses. *Current Oncology Reports, 9,* 147–151. doi:10.1007/s11912-007-0013-4

Schneider, D.F., & Chen, H. (2013). New developments in the diagnosis and treatment of thyroid cancer. *CA: A Cancer Journal for Clinicians, 63,* 374–394. doi:10.3322/caac.21195

Sheth, S. (2006). Chemoprevention for the treatment of head and neck cancers. *U.S. Pharmacist, 1,* 16–21. Retrieved from http://www.uspharmacist.com/content/d/trendwatch/c/11729

Shin, D.M., & Saba, N.F. (2014). Chemoprevention and screening in oral dysplasia and squamous cell head and neck cancer [UpToDate]. Retrieved from http://www.uptodate.com/contents/chemoprevention-and-screening-in-oral-dysplasia-and-squamous-cell-head-and-neck-cancer

Silva, J.H., Sá, B.C., Avila, A.L., Landman, G., & Duprat Neto, J.P. (2011). Atypical mole syndrome and dysplastic nevi: Identification of populations at risk for developing melanoma—Review article. *Clinics (Sao Paulo), 66,* 493–499. doi:10.1590/S1807-59322011000300023

Skin Cancer Foundation. (2014). What is actinic keratosis? Retrieved from http://www.skincancer.org/skin-cancer-information/actinic-keratosis/what-is-actinic-keratosis

Skin Cancer Foundation. (2015). Dysplastic nevi (atypical moles). Retrieved from http://www.skincancer.org/skin-cancer-information/dysplastic-nevi

Smith, W., & Saba, N.F. (2005). Retinoids as chemoprevention for head and neck cancer: Where do we go from here? *Critical Reviews in Oncology/Hematology, 55,* 143–152. doi:10.1016/j.critrevonc.2005.02.003

Straif, K., Benbrahim-Tallaa, L., Baan, R., Grosse, Y., Secretan, B., El Ghissassi, F., ... WHO International Agency for Research on Cancer Monograph Working Group. (2009). A review of human carcinogens—Part C: Metals, arsenic, dusts, and fibres. *Lancet Oncology, 10,* 453–454. doi:10.1016/S1470-2045(09)70134-2

Stratigos, A.J., & Katsambas, A.D. (2009). The value of screening in melanoma. *Clinics in Dermatology, 27,* 10–25. doi:10.1016/j.clindermatol.2008.09.002

Syrjänen, S., Lodi, G., von Bültzingslöwen, I., Aliko, A., Arduino, P., Campisi, G., ... Jontell, M. (2011). Human papillomaviruses in oral carcinoma and oral potentially malignant disorders: A systematic review. *Oral Diseases, 17*(Suppl. 1), 58–72. doi:10.1111/j.1601-0825.2011.01792.x

Travis, L.B., Rabkin, C.S., Brown, L.M., Allan, J.M., Alter, B.P., Ambrosone, C.B., ... Greene, M.H. (2006). Cancer survivorship—Genetic susceptibility and second primary cancers: Research strategies and recommendations. *Journal of the National Cancer Institute, 98,* 15–25. doi:10.1093/jnci/djj001

Tsao, A.S., Kim, E.S., & Hong, W.K. (2004). Chemoprevention of cancer. *CA: A Cancer Journal for Clinicians, 54,* 150–180. doi:10.3322/canjclin.54.3.150

Tsao, S.W., Yip, Y.L., Tsang, C.M., Pang, P.S., Lau, V.M., Zhang, G., & Lo, K.W. (2014). Etiological factors of nasopharyngeal carcinoma. *Oral Oncology, 50,* 330–338. doi:10.1016/j.oraloncology.2014.02.006

Turner, J.H., & Reh, D.D. (2012). Incidence and survival in patients with sinonasal cancer: A historical analysis of population-based data. *Head and Neck, 34,* 877–885. doi:10.1002/hed.21830

van der Waal, I. (2014). Oral potentially malignant disorders: Is malignant transformation predictable and preventable? *Medicina Oral, Patologia Oral y Cirugia Bucal, 19,* e386–e390. doi:10.4317/medoral.20205

Walsh, T., Liu, J.L., Brocklehurst, P., Glenny, A.M., Lingen, M., Kerr, A.R., ... Scully, C. (2013). Clinical assessment to screen for the detection of oral cavity cancer and potentially malignant disorders in apparently healthy adults. *Cochrane Database of Systematic Reviews, 2013*(11). doi:10.1002/14651858.CD010173.pub2

Wang, Y., Zhang, Y., & Ma, S. (2013). Racial differences in nasopharyngeal carcinoma in the United States. *Cancer Epidemiology, 37,* 793–802. doi:10.1016/j.canep.2013.08.008

Warnakulasuriya, S., Johnson, N.W., & van der Waal, I. (2007). Nomenclature and classification of potentially malignant disorders of the oral mucosa. *Journal of Oral Pathology and Medicine, 36,* 575–580. doi:10.1111/j.1600-0714.2007.00582.x

Woods, R.S., O'Regan, E.M., Kennedy, S., Martin, C., O'Leary, J.J., & Timon, C. (2014). Role of human papillomavirus in oropharyngeal squamous cell carcinoma: A review. *World Journal of Clinical Cases, 2,* 172–193. Retrieved from http://www.ncbi.nlm.nih.gov/pmc/articles/PMC4061306

World Health Organization. (2015). Risk factors. Retrieved from http://www.who.int/topics/risk_factors/en

Wyss, A., Hashibe, M., Chuang, S.C., Lee, Y.C., Zhang, Z.F., Yu, G.P., ... Olshan, A.F. (2013). Cigarette, cigar, and pipe smoking and the risk of head and neck cancers: Pooled analysis in the International Head and Neck Cancer Epidemiology Consortium. *American Journal of Epidemiology, 178,* 679–690. doi:10.1093/aje/kwt029

CHAPTER 5

Patient Assessment

Cindy J. Dawson, RN, MSN, CORLN

Introduction

The majority of head and neck malignancies arise from the mucosal lining of the upper aerodigestive tract and the adjacent salivary glands. Presenting symptoms are site dependent. Histologically, squamous cell carcinoma (SCC) accounts for 90% of all head and neck cancers worldwide (Cardesa & Nadal, 2014). SCC of the mucosal membranes usually appears as a whitish plaque (leukoplakia), a velvety red area (erythroplasia), or an ulcer. These tumors spread in area and depth and eventually invade adjacent and underlying structures. The most frequent signs and symptoms associated with head and neck cancer are

- Sore throat that does not heal (the most common symptom)
- Red or white patch in the mouth
- Lump or mass in the head and neck area (with or without pain)
- Foul mouth odor not explained by hygiene
- Hoarseness or change in voice
- Nasal obstruction or persistent nasal congestion
- Frequent nosebleeds or unusual nasal discharge
- Difficulty breathing
- Double vision
- Numbness or weakness of a body part in the head and neck region
- Pain or difficulty chewing, swallowing, or moving the jaws or tongue
- Ear pain
- Blood in the saliva or phlegm (mucus discharged in mouth from respiratory passages)
- Loosening of teeth
- Dentures that no longer fit
- Unexplained weight loss
- Fatigue.

Care of patients with head and neck cancer is best provided by a multidisciplinary team of healthcare providers that includes head and neck surgeons, radiation oncologists, medical oncologists, radiologists, pathologists, dental prosthodontists, clinical nurse specialists, specialized nurses, speech-language pathologists, and dietitians (Friedland et al., 2011; Wheless, McKinney, & Zanation, 2010).

Multiple factors affect the care of patients with head and neck cancer, and conducting a thorough assessment to ensure a holistic approach is important prior to treatment. Patients should complete a comprehensive medical history questionnaire detailing the chief complaint for seeking care, past medical history, medications, allergies, social history, family history, and review of systems. They will receive information regarding privacy and sign necessary consent forms. Vital signs—height, weight, temperature, pulse, blood pressure, respirations, and, when indicated, pulse oximetry—are obtained. A specific tobacco use history is obtained, and if the patient is currently using tobacco, the nurse should explain the importance of stopping tobacco use and provide support to the patient. Tobacco use history includes information on whether the patient currently uses tobacco, is a former user, or has never used. The tobacco user (past or present) defines the type, amount, and duration of use. Expression of cigarette tobacco abuse as "pack-years" can help to quantify the risk for medical complications. Pack-year is calculated by multiplying the number of cigarette packs by the number of years smoked (National Cancer Institute, n.d.). For example, a patient with a 10 pack-year history could have smoked one pack per day for 10 years or 10 cigarettes (half a pack) per day for 20 years.

The nurse should evaluate patients for the presence of pain at the initial encounter and every subsequent visit. It is important to capture the pain intensity using a standardized tool, such as the 0–10 verbal numeric scale or the face diagram pain rating scale. A positive pain response triggers a comprehensive assessment of location, intensity, timing (e.g., onset, duration, course, persistent or intermittent), interference with activities, description or quality of the pain, and aggravating and alleviating factors, including any measures taken to relieve the pain and their effectiveness (National Comprehensive Cancer Network®, 2015). Depending on the response, therapeutic intervention may be required. This often is the first step in caring for patients with cancer and aids in developing trust with the clinical team.

Patients with head and neck cancer are often malnourished secondary to pain and may have difficulty swallowing, alcohol and/or tobacco abuse, tumor interference, or treatment sequelae affecting dietary intake. Stratton and colleagues (as cited in von Meyenfeldt, 2005) reported a malnutrition prevalence of 65%–75% of patients with head and neck cancer. Many patients present malnourished at first encounter; Varkay, Tang, and Tan (2010) noted that 40% of patients with head and neck cancer are malnourished at presentation. Malnutrition negatively affects morbidity and mortality of patients with cancer (Gourin, Couch, & Johnson, 2014; Tan et al., 2015). A nutritional assessment is essential to identify and quantify any current or potential problems (e.g., weight loss, dysphagia, food intolerances). Weight and height measurements are essential baseline values, but it also is important to complete an oral cavity assessment and nutritional screening.

Use of a standardized tool when assessing the oral cavity is critical both pre- and post-treatment (Farrington, Cullen, & Dawson, 2010). Many tools are available for this intervention and are based on the visual inspection of the oral cavity. During the initial visit of a patient with head and neck cancer, some sample assessment questions include
- "How would you describe your diet and nutritional status: Poor, probably inadequate, adequate, or excellent?"
- "Have you experienced a weight loss over the past two to three months? If yes, was the weight loss intentional?"
- "Do you have difficulty or pain when chewing or swallowing your food? If yes, has this caused you to change the types or consistency of the food you eat? What do you eat in a normal day?"

Patients undergoing treatment or post-treatment will require the following nursing interventions.
- Monitor weight on every clinic evaluation.
- Perform oral cavity assessment.
- If weight loss has occurred, assess diet, noting any difficulty eating, swallowing, or complications with enteral feedings.
- Provide intervention as needed (e.g., consult dietitian, use written nutritional materials, assess need for supplements).

An educational assessment is performed to evaluate patients' readiness to learn, potential barriers to learning, level of education, reading level, and preferred style of learning. Patient education begins with the initial visit and continues throughout treatment. Examples of educational assessments are available in *The Joint Commission Guide to Patient and Family Education* (Joint Commission Resources, 2010). Defining the barriers (e.g., cognitive, religious, cul-

tural, language, communication, financial, physical, emotional), educational preferences (e.g., reading, listening, doing, observing), and readiness for the treatment regimen is imperative at the initial encounter and during subsequent visits. Patients should receive verbal and written information regarding treatment modalities at a reading level they are able to understand. The U.S. Department of Health and Human Services Office of Disease Prevention and Health Promotion (n.d.) provides a number of recommendations in the *Quick Guide to Health Literacy*, including
- Organize information so that the most important points appear first.
- Break complex information into understandable sections, limiting the number of messages at one time.
- Communicate in plain and simple language, avoid medical jargon, and explain medical terminology.
- Supplement instructions with pictures.
- Evaluate the patient's understanding by asking open-ended questions.
- Encourage the patient to ask questions.

In addition to the educational assessment, patients' potential knowledge deficits and learning needs are identified during this session. Examples include instruction on basic health practices, issues of self-care, patient safety, infection control, the use of medical equipment, and available community resources.

There is growing concern about medical care provided to patients who are unable to make decisions alone. Advances in medical technology now provide a number of treatments that may prolong life. Some patients do not want these treatments, whereas others wish to take advantage of every procedure available. The nurse should inquire if the patient has an advance directive or durable power of attorney for healthcare decisions. These legal documents will help to guide healthcare providers and caretakers in further medical treatment when the patient is unable to participate in decision making. A copy of the advance directive or durable power of attorney should be placed in the patient's medical record. If these documents are not available, the physician should note any conversations with the patient identifying his or her wishes. Information on obtaining advance directives should be made available to the patient and family.

Comprehensive Health History

Present Illness

The history of the present illness for head and neck cancer is similar to a general patient history. A careful and deliberate search for the onset, location, quality, severity, timing/duration, context, and positive and negative modifying factors of the patient's complaint is completed. Pertinent information regarding the signs and symptoms related to head and neck cancer is obtained. A listing of pertinent negatives and positives can help to gauge the tumor size and clinical stage of the tumor. For example, a small laryngeal cancer may cause hoarseness without aspiration, dysphagia, or cough. Using a process of active listening may aid the healthcare provider in establishing rapport with patients. A process of listening that repeats and verifies clinical information will enhance the accuracy of the history and will increase patients' trust with the clinician.

Past Medical History

A list is prepared of current medications, including prescription and over-the-counter drugs, vitamins, and herbal preparations, and allergies, including inhalants, drugs, and latex. Patients should be questioned about any past medical conditions, with emphasis on major illnesses or injuries, hospitalizations, and surgeries. Record any implants (e.g., artificial heart valves, hip prosthesis) or external devices used. Specifically ask if they have been instructed to routinely take antibiotics prior to a procedure, such as dental work.

Psychosocial and Cultural History

A psychosocial assessment includes information about patients' lifestyles, occupations, activities of daily living, and religious beliefs. Responses are recorded on the patient medical questionnaire. The use of tobacco, alcohol, and other substances is reviewed. Often, patients are unwilling to provide an accurate estimate of alcohol consumption. The nurse should guide the discussion and question patients about the frequency of use and amounts of beer, liquor, or wine. Nonjudgmental questioning with the intentional use of high estimates may yield more accurate information. The nurse also should determine whether patients are at risk for AIDS (e.g., homosexual activity, IV drug use, previous blood transfusion). According to Ridge, Mehra, Lango, and Feigenberg (2013), high-risk behaviors associated with HPV 16 infection need to be ascertained (e.g., sexual activity, oral lesions). Assess patients' occupations for any contributing role they may play in the diagnosis. The implication of the diagnosis and treatment of cancer on patients' return to work and the effect on the family should be addressed, as they are foremost on the minds of both patients and families. Patients' cultural background may play a role in the diagnosis and treatment of head and neck cancer. Cultural beliefs could influence their willingness to accept the diagnosis and proposed treatment.

Family Medical History

The family history completes patients' medical picture, as documented in the medical record. The nurse should question patients about any family members who have been diagnosed with cancer or other comorbidities, including cardiac, pulmonary, renal, and endocrine disorders.

Review of Systems

A review of systems of the body can provide valuable information regarding concomitant medical diagnoses and may raise suspicions of metastatic disease. A common review of systems includes the following elements (DeGowin, 1994).
- Skin, hair, and nails
- Lymph nodes
- Bones, joints, and muscles
- Hematopoietic system
- Endocrine system
- Allergic and immunologic history
- Head
- Eyes
- Ears
- Nose
- Mouth
- Throat
- Neck
- Breasts
- Respiratory system
- Cardiovascular system
- Gastrointestinal system
- Genitourinary system
- Nervous system
- Pregnancy
- Mental status

Physical Examination

A comprehensive head and neck examination is performed by inspection, auscultation, and palpation to evaluate potential physical causes of a patient's complaints. The following are included in a complete physical examination.
- Vital signs
  - Blood pressure—sitting, standing, and lying
  - Pulse rate and regularity
  - Respiration
  - Temperature
  - Height
  - Weight
  - Pulse oximetry (when indicated)
- General assessment
  - Development
  - Nutrition
  - Body habitus (i.e., physique, general description of appearance)
  - Grooming
  - Ability to communicate

- Head and face
  - Inspect the head and face. Note scars, lesions, masses, skin texture, and color.
  - Survey the facial skeleton. Note symmetry, crepitus, step-offs, or unusual features or proportions.
  - Palpate the face. Note tenderness over the sinuses.
  - Examine the salivary glands. Note the amount and consistency of saliva.
  - Assess the facial nerve. Note facial symmetry and strength.
- Eyes
  - Observe extraocular movement, evidence of nystagmus, and primary gaze alignment.
  - Note the pupil size and reactivity to light.
- Ears
  - Inspect the skin of the external ear for lesions, scars, and masses.
  - Inspect the external auditory canals and tympanic membranes using an otoscope. Note any drainage.
  - Evaluate the mobility of the tympanic membrane using a pneumatic otoscope.
  - Assess hearing with tuning forks, whispered voice, and finger-rub thresholds.
- Nose
  - Inspect the external nose for lesions, masses, and scars.
  - Examine the nasal mucosa, septum, and turbinates for inflammation, mucus, yellowish drainage, polyps, and obstruction.
- Oral cavity, larynx, and nasopharynx
  - Inspect the lips, teeth, and gingiva.
  - Examine the oral mucosa, hard and soft palate, tongue, floor of the mouth, retromolar trigone, and tonsillar pillars, looking for asymmetry and lesions.
  - Evaluate the hydration of the mucosal surfaces.
  - Palpate the oral cavity for masses.
  - Examine the pharyngeal walls and pyriform sinuses for pooling of saliva, asymmetry, and lesions.
  - Perform an indirect mirror examination of the larynx, giving special attention to the mucosa, mobility, and symmetry of the true vocal folds and appearance of the false cords and epiglottis.
  - Perform a mirror examination of the nasopharynx, noting the appearance of the mucosa, adenoids, posterior choanae, or nares, and opening of the eustachian tube.
- Neck
  - Examine the neck for overall appearance and symmetry.
  - Palpate the neck for masses, tracheal position, and crepitus.
  - Palpate the lymph nodes, noting seven levels of the nodes bilaterally.
  - Palpate the thyroid, noting enlargement, tenderness, and masses.
- Neurologic examination
  - Test cranial nerves and note any deficits.

- Perform a brief mental status assessment, especially noting orientation to time, person, and place and the patient's mood and affect.
- Perform a gross assessment of hearing and balance. Ask patient if he or she can hear a normal voice and walk without difficulty.
- Respiratory system evaluation
  * Inspect the chest, noting symmetry, expansion, and respiratory effort.
  * Auscultate the lungs, especially noting breath sounds, adventitious sounds, and rubs.
- Cardiovascular examination: Auscultate the heart with special attention to abnormal sounds and murmurs.

If a suspicious lesion is found during the examination, document the appearance, location, character (e.g., ulcerated, encapsulated, smooth), size, and extent of the growth. Further workup, including radiologic studies, will determine treatment. The size of the tumor, extension to adjacent structures, evidence of spread into the cervical lymphatics, and clinical evidence of distant metastasis form the basis for the clinical staging of the tumor.

A comprehensive physical examination of patients suspected of having a head and neck malignancy will require a flexible fiber-optic endoscopic examination of the upper aerodigestive tract. This will allow the examiner to view the nasopharynx, oropharynx, hypopharynx, larynx, and opening of the esophagus. The procedure is usually well tolerated and is performed in the office setting.

Photographic or digital image documentation of the physical findings is an important adjunct tool used during the pretreatment physical examination. Images of superficial intraoral or pharyngeal lesions are easily obtained, and nasopharyngeal, hypopharyngeal, and laryngeal images are obtained during the flexible fiber-optic examination. Lesions of the esophagus or hypopharyngeal lesions at the esophageal inlet may be better visualized using esophagoscopy.

After completion of the history and physical examination, a preliminary differential diagnosis can be made. A presentation of the findings can be made to a tumor board as needed but may be delayed until after a histologic diagnosis.

Diagnostic Evaluation— Histologic Diagnosis

Biopsy

In some situations, a biopsy of suspicious lesions can be performed in the office or clinic. A computed tomography (CT) scan, magnetic resonance imaging (MRI) scan, or other radiographic procedure may be performed to define the lesion and surrounding anatomy without the potential distortion produced by the biopsy.

A fine needle aspiration biopsy (FNAB) of masses in the oral cavity or neck can be useful in making a diagnosis. FNAB provides cells for histologic evaluation of salivary gland neoplasms and enlarged lymph nodes. The pathologist may be able to differentiate inflammatory, reactive, benign, and neoplastic processes with FNAB. FNAB uses a fine needle (22- to 25-gauge), does not seed tumor cells, and may provide a quick diagnosis.

An open biopsy of a neck mass may be done when FNAB proves to be nondiagnostic. Good practice is to avoid an open biopsy of a neck mass as an initial step in evaluation because of the concern that the open biopsy could spread tumor cells into the neck or potentially complicate a subsequent imaging examination. However, as long as timely and appropriate treatment is initiated, it is not clear whether an open biopsy of a malignant neck mass compromises survival (Hoffman, 2013).

Panendoscopy

Panendoscopy of the upper aerodigestive tract is required to obtain tissue for diagnosis, screen for multiple lesions, and stage the disease. Panendoscopy usually is performed under general anesthesia in an outpatient procedure area. The procedures included in a panendoscopy are

- Nasopharyngoscopy
- Rhinoscopy
- Direct laryngoscopy
- Esophagoscopy
- Bronchoscopy
- Inspection and bimanual palpation of the oral cavity and neck
- Deep palpation of the base of the tongue.

Directed biopsies are done at the sites most likely to harbor a neoplasm and to map the extent of any suspicious lesion (Hoffman, 2013). Following the endoscopic procedures and biopsies, patients are instructed to notify the physician of shortness of breath, chest pain, or hemoptysis, which may indicate a complication. Written instructions in addition to verbal communication regarding postprocedure care are standard practice.

Imaging and Other Studies

Various imaging studies can be useful in evaluating suspected head and neck malignancies. Chest x-ray is obtained to evaluate cardiopulmonary status and to review for second primary or metastatic lung tumors. CT scan with contrast is used to evaluate the extent of disease at the primary site and to evaluate regional node status and assess adjacent bony structures. MRI is used to evaluate tumor and lymph node status, especially in patients with poor renal function or allergy to the contrast medium. MRI is most useful in defining tumor and soft tissue relationships but does not define bony involvement well because of the low density of protons in bone. Positron-emission tomography scan is used to assess the extent of the primary lesion and determine distant metastasis. It is also used to determine the existence of recurrence after therapy. Ultrasound may be helpful for evaluating selected neck masses, especially a tumor adjacent to a vascular structure, such as the carotid artery, or a thyroid mass. The sound wave image produced by an ultrasound does not provide the level of anatomic detail visualized by other radiographic studies. It provides little information about the evaluation of a tumor's relationship to bone and cartilaginous structures. Ultrasound is not as comprehensive or definitive as a CT or MRI scan.

Laboratory and Evaluation Testing

A number of laboratory tests can aid in diagnostic evaluation.

- **Complete blood count with differential**—assesses hemoglobin and hematocrit levels, white blood cell count, especially neutrophil and lymphocyte counts, and platelets.
- **Electrolytes and liver function tests**—detect changes in liver enzymes, electrolytes, and renal function; useful in monitoring for drug toxicities.
- **Thyroid function tests**—specific thyroid-stimulating hormone T4 assesses the status of thyroid function prior to treatment of a thyroid tumor. Many types of cancer treatment can affect the function of the thyroid gland; therefore, obtaining a baseline status is important.
- **Glucose (fasting)**—screens for diabetes mellitus.
- **Blood urea nitrogen/creatinine**—assesses renal function prior to IV contrast during CT scan.
- **HPV serotype and Epstein-Barr virus of tissue biopsy specimens**—suggested for squamous cell or undifferentiated histology.
- **Coagulation studies**—assess bleeding tendency prior to therapy.
- **Prostate-specific antigen test**—may be performed on a male with an unknown primary adenocarcinoma that is metastatic to the neck.
- **Urinalysis**—detects proteinuria, pyuria, or urinary tract infection.
- **Electrocardiogram**—performed in men older than age 45 or women older than age 50 with a history of heart problems.
- **Pulmonary function testing**—performed on patients at risk for perioperative complications or potential lung disease.

Diagnostic Evaluation—Consultations

Concomitant medical diagnoses are addressed as part of the complete diagnostic evaluation. Consultations that may be required include the following.

- **Internal medicine**—assists in the management of general medical problems (e.g., chronic obstructive pulmonary disease, hypertension, diabetes mellitus) prior to, during, and after the cancer treatment.
- **Anesthesia**—evaluates patients for prolonged and extensive anesthesia that is needed during ablative and reconstructive surgery.
- **Radiation oncology**—evaluates the role of radiation therapy in the cancer treatment.
- **Medical oncology**—determines the role of systemic medical therapies (e.g., chemotherapy, biotherapy) in the overall treatment plan.
- **Nutrition services**—assesses patients' nutritional status and makes recommendations of ways to optimize outcomes before, during, and after cancer treatment.
- **Social services**—provides supportive services to patients and families; offers suggestions for assistance with financial, travel, and housing needs; counsels patients regarding adjustment to illness; and assists nurses and physicians with discharge planning.
- **Audiology services**—evaluates patients' hearing pretreatment, especially if ototoxic chemotherapy is planned.
- **Speech pathology**—provides counseling and instruction for postoperative speech and swallowing problems.
- **Dental/prosthodontics**—evaluates and treats dental problems; counsels patients regarding essential oral hygiene that will be required before, during, and after radiation therapy; and collaborates with the surgeon to develop prosthetic devices for reconstruction of defects.

Other referrals and evaluations that may be useful depending on the surgical procedure include the following.
- **Ophthalmology**—assesses eye/vision function with sinus tumors, for tumors in adjacent structures, or when radiation may affect orbits.
- **Neurology/neurosurgery**—evaluates tumors adjacent to skull base.
- **Vascular surgery**—performs assessment if suspicion of direct vascular involvement of the tumor or if reconstruction is necessary following surgical resection.
- **Oral surgery**—evaluates for dental extraction/therapy prior to radiation.

Tumor Staging

Tumor-Node-Metastasis Classification

Accurate staging of cancer is important in determining treatment and prognosis. The tumor-node-metastasis (TNM) classification system developed by the American Joint Committee on Cancer (AJCC) (Edge et al., 2010) is based on the premise that cancers of the same anatomic site and histologic type share similar patterns of growth and outcomes. The stage of the cancer correlates with the extent of the disease and prognosis for the patient.

- **T** defines the extent of the primary tumor.
- **N** is the absence or presence and extent of regional lymph node metastasis.
- **M** is the presence or absence of distant metastases.

The use of numerical subsets of the TNM components indicates the progressive enlargement or worsening of the malignant disease (Edge et al., 2010).
- **Primary tumor (T)**
  - TX—Primary tumor cannot be assessed.
  - T0—No evidence of primary tumor
  - Tis—Carcinoma in situ
  - T1, T2, T3, T4—Increasing size and/or local extension of the primary tumor
- **Regional lymph nodes (N)**
  - NX—Regional lymph nodes cannot be assessed.
  - N0—No regional lymph node metastases
  - N1, N2, N3—Increasing number or extent of regional lymph nodes: unilateral, ipsilateral, and bilateral
- **Distant metastasis (M)**
  - M0—No evidence of distant metastases
  - M1—Distant metastases present

Further subsets of classification (e.g., T1 N2b M0) are defined based on site-specific characteristics of the tumor and biologic aggressiveness in the neck (Edge et al., 2010).

The TNM classification system is a shorthand method for describing the presentation of the malignant tumor. Edge et al. (2010) recommended the following rules.
- All patients should be followed through the initial course of surgery or for four months, whichever is longer.
- All tumors must be confirmed microscopically.
- Five TNM staging classifications are described.
  - Clinical classification, designated as cTNM or TNM
  - Pathologic classification, designated as pTNM
  - Post-therapy classification, designated as ycTNM or ypTNM
  - Retreatment classification, designated as rTNM
  - Autopsy classification, designated as aTNM

Clinical Staging Classification

Clinical assessment uses the information available before the first definitive treatment, including but not limited to the physical examination, imaging, endoscopy, biopsy, and surgical exploration. Clinical stage is assigned prior to any cancer-related treatment and is not changed on the basis of subsequent information. Based on AJCC guidelines, the clinical stage is essential for selecting and evaluating primary therapy for head and neck cancer (Edge et al., 2010).

Pathologic Staging Classification

Pathologic staging uses the evidence acquired prior to treatment and is supplemented or modified by the evidence acquired from surgery, particularly the pathologic examination. The pathologic stage provides additional data used for estimating the patient's prognosis and calculating end results.

Reasonable efforts to reconstruct the tumor size (pT) may be required if there have been previous biopsies or partial excision of the cancer prior to definitive surgery. The complete assessment of the regional lymph nodes (pN) ideally involves the removal of a sufficient number of lymph nodes to evaluate the highest pN status. Pathologic staging is essential to define the extent of the primary tumor and the status of regional lymph nodes. Pathologic staging depends on the proven anatomic extent of disease and whether the primary lesion has been completely removed.

Post-Therapy Staging Classification

This new classification represents cases when systemic or radiation therapy is given before surgery, or no surgery is performed and the extent of the cancer is evaluated at the conclusion of the therapy. Post-therapy staging classification is useful because the response to therapy may provide information and help direct the clinician's decision making regarding the extent of surgery or requirement for additional systemic or radiation therapy.

Retreatment Staging Classification

This classification is made when further treatment, such as chemotherapy, is planned for a cancer that recurs following a disease-free interval. All information available at the time of retreatment should be used in determining the stage of the recurrent cancer, rTNM. Biopsy confirmation of the recurrence is useful, but with pathologic proof of the primary site, clinical evidence of distant metastases may be used.

Autopsy Staging Classification

This classification occurs during postmortem examination of the patient when the disease process was not evident prior to the patient's death.

Stage Grouping

Cancer staging is a universal method used to describe the extent of the cancer. The TNM classification *c* or *p* is used to assign a patient to a specific clinical stage of disease. The larger and more disseminated the tumor, the higher the stage and the worse the prognosis. The *AJCC Cancer Staging Manual* (Edge et al., 2010) provides information that can be used to assign the clinical stage of a cancer based on the anatomic site and TNM classification. Level 0 of TNM classification associated with a clinical stage varies for different anatomic sites. Staging is an important step that assists in the determi-

nation of appropriate treatment and estimation of prognosis of the individual patient (National Cancer Institute Surveillance, Epidemiology, and End Results Program, n.d.).

Histopathologic Type of Cancer

The World Health Organization's International Histological Classification of Tumours is used to type the cancer (Edge et al., 2010). The histologic tumor type is a qualitative assessment that is categorized according to the tissue or cell type it most closely resembles (e.g., hepatocellular, SCC) (Edge et al., 2010). A list of international classification of disease codes is presented in anatomic site-specific editions from the World Health Organization and can be found in the *AJCC Cancer Staging Manual* (Edge et al., 2010).

Histologic Grade

The histologic grade of a cancer is a qualitative assessment of the differentiation of the tumor expressed as the extent to which a cancer resembles the normal tissue at that site and is an indicator of the aggressiveness of a tumor. Grading systems can vary depending on the tumor type. Tumor grade is assigned based on the degree of differentiation from normal tissue, generally grade 1, 2, 3, or 4 (Edge et al., 2010).

Cancer Staging Systems Summary

The clinical assessment of patients with cancer can best guide treatment and prognosis when the following information has been determined.
• Anatomy—primary site
• Regional lymph node status
• Metastatic sites, if present
• Tumor staging using clinical and pathologic TNM classification and site-specific parameters
• Histopathologic type
• Histologic grade

The clinical cancer staging assessment is an important part of a patient's medical record indicating the anatomic extent of disease. It complements a thorough history and physical examination and provides the basis for subsequent treatment and follow-up (see Figure 5-1).

Treatment

Tumor Board

After completion of the primary evaluation, all new patient cases should be presented at a multidisciplinary tumor board conference, as this may affect diagnostic and treatment decisions (Wheless et al., 2010). As outlined in

---

Figure 5-1. Head and Neck Tumor Sites

- **Oral cavity**—mucosal lip, buccal lip, lower alveolar ridge, upper alveolar ridge, retromolar gingiva (retromolar trigone), floor of the mouth, hard palate, and anterior two-thirds of the tongue (oral tongue)
- **Pharynx**—nasopharynx, hypopharynx, and oropharynx (posterior one-third of tongue, tonsil, base of tongue)
- **Larynx**—supraglottis, glottis, and subglottis
- **Nasal cavity and paranasal sinuses**
- **Major salivary glands**—parotid, submandibular, and sublingual
- **Thyroid gland**

---

the *Iowa Head and Neck Protocols* (Hoffman, 2013), the goals of a tumor board are the following.

- Gather all pertinent diagnostic material regarding individual cases to permit review.
- Assign a recommended treatment plan and offer reasonable alternatives.
- Assign definitive staging.
- Create an interactive environment to foster communication between specialties.
- Teach the participating staff, fellows, and resident physicians.
- Teach medical students.
- Provide a forum in which second opinions are routinely offered.
- Develop or add to a detailed cancer database.

The attendees include all specialized team members who have evaluated the patient. Core members of the tumor board for all cases presented are head and neck surgeons, radiation oncologists, diagnostic radiologists, pathologists, dental prosthodontists, medical oncologists, oncology nurses, oncology social workers, and speech-language pathologists. The team provides input regarding the best treatment plan for the patient. A TNM staging form is completed for the primary site of the tumor with the pathology defined for T, N, M, and stage. A consensus for treatment is gathered from all tumor board members for presentation to the patient and family. Treatment options may include surgery, radiation, chemotherapy, or a combination of any of the three. The consequences of no further treatment are also discussed.

Patient and Family Counseling

The head and neck surgeon presents the results of the diagnostic evaluation and tumor board recommendations to patients and families in a compassionate but direct fashion. A review of the treatment options is presented with an emphasis on a balanced and complete picture of all treatment modalities—surgery, radiation therapy, chemotherapy, or combined modalities. A thorough and impartial appraisal of treatment options and alternatives is essential to reduce

any "framing bias" about the risks and benefits of therapy for a patient's cancer (Gordon-Lubitz, 2003). Risk perception is affected not only by patient factors (e.g., gender, prior beliefs, past experience), but also by how the treatment information is presented. A combination of visual displays, statistical information with individualized risk estimates, and qualitative explanations of therapy is necessary to obtain informed consent.

A description of the result of surgical intervention, including anatomic alterations, should be followed by the benefits of reconstructive interventions. Informed consent processes should be regarded as a crucial interactive educational tool that encourages patients to accept certain responsibilities. When properly communicated, an informed consent can place patients' expectations at a more manageable and realistic level. The consent process can reduce the risk of liability from the potentially disfiguring surgery by educating patients and families about the complications that can occur and the importance of deciding whether the offered procedure is worth the risk. Should a patient decide on no further treatment, a thorough discussion about the natural progression of the cancer is necessary. The gravity of this discussion warrants the involvement of family or significant others. Often, it is desirable to schedule a follow-up appointment to repeat the information and answer subsequent questions once the patient and family have had time to evaluate the options. The need to obtain a second opinion should be balanced against the nature or extent of the cancer and the desire for the timely treatment of the cancer. If the tumor is advanced, a delay in treatment to obtain a second opinion may compromise patient survival. The amount of information that is shared often makes it difficult for both patients and physicians to remember; a checklist may be helpful to document that the patient received the necessary information during the assessment (see Figure 5-2). Many physicians have a nurse witness the informed consent procedure. It is the nurse's role to review the informed consent process and operative consent form and to ask patients and families questions (preferably open-ended) with repeat-back technique. Examples of questions that can be asked are

- "Have you read this form or has it been read to you, and can you share with me what it says?"
- "Can you tell me what you understood from your physician about the planned treatment/procedure?"
- "Do you have any further questions?"

By reviewing this form, the nurse witness specifically verifies that the patient read the form, understood it, and had all of his or her questions answered.

The head and neck oncology nurse specialist coordinates and facilitates patient care among multiple disciplines within the healthcare facility and the local community, including home health agencies, referring physician, and other community support services. As an educator, the nurse initially provides information to patients and family members on

Figure 5-2. Sample Check-Off Sheet

Check-Off Sheet	Document	Date	Initials
Document the written/verbal teaching and diagnosis materials provided and recommendations.	Summary of tumor board		
	Clinical indicators reviewed		
	Teaching material provided		
	Illustration of surgery		
	Smoking cessation and substance abuse information		
Complete these documents as the patient proceeds through cancer workup and treatment.	Surgical plan reviewed		
	Post-op care instructions		
	Informed consent		
	Witness		
	Second opinion		

the cancer diagnosis, risk factors, diagnostic tests and procedures, recommended therapy, consequences, and side effects. During treatment and follow-up, education focuses on changes to body image, nutrition, functional support, quality of life, and symptom management. A major nursing role is coordinating and attending weekly tumor board conferences. In coordinating the head and neck tumor board, the nurse specialist reviews the patient list, confirms attendance with pertinent specialties, compiles cancer-staging decisions, arranges pretreatment consultation, and serves as a resource for patients and families. Another role is attending multidisciplinary rounds on the inpatient unit along with speech pathology and dietary. These rounds address patient progress, discharge-planning issues, and follow-up needs. The nurse is an integral participant in research activities in head and neck oncology. The head and neck nurse specialist helps to identify potential patient participants for studies and implements the protocol into the patient's treatment plan.

Treatment Modalities

The desired outcome of treatment may be to either cure or control the disease. According to Rodriguez and Adelstein (2010), the definitive or curative treatment modalities for early and locally advanced head and neck disease are surgery and radiation. Chemotherapy is another treatment modality but is not curative alone. Combining chemotherapy and radiation has been shown to improve outcomes. Curative options are not available for patients with metastatic head and neck cancer. Treatment goals for these patients are disease control and palliation of symptoms. Patients who have had surgery or radiation early in the treatment process can be offered palliative care with chemotherapeutic agents, and positive responses have been reported (Rodriguez & Adelstein, 2010).

Considerations for treatment are based on factors regarding the tumor, such as anatomic site, stage, and grade. Patient factors, such as general health, age, occupation, comorbidities, previous therapy, patient's wishes, social habits, and patient reliability for follow-up also are considered when determining treatment options. Treatment plans for surgical resection or radiation should include complete removal of the cancer, satisfactory post-treatment functioning, and acceptable cosmetic result.

Summary

The clinical presentation, diagnostic evaluation, tumor staging, and treatment recommendations for patients with head and neck cancer is a complex and comprehensive process. A flow chart delineating the assessment pathway of the typical patient is presented in Figure 5-3. A comprehensive evaluation and treatment recommendation provides patients and families with the best treatment options for a difficult and complicated disease.

References

Cardesa, A., & Nadal, A. (2011). Carcinoma of the head and neck in the HPV era. *Acta Dermatovenerologica Alpina, Pannonica, et Adriatica, 20*, 161–173.

DeGowin, R.L. (1994). *DeGowin and DeGowin's diagnostic examinations* (6th ed.). New York, NY: McGraw-Hill.

Figure 5-3. Patient Assessment Flow Chart

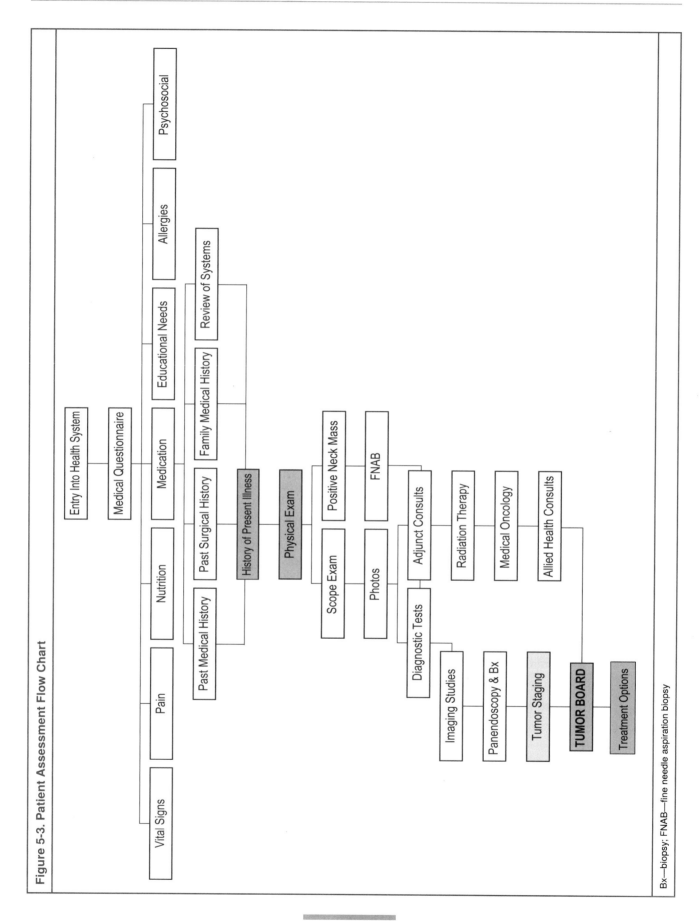

Bx—biopsy; FNAB—fine needle aspiration biopsy

Edge, S.B., Byrd, D.R., Compton, C.C., Fritz, A.G., Greene, F.L., & Trotti, A. (Eds.). (2010). *AJCC cancer staging manual* (7th ed.). New York, NY: Springer.

Farrington, M., Cullen, L., & Dawson, C. (2010). Assessment of oral mucositis in adult and pediatric oncology patients: An evidence-based approach. *ORL—Head and Neck Nursing, 28*(3), 8–15.

Friedland, P.L., Bozic, B., Dewar, J., Kuan, R., Meyer, C., & Phillips, M. (2011). Impact of multidisciplinary team management in head and neck cancer patients. *British Journal of Cancer, 104,* 1246–1248. doi:10.1038/bjc.2011.92

Gordon-Lubitz, R.J. (2003). Risk communication: Problems of presentation and understanding. *JAMA, 289,* 95. doi:10.1001/jama.289.1.95

Gourin, C.G., Couch, M.E., & Johnson, J.T. (2014). Effect of weight loss on short-term outcomes and costs of care after head and neck cancer surgery. *Annals of Otology, Rhinology and Laryngology, 123,* 101–110. doi:10.1177/0003489414523564

Hoffman, H. (2013). Iowa head and neck protocols. Retrieved from https://iowaheadneckprotocols.oto.uiowa.edu

Joint Commission Resources. (2010). *Advancing effective communication, cultural competence, and patient- and family-centered care: A roadmap for hospitals.* Oakbrook Terrace, IL: Author.

National Cancer Institute. (n.d.). NCI dictionary of cancer terms. Retrieved from http://www.cancer.gov/dictionary?CdrID=306510

National Cancer Institute Surveillance, Epidemiology, and End Results Program. (n.d.). Cancer registration and surveillance modules: Staging a cancer case. Retrieved from http://training.seer.cancer.gov/staging

National Comprehensive Cancer Network. (2015). *NCCN Clinical Practice Guidelines in Oncology (NCCN Guidelines®): Adult cancer pain* [v.1.2015]. Retrieved from http://www.nccn.org/professionals/physician_gls/pdf/pain.pdf

Ridge, J.A., Mehra, R., Lango, M.N., & Feigenberg, S. (2013). Head and neck tumors. Cancer management. Retrieved from http://www.cancernetwork.com/head-and-neck-tumors

Rodriguez, C.P., & Adelstein, D.J. (2010). Head and neck cancer. Retrieved from http://www.clevelandclinicmeded.com/medicalpubs/diseasemanagement/hematology-oncology/head-and-neck-cancer/Default.htm

Tan, C.S., Read, J.A., Phan, V.H., Beale, P.J., Peat, J.K., & Clarke, S.J. (2015). The relationship between nutritional status, inflammatory markers and survival in patients with advanced cancer: A prospective cohort study. *Supportive Care in Cancer, 23,* 385–391. doi:10.1007/s00520-014-2385-y

U.S. Department of Health and Human Services Office of Disease Prevention and Health Promotion. (n.d.). Quick guide to health literacy. Retrieved from http://www.health.gov/communication/literacy/quickguide/quickguide.pdf

Varkey, P., Tang, W.R., & Tan, N.C. (2010). Nutrition in head and neck cancer patients. *Seminars in Plastic Surgery, 24,* 325–330. doi:10.1055/s-0030-1263074

von Meyenfeldt, M. (2005). Cancer-associated malnutrition: An introduction. *European Journal of Oncology Nursing, 9,* S35–S38. doi:10.1016/j.ejon.2005.09.001

Wheless, S.A., McKinney, K.A., & Zanation, A.M. (2010). A prospective study of the clinical impact of a multidisciplinary head and neck tumor board. *Otolaryngology—Head and Neck Surgery, 143,* 650–654. doi:10.1016/j.otohns.2010.07.020

CHAPTER 6

Surgical Management

Raymond Scarpa, DNP, APNC, AOCN®, and Joanne Lester, PhD, CNP, AOCN®

Introduction

Surgery remains an integral treatment modality in primary cancers of the head and neck. The goals of surgical management are to remove the tumor, restore functions, preserve cosmetic appearance, and extend disease-free survival. Successful surgical outcomes can be limited by the extent of tumor, defects secondary to previous surgery, and required skills and experiences of the surgical team (Zafereo, 2013).

Novel approaches to the surgical management of head and neck cancer include the use of new imaging techniques that can improve morbidity and mortality by guiding initial diagnosis, extent of disease, and subsequent treatment of malignancy (Shukla-Dave et al., 2012). Directed surgical approaches that use laparoscopy or robotic-assisted procedures have the potential to reduce the extent of surgery, improve morbidity and mortality rates, and increase patient satisfaction associated with most head and neck cancers (Tae et al., 2014).

This chapter will discuss various evidence-based surgical and reconstructive procedures for selected tumors in the head and neck. Personalized surgical care will be reviewed with attention to tumor type, biologic or molecular markers, and personal characteristics. Surgical issues relevant to the geriatric population will be highlighted. Potential functional and cosmetic outcomes of various procedures will be discussed with recommended nursing interventions.

Tumor Resection

Surgical resection of early-stage head and neck malignancies (e.g., T1 or T2 lesions) is performed for locoregional control and curative intent (Dik et al., 2014). These surgical procedures typically result in favorable cosmetic and functional outcomes, but they may negatively affect patient satisfaction (Al-Dhahri, Mubasher, Mufarji, Allam, & Terkawi, 2014; Ringash et al., 2015).

Multimodality Approach

Patients with locally advanced disease (e.g., T3 or T4 lesions) or lymphatic nodal metastases may require combined-modality treatment involving surgery, chemotherapy, radiation therapy, or biologic therapy (Cohen et al., 2014). Surgery remains part of the primary treatment, but it may not be the first treatment the patient receives if neoadjuvant chemotherapy and radiation therapy are necessary for tumor reduction (Cohen et al., 2014). Modified or radical surgical neck resections, often required in T3 and T4 disease, can result in significant cosmetic and functional defects (Checcoli et al., 2013; Sheikh, Shallwani, & Ghaffar, 2014; Xue, Wang, & Chen, 2013) with significant negative effects on patient satisfaction (Ringash et al., 2015). Patients should be offered treatment at institutions that provide reconstructive surgical procedures using microvascular tissue flaps and grafts to provide restorative improvement in acquired defects (Choi, Lee, & Oh, 2013; Moubayed, Rahal, & Ayad, 2014).

Palliative Surgery

Palliative debulking surgery may be indicated as a secondary treatment for advanced disease to provide functional or symptomatic relief from lesions that invade or compress vital structures in the head and neck (Kamisetty, Mayland, Jack, Lowe, & Rogers, 2014; Roland & Bradley, 2014).

Personalized Approach to Tumor Resection

While surgery remains a cornerstone in the treatment of head and neck cancers, individualized therapies are emerging that require a personalized approach based on pathologic findings, host characteristics, and molecular profiles (Lucs, Saltman, Chung, Steinberg, & Schwartz, 2013). Today, extensive data about tumor type (e.g., presence or absence of human papillomavirus [HPV]), patient-specific indications, environment (e.g., tobacco use, chemical exposure), clinical profile, oncologic markers, and genetic variations of the tumor and host are available and should be considered prior to any treatment beyond diagnostic procedures and biopsy (Barry et al., 2014; Jessri & Farah, 2014; Lucs et al., 2013).

Surgical-related trends include surgery de-escalation with acceptance of closer margins, specifically in early-stage (i.e., stage I or II) oral cavity squamous cell carcinoma (Barry et al., 2014). A personalized approach is necessary to determine the safety of surgical de-escalation in these tumors with attention to cervical lymph node pathology and the presence or absence of extracapsular spread (Barry et al., 2014). HPV-positive tumors in young nonsmoking patients often respond better to chemotherapy and radiation therapy (Peacock et al., 2014).

Geriatric Issues

Attention to chronologic age alone may result in less aggressive treatment or negate referral to appropriate cancer resources (Korc-Grodzicki et al., 2014; Walko & McLeod, 2014). Careful selection of appropriate geriatric operative candidates may ensure maintenance of health status and improved disease-free survival (Shuman et al., 2013). The presence of early or progressive dementia may result in difficult decision making for complex surgical treatment.

Review of geriatric oncology guidelines (Hurria et al., 2014; National Comprehensive Cancer Network® [NCCN®], 2015) with incorporation of a geriatric oncology clinic may be useful to rapidly and accurately identify any issues that may delay surgery or lead to surgical complications. Preadmission assessment or interventions for cardiopulmonary status and medical optimization may result in improved postsurgical outcomes (Shuman et al., 2013). Geriatric issues, such as comorbidities, cognitive status, psychological state, fragility, functional status, mobility, fall risk, nutritional status, fatigue, polypharmacy, social support, and home environment, should be assessed pre- and postoperatively with appropriate preadmission testing, inpatient care, referrals, and discharge planning (Extermann & Hurria, 2007; Shuman et al., 2013; Wildiers et al., 2014).

Nursing Interventions

Registered and advanced practice nurses are integral to patient-family-physician communication and assistance with complex treatment decision making (Shuman et al., 2013). Attention to medication adherence, falls, mobility, safety, and comorbid conditions may guide preadmission assessment, discharge planning, and rehabilitation referrals (Korc-Grodzicki et al., 2014). Patients who undergo surgical resec-

tion of advanced tumors are discharged from the hospital with multiple long-term or permanent needs. Patients should be critically reviewed to determine if home discharge is feasible and what needs exist in regard to home care or if rehabilitative or extended-care facilities are necessary. Readmission rates should be reviewed to determine pre-, peri-, and postoperative needs that can be further addressed. In geriatric patients, systems should be evaluated as described previously from diagnosis to rehabilitation (Korc-Grodzicki et al., 2014).

Removal of the larynx or significant surgical alterations of the oropharynx, auditory nerves, or neck may require assistive devices such as language processors to enhance or enable verbal communication. Preoperative assessment of language or hearing issues and postoperative auditory, verbal, and social environment outcomes are necessary to promote successful outcomes (Li, Vikani, Harris, & Lin, 2014).

Psychological Issues

Patients with head and neck malignancies often have significant psychological and emotional issues secondary to their diagnoses and personal habits, with frequent tobacco and alcohol abuse (Chang et al., 2013). The presence of substance abuse is discussed with recommendations for prompt cessation. Smoking cessation is extremely important, as continuation of any tobacco product may increase the risk of surgical, reconstructive, or healing complications; local recurrence rate; or cancer death (Fiorini, Deganello, Larotonda, Mannelli, & Gallo, 2014; Sharp, McDevitt, Carsin, Brown, & Comber, 2014). Cessation of alcohol use is also recommended (Chang et al., 2013; Genther & Gourin, 2012). Abrupt or even gradual cessation of smoking or alcohol intake can be very difficult and may increase complications, length of hospital stay, comorbid conditions, and mortality (Chang et al., 2013). Cessation of substance abuse also may affect family and friend support. Symptoms related to withdrawal, such as hallucinations and increased anxiety, irritability, and sensitivity, can be difficult for patients and their families or friends to manage or support. Provisions are needed to enhance an environment that promotes successful patient outcomes and cancer prevention initiatives. Recurrent tobacco use in patients within one year of diagnosis is greater than 50% (Simmons et al., 2013); therefore, patients require continual encouragement and interventions from the healthcare team.

Patients often are faced with life-altering decisions that may result in transient or permanent changes in oral intake and air exchange, with visible scars and appliances. Quality of life can be favored over quantity of life in early decision making, although most patients and their families agreed about treatment priorities and were without regret at six months post-treatment (Gill et al., 2011). According to Gill et al. (2011), the top six priorities of agreement between patients and their families included (1) being cured of cancer, (2) living as long as possible, (3) having no pain, (4) being able to swallow all foods, (5) having normal energy, and (6) returning to normal activities. Patients also ranked other items, such as having an easily understood speech, keeping a natural voice, having a comfortably moist mouth, maintaining their appearance, and being able to chew normally, as further priorities as compared to their families' rankings of these same items (Gill et al., 2011).

Neck Dissection

The term *neck dissection* refers to the unilateral (e.g., ipsilateral) or bilateral (e.g., ipsilateral and contralateral) surgical removal of cervical lymph nodes in the neck (see Figure 6-1). Nodal levels are classified as the following (Dubner, 2013).
- I: Submental and submandibular
- II: Upper jugular
- III: Middle jugular
- IV: Lower jugular
- V: Posterior triangular
- VI: Anterior, central, or compartmental lymph nodes

Neck dissections generally are performed in conjunction with initial surgical resection of primary tumors in the upper aerodigestive tract, although they may require a second surgery after evaluation of pathology results of initial tumor resection (Xue et al., 2013).

Lymph node status is a significant prognostic factor, especially in non–HPV-associated disease (Peng et al., 2014). In patients with squamous cell carcinoma of the tongue and a clinical presentation of T1 N0 (e.g., small tumor size, clinically negative lymph nodes) disease, a neck dissection is not typically indicated. In patients with papillary thyroid cancer, a prophylactic modified node dissection may be recommended in patients who have at least two of the following: male gender, 55 years of age or older, tumor size greater than 3 cm, or significant extrathyroid tumor extension (Xue et al., 2013).

Neck Dissection Indications

Indications for a neck dissection include the size, location, pathology, and oncogenetics of the primary tumor and the potential lymphatic drainage pattern associated with that site. Clinical evidence of disease in the cervical nodes (e.g., palpable lymph nodes, radiographic evidence of multiple enlarged nodes) may warrant a preoperative needle biopsy with or without ultrasound guidance (Xue et al., 2013). If a cervical lymph node is positive, a neck dissection may be warranted, or surgery may be delayed in favor of combined chemotherapy and radiation therapy. Intraoperative removal of an enlarged node with frozen section may likewise be necessary prior to performing a modified or radical neck dissection. In the absence of clinical evidence, a sentinel lymph node biopsy may be performed in the jugular carotid chain of the lateral neck compartment at the time of surgery (Xue et al., 2013) with an intraoperative frozen section. If positive for disease,

Figure 6-1. Node Groups and Lymphatic Drainage

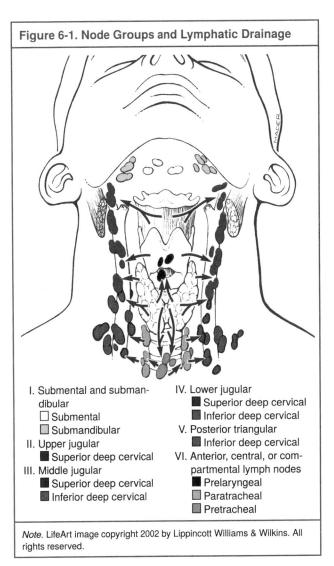

I. Submental and subman-
   dibular
   ☐ Submental
   ☐ Submandibular
II. Upper jugular
   ■ Superior deep cervical
III. Middle jugular
   ■ Superior deep cervical
   ■ Inferior deep cervical

IV. Lower jugular
   ■ Superior deep cervical
   ■ Inferior deep cervical
V. Posterior triangular
   ■ Inferior deep cervical
VI. Anterior, central, or com-
   partmental lymph nodes
   ■ Prelaryngeal
   ■ Paratracheal
   ■ Pretracheal

Note. LifeArt image copyright 2002 by Lippincott Williams & Wilkins. All rights reserved.

then the neck dissection is subsequently performed to evaluate the extent of regional disease (Xue et al., 2013).

Modified Radical Neck Dissection

A modified radical neck dissection includes removal of levels II through V cervical lymph nodes. Often, level VI lymph nodes are removed as well, with preservation of nonlymphatic structures. This procedure is indicated in cases of metastatic disease that do not involve or are nonadherent to any nonlymphatic structures in the neck. Modified neck dissection is designed to reduce the cosmetic and functional limitations associated with radical neck dissections without compromising the oncologic treatment or disease-free outcomes.

Central Neck Dissection

A central neck or central compartment dissection involves surgical removal of level VI cervical lymph nodes, which are bound by the hyoid bone, innominate vein, and carotid sheaths. This procedure is most commonly performed in patients with thyroid cancer who present with metastatic nodal disease or who later develop metachronous central nodal disease (Xue et al., 2013).

Surgical Approach

Multiple surgical approaches can be used when performing a modified or radical neck dissection. Most commonly, an incision is made at the level of the mastoid process that extends two fingerbreadths below the angle of the mandible to the anterior part of the mandible. A second incision is made at the midpoint of the first incision over the posterior aspect of the sternocleidomastoid in a lazy "S" fashion downward to the mid-clavicle. This is referred to as the Crile technique and allows access to the submandibular area. A second parallel incision is made from the sternoclavicular joint to the anterior border of the trapezius (Tubachi, Jainkeri, Gadagi, & Gunari, 2013). The standard radical neck dissection removes the fascia and lymphatic tissue deep to the platysma en bloc from levels I–V. It also removes all the aforementioned nonlymphatic structures (Dubner, 2013) (see Figure 6-2).

The endoscopic approach for organ removal in head and neck malignancies is emerging as a preferred option to open resection with visible scars. Endoscopic surgery for thyroid malignancies can reduce skin paresthesias and improve cosmetic results (Lee & Chung, 2013). The robotic-guided surgical approach improves visibility, decreases movement, improves dexterity, and enhances the ability of the surgeon to perform a neck dissection (Lee & Chung, 2013).

Radical Neck Dissection

Radical neck dissection can be performed in an ipsilateral or bilateral fashion and involves removal of all lymph nodes from levels I–V: fascia; internal jugular vein; submandibular gland; spinal accessory; greater auricular nerves; and sternocleidomastoid, digastric, and stylohyoid muscles (Dubner, 2013; Popescu, Berteşteanu, Grigore, Scăunaşu, & Popescu, 2012; Xue et al., 2013). This procedure is indicated for N3 disease (e.g., extracapsular extension of lymph nodes) or when other metastatic disease is found in the neck, including direct extension to any structure (Dubner, 2013; Scarpa, 2014).

Extended Radical Neck Dissection

Extended radical neck dissection removes all structures included in the radical neck dissection with the removal of additional lymphatic and nonlymphatic structures, including the mediastinal, parapharyngeal, or paratracheal lymph nodes; carotid artery; skin; and vagus and hypoglossal nerves (Forastiere et al., 2008; Xue et al., 2013). Extended radical neck dissection can leave the patient with significant functional and cosmetic impairments. The degree of impairment

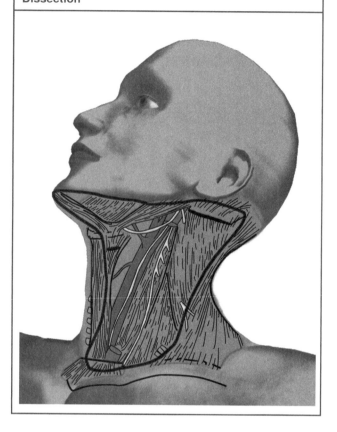

Figure 6-2. Surgical Incision for Radical Neck Dissection

will vary depending on the full extent of surgery and specific structures removed.

Selective Neck Dissection

Selective neck dissection involves preservation of one or more lymph node groups that would normally be removed in a radical neck dissection. The basis for selective removal or preservation of various lymphatic groups depends on the primary tumor site and the predicted pattern of lymphatic spread (Dubner, 2013). This term and the specific levels of lymphatics removed are now used to describe these procedures (e.g., selective neck dissection levels I–III).

In 2002, the Committee for Head and Neck Surgery and Oncology revised its previous classification of selective neck dissections and now requires documentation of all levels of lymphatics removed during surgery. Of note, any bilateral anatomic structures in the neck that are divided as "A" or "B" must be clearly documented as preserved or excised tissue in a selective neck dissection. A selective neck dissection of level I–III cervical lymph nodes, previously termed a supraomohyoid neck dissection, is indicated for primary malignant lesions in the oral cavity with either N0 or N1 neck disease. It can also include level IV, especially if the tongue is involved. This procedure involves removal of lymphatic tissue in the submental area, the submandibular gland, and lymphatic tissue along the internal jugular vein (see Figure 6-3). It also includes the fascia that covers the sternocleidomastoid and preserves the spinal accessory nerve (Mitzner, 2013).

The selective neck dissection of level II–IV cervical lymph nodes, previously termed a lateral neck dissection, is indicated for primary tumors found in the oropharynx, hypopharynx, or larynx. Lymphatic tissue is removed from the level of the clavicle up to the base of skull. Tissue from the posterior border of the sternocleidomastoid is removed posteriorly to the anterior sternohyoid muscle (Mitzner, 2013).

The selective neck dissection of the level VI cervical lymph nodes was previously termed the anterior neck dissection (see Figure 6-4). The hyoid bone, suprasternal notch, and carotid sheath are the superior, inferior, and lateral borders of the dissection, respectively. The anterior compartment neck dissection is indicated for primary tumors of midline neck structures, such as the thyroid or parathyroid glands, hypopharynx, cervical trachea, cervical esophagus, glottis, and subglottic areas of the larynx (Mitzner, 2013).

The selective neck dissection with dissection of cervical node levels II–V, previously termed posterior lateral neck dissection, is indicated for cutaneous lesions on the scalp and postauricular or suboccipital areas of the head and neck. It involves removal of the lymph nodes in these regions in addition to lymphatic tissue aside the jugular

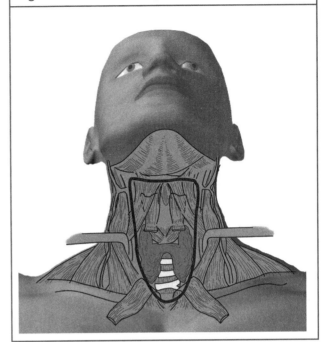

Figure 6-4. Anterior Neck, Level VI

chain or posterior triangle located superior to the accessory nerve. In cases of malignant lesions located in the preauricular area, frontal area of the scalp, or temporal area, a selective neck dissection (see Figure 6-5), including levels II, III, and V, is indicated (Mitzner, 2013).

Geriatric Issues

Most cancer surgeries, including head and neck, are not elective in nature, although surgical approaches may differ, as can the extent of the surgery. Each geriatric patient should be evaluated on an individual basis to determine the potential goals of the surgery, risk stratification for perioperative morbidity and mortality (Korc-Grodzicki et al., 2014), and what will be gained or lost if the surgical plan is modified. Considerations of anesthesia time, recuperation, social and living status, potential treatment beyond surgery, and other issues must be discussed preoperatively with the patient and family (Korc-Grodzicki et al., 2014). Chronologic age alone should not guide these decisions. Geriatric issues, as previously described, need to be evaluated in a geriatric clinic to minimize their impact on function, form, and quality of life (Korc-Grodzicki et al., 2014).

Nursing Indications

Cancers of the head and neck pose some significant issues, including limitations of upper body and head mobility and a decrease in neck and shoulder range of motion (Sheikh et

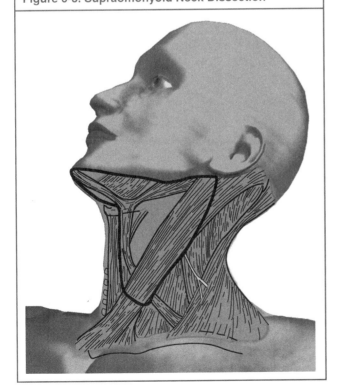

Figure 6-3. Supraomohyoid Neck Dissection

Figure 6-5. Posterior Lateral Neck Lymph Nodes

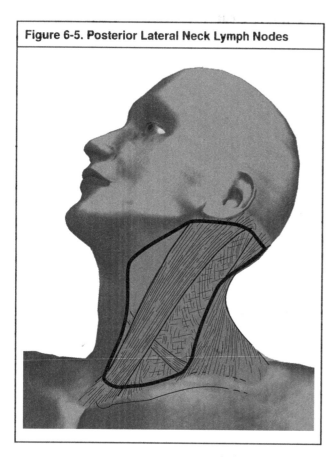

improve treatment plans (Pellini et al., 2014). Personalized care can be provided with directed, individualized treatment plans. Less-invasive surgical procedures that use endoscopic approaches may decrease short- and long-term side effects without compromising outcomes (Fan et al., 2014).

Cancer of the Larynx

The larynx (see Figure 6-6) is a complex neuromuscular organ that is divided into three regions: supraglottic, glottic, and subglottic. The supraglottic larynx starts at the superior tip of the epiglottis and extends to include the false vocal cords. This area acts as a passageway for air and protects the airway. Malignant lesions in these regions tend to present in advanced stages that cause symptoms such as dysphagia or aspiration of secretions or food particles, with resulting pneumonia.

The glottic area of the larynx is composed of the true vocal cords and the anterior and posterior commissures. The vocal cords protect the airway during swallowing and vibrate as air passes over them. Vibrations and the pressure of the cricothyroid and thyroarytenoid muscles create vocal sounds (Titze, 2014). The subglottic area extends from the inferior edge of the true vocal cord to the lower border of the cricoid cartilage.

Etiology

Laryngeal cancers are more common in men than in women and are associated with smoking (70%–85%) and

al., 2014). Patients should be assessed for pre- and postoperative restrictions and the potential impact on safety, eating, and activities of daily living. Assessment tools, such as the Disabilities of the Arm, Shoulder, and Hand (DASH) questionnaire, may be helpful in measuring regress or progress (Goldstein et al., 2015). Dietary specialists should be involved in the assessment of pre- and postoperative nutritional status, addressing potential weight loss, protein loss, and alternative means of nourishment.

Feelings of guilt related to the etiology of their disease (e.g., smoking or alcohol abuse) coupled with the fear of a cancer diagnosis and potentially disabling and disfiguring treatment can be difficult for patients and family members to handle alone. Communication challenges may be overwhelming for patients and caregivers. Discussion of these feelings and referral to a mental health clinical nurse specialist or psychologist may be helpful.

In summary, neck dissection can have both therapeutic and diagnostic values. While the surgical intent is to remove the disease, the pathologic information obtained from a neck dissection may help guide staging and future treatment. The ability to diagnose and treat head and neck malignancies with combined modalities has led to improved patient outcomes. The development of enhanced diagnostic tests, such as positron-emission tomography scans, continues to direct and

Figure 6-6. Levels of the Larynx

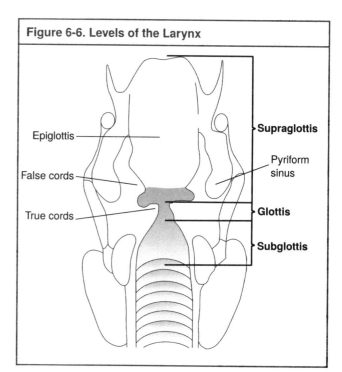

excessive alcohol use (25%), with a combined smoking and alcohol etiology of 89% (Boing et al., 2011; Santi, Kroll, Dietz, Becher, & Ramroth, 2014). The etiology of laryngeal cancers is further explained by influential factors of job classification, socioeconomic status, and exposure to carcinogenic agents (Santi et al., 2014). HPV infection is an emerging prognostic and etiologic factor of laryngeal cancers (27%) with a potential independent or covariate effect (Haws & Haws, 2014). Associations between genetic polymorphisms and known etiologic factors may aid in the prediction of personal significant risk of laryngeal cancer development and survival (Lu et al., 2014).

Approximately 75% of all laryngeal tumors arise from glottis vocal cords, then the supraglottis, and few subglottic cancers (Haws & Haws, 2014). The majority of laryngeal tumors are squamous cell carcinomas with further subsite categorization for staging purposes (Haws & Haws, 2014). Persistent hoarseness or a nonproductive cough for more than two weeks can be an early warning sign and often leads patients to seek evaluation.

The overall survival and prognoses of patients with laryngeal cancer are largely dependent on the subsite of origin. Tumors that originate in the supraglottic area tend to have a poorer prognosis and are also more likely to be high-grade malignancies (Haws & Haws, 2014). The presence or absence of extracapsular spread and regional lymph node metastases are the two most important prognostic indicators in supraglottic cancer (Haws & Haws, 2014).

Treatment of Laryngeal Cancers

Early-stage laryngeal cancers usually are treated with radiation therapy alone with excellent functional outcomes and a high potential cure rate. Locally advanced or recurrent laryngeal cancers often require combination therapy with chemotherapy, radiation therapy, or organ removal (Qian et al., 2014) with a rerouted airway. Treatment options are dependent on the extent of tumor, clinical presentation, overall general health (Mannelli et al., 2014), and preexisting comorbid conditions. Preoperative imaging with computed tomography or magnetic resonance imaging scans and use of intraoperative endoscopic guidance has significantly improved treatment planning (Allegra et al., 2014; Mannelli et al., 2014). A modified or radical neck dissection is indicated with clinical or imaging evidence of metastatic cervical lymph nodes (Yu, Wang, Xu, & Wu, 2014).

Surgical approaches include hemilaryngectomy or total laryngectomy using a variety of surgical techniques and reconstructive procedures. The most common procedures are supraglottic laryngectomy, supracricoid laryngectomy with cricohyoidopexy, and supracricoid laryngectomy with cricohyoidoepiglottopexy (Yu et al., 2014). Surgical access is gained through an anterior incision on the neck (e.g., in a natural skin fold) and provides for excellent healing (Duke,

Chaung, & Terris, 2014). Intraoperative frozen sections of surgical margins enable removal of cancerous tissue with preservation of benign essential structures (Mannelli et al., 2014).

Conversely, a total laryngectomy with a permanent tracheostoma is a life-altering surgery with significant comorbidity and lifelong challenges (Haws & Haws, 2014). Organ preservation may be achieved in advanced laryngeal cancers with the use of chemotherapy, radiation therapy, and molecular-targeted therapy (Denaro, Russi, Adamo, & Merlano, 2014). Although this approach may avoid a debilitating surgery, the larynx remains a nonfunctioning organ. Airway and nutrition issues may still persist, necessitating a permanent tracheostomy and feeding tube. If preservation of the larynx does not equal successful preservation of laryngeal function (e.g., persistent hoarseness, dysphagia, aspiration, or dyspnea), definitive surgical treatment (i.e., total laryngectomy) should be considered (Qian et al., 2014).

Preservation of the Larynx

The Cooperative Studies Program of the Veterans Affairs Laryngeal Cancer Study Group (1991) focused on organ preservation in advanced laryngeal cancers. This landmark study examined (1) survival rates of patients with locally advanced laryngeal cancer treated with chemotherapy and radiation and (2) surgical salvage for nonresponders versus surgery with total laryngectomy and radiation. The two-year survival rate for both groups was 68%. The larynx was preserved in 66% of the surviving patients and 31% of the entire group. At three years, 40% of the chemotherapy/radiation group remained alive and disease free with an intact larynx (Department of Veterans Affairs Laryngeal Cancer Study Group, 1991).

Several potential options for organ preservation of the larynx exist, including multimodality treatment with chemotherapy and radiation therapy, a partial laryngopharyngectomy with or without tissue flap, or transoral surgery (Tomifuji et al., 2014). In select cases, transoral laser surgery may be a viable approach to laryngeal tumors with preservation of organ and vocal function and patent airway (Breda, Catarino, & Monteiro, 2014). Transoral surgery is less invasive and typically preserves swallowing function because it is less disruptive to the nerve and muscle anatomy and also because the absence of tracheotomy results in normal laryngeal elevation (Tomifuji et al., 2014).

Surgical Approaches

Total Laryngectomy

The total laryngectomy is indicated for stage III and IV laryngeal carcinomas or stage II tumors unsuitable for partial laryngectomy (e.g., larger than 1.5 cm). The total laryngectomy is also indicated for carcinoma at the base of the tongue extending beyond the circumvallate papillae, for subglottic or glottic carcinomas with subglottic extension into the larynx, or as salvage surgery for recurrent tumor due to failed irradiation. A total laryngectomy is also performed in conjunction with removal of the entire hypopharynx for surgical management of hypopharyngeal tumors (Haw & Haw, 2014).

Total laryngectomy involves removal of the entire larynx, thyroid and cricoid cartilages, and hyoid bone. To create an airway, a permanent stoma is made by suturing the trachea to the skin of the anterior neck. Following a total laryngectomy, air can enter the mouth but no longer enters the upper aerodigestive tract. Patients lose their sense of smell, which in turn diminishes their sense of taste. Patients can no longer sneeze, sniff, or blow their nose.

Voice rehabilitation is an essential component of postoperative management after total laryngectomy. Various options are available to rehabilitate the voice, including the learning and development of esophageal speech or use of a tracheoesophageal voice prosthesis or electrolarynx. Esophageal speech is produced by compressing air into the esophagus and then releasing it in a controlled fashion, similar to a burp. This results in vibratory movement of the pharyngeal-esophageal segment. This method is difficult to learn and often produces an undesirable type of voice.

Esophageal speech has largely been replaced by tracheoesophageal puncture (Guttman et al., 2013). The prosthesis is inserted into a surgically created tracheoesophageal fistula. Pulmonary air is diverted through a one-way valve in the device causing vibration of the pharyngeal-esophageal segment and voice production. This procedure provides superior voice intelligibility when compared to any other method of voice rehabilitation (Guttman et al., 2013). The tracheoesophageal puncture can be performed at the time of surgery or as a separate postoperative procedure.

Partial Laryngectomy

A partial laryngectomy is used to resect malignant lesions confined to the true vocal cords and includes procedures of cordectomy, vertical partial laryngectomy, or hemilaryngectomy. The partial laryngectomy is performed to preserve three important laryngeal functions: swallowing, phonation, and breathing (Ruberto et al., 2014).

A cordectomy consists of a limited excision of the true vocal cords and uses a midline thyrotomy (e.g., incision through the thyroid cartilage). This procedure is indicated for limited lesions without extension to the anterior commissure or involvement of the arytenoid cartilage.

A vertical partial laryngectomy, or hemilaryngectomy, is performed when the tumor involves the anterior commissure or the lesion extends into the vocal process of the arytenoids, superficial transglottic lesions, and areas of recurrence post-radiation therapy (Xue et al., 2013). A partial laryngec-

tomy should not be performed when the tumor extends to the posterior commissure, when it invades the bilateral thyroid or arytenoid cartilages, or with findings of a fixed vocal cord due to tumor involvement. Reconstructive techniques are various and often utilize a sternohyoid muscle flap (Yu et al., 2014).

The supraglottic laryngectomy is a horizontal resection of the upper part of the larynx and the area superior to the true vocal cords and epiglottis with a horizontal incision just above the vocal cords (Xue et al., 2013). This surgery is indicated for the treatment of T1, T2, and some T3 primary tumors of the supraglottic area, involving the laryngeal surface of the epiglottis, infrahyoid and suprahyoid epiglottis, ventricular folds, and aryepiglottic folds. Because the true vocal cords are preserved, this surgical approach allows for the maintenance of laryngeal function. Patients will have a temporary tracheotomy until postoperative edema of the surgical site resolves (Xue et al., 2013).

The standard transcervical approach to the supraglottic laryngectomy is an incision that extends through the vallecula superiorly, the aryepiglottic folds posteriorly, the apex of the ventricle inferiorly, and the thyroid cartilage anteriorly. The upper part of the larynx is removed with reconstruction of the aerodigestive area (a suture between the residual thyroid cartilage and hyoid bone) (e.g., thyrohyoidopexy) (Ruberto et al., 2014). This resection can include the hyoid bone, epiglottis, superior half of the thyroid cartilage, aryepiglottic folds, and the false folds to the arytenoids. Occasionally, one or both arytenoid cartilages are removed. Contraindications for a transcervical supraglottic laryngectomy include tumors that extend to the interarytenoid space, postcricoid mucosa, and true vocal folds. Tumors that result in vocal cord fixation are a contraindication for supraglottic laryngectomy (Xue et al., 2013).

Aspiration is a major concern in patients who have undergone a supraglottic laryngectomy. Careful assessment of pulmonary function status should be performed before, during, and after this procedure. Patients who have less than optimal pulmonary function may be more appropriately treated with a total laryngectomy.

The supracricoid laryngectomy with cricohyoidopexy is a horizontal partial laryngeal surgical procedure that allows patients with advanced supraglottic and transglottic cancers to safely avoid a total laryngectomy (Ruberto et al., 2014). The supracricoid laryngectomy with cricohyoidopexy is indicated for T2 and T3 supraglottic lesions that invade or extend into the glottic level, the anterior commissure, the floor of the ventricle, or the paraglottic space. Tumors with vocal cord fixation also may be treated with this procedure if some level of arytenoid function is present.

The resection includes the supracricoid larynx excluding the epiglottis stump, vocal cords, thyroid cartilage, and one arytenoid cartilage (Ruberto et al., 2014). The reconstruction involves securing the cricoid to the residual epiglottic stump and hyoid bone (e.g., cricohyoidoepiglottopexy) (Ruberto et al., 2014). The superior laryngeal nerve must be preserved to enable effective swallowing.

The aforementioned surgical procedures are reserved for select patients who present with limited- or early-stage disease, few comorbid conditions, and good support systems. Patients need to be motivated to undergo lifestyle changes in the postoperative period (e.g., cessation of tobacco and alcohol use, voice therapy).

Rehabilitation

Rehabilitation of patients who have undergone any type of partial laryngectomy is necessary to ensure optimal outcomes. Partial laryngectomy should result in a hoarse but serviceable voice, functional swallowing, and the ability to breathe without a permanent tracheotomy.

Within a few days after surgery, the cuffed tracheotomy tube should be removed and replaced with a fenestrated tracheostomy tube (Ruberto et al., 2014). Within one week after surgery, a referral to speech and language specialists is necessary to assess and teach swallowing techniques and speech rehabilitation. Semisolid and soft foods are gradually introduced; liquids are reserved for last because of the potential difficulty with swallowing (Ruberto et al., 2014).

Decannulation of the tracheostomy should begin to avoid formation of granulation tissue or subcutaneous emphysema. Edema that persists for more than six to eight weeks may indicate tumor regrowth and should be appropriately assessed. Patients who received preoperative radiation therapy are at increased risk for persistent edema and may require longer use of an airway.

Dysphagia remains one of the most common postoperative symptoms due to restoration of swallowing; persistent dysphagia may indicate detachment of the reconstructed pexy (Ruberto et al., 2014). Observed bleeding from the site should be rapidly assessed, as emergency surgery may be required in the event of suture loosening of a ligated vessel. This serious complication typically occurs with patient-induced, Valsalva-type pressure and is reversible if assessed prior to significant blood loss (Ruberto et al., 2014).

Minimally Invasive Techniques

Endoscopic transoral surgery has evolved as a treatment modality for early to moderately advanced laryngeal carcinomas (Lallemant et al., 2013). The laparoscopic approach with remote access eliminates the neck incision, thus improving cosmesis (Duke et al., 2014). Several noninvasive approaches are available, including transoral videolaryngoscopic surgery, transoral laser microsurgery, and transoral robotic surgery.

During videolaryngoscopic surgery, an endoscope is introduced into the tumor area as a visual guide. Using screen images, the surgeon employs endoscopic instruments to remove the tumor en bloc. In cases of positive lymph nodes, a neck dissection is also performed (Tomifuji et al., 2014). A tracheostomy is not routinely performed except for bilateral disease, large tumors, difficult intubation, or postoperatively for brief management. Persistent dysphagia may be a significant side effect after a transoral approach because the procedure may require placement of a percutaneous endoscopic gastrostomy tube (Tomifugi et al., 2014).

Transoral robotic surgery is dependent on a normal tongue size and appearance (e.g., absence of macroglossia), absence of retrognathic mandible, and an adequate oral opening to enable introduction of the endoscopic and two instrument arms (Iloreta, Anderson, & Miles, 2014). In patients who would significantly benefit from this minimally invasive approach, unilateral or bilateral mandibular osteotomy can be performed to expand the transoral route (Iloreta et al., 2014). Patients who require salvage surgery but are unable to undergo transoral robotic surgery because of radiation-induced fibrosis may benefit from transoral laser microsurgery (Iloreta et al., 2014).

Transoral laser microsurgery provides another minimally invasive approach to the surgical treatment of laryngeal cancers. This approach offers similar survivorship outcomes as laryngectomy yet provides preservation of the larynx with acceptable functionality (Breda et al., 2014). A laser-safe nasoendotracheal tube is necessary for this procedure. A 3–4 cm vertical mouth opening provides an optimal transoral view for the surgical team. The surgeon operates the controls as the surgical team stabilizes and moves endoscopic trocars (Breda et al., 2014). The carbon dioxide laser creates an incision around the tumor with 10 mm visual margins. The tumor is excised from the laryngeal attachments and removed en bloc with minimal blood loss (Breda et al., 2014).

Transoral robotic surgery is another innovative approach to minimally invasive surgery. The da Vinci® Surgical System provides a magnified, high-resolution, and three-dimensional view (Weinstein et al., 2012) that enables the surgeon to see far more than the traditional two-dimensional operative field (Lallemant et al., 2013). Additionally, the surgeon is able to operate remotely using the system's joystick controls, which provides precise movements of the instruments (Weinstein et al., 2012). The combination of transoral laser microsurgery and robotic surgery may be ideal to enhance minimally invasive surgery (Vicini et al., 2014), although randomized phase III studies that compare endoscopic robotic surgery, traditional surgery, and radiation therapy are necessary to fully measure the potential of minimally invasive approaches (Nichols et al., 2013).

Cancers of the Sinonasal Tract

Malignancies of the sinonasal tract characterize less than 1% of all malignant tumors and 3%–5% of all head and neck tumors (Llorente, López, Suárez, & Hermsen, 2014). The most common site for malignant tumors of the sinonasal tract is the maxillary sinus; squamous cell carcinoma is the most common pathologic finding (Llorente et al., 2014). Adenocarcinomas are found in the ethmoid sinus and nasal cavity. The remaining 20% are tumors with clinical, etiologic, pathologic, and genetic features different from head and neck tumors (Llorente et al., 2014). Sinonasal tract malignancies are twice as common in men as in women and more common in White men 50–70 years old (Llorente et al., 2014). Sinonasal malignancies are considered an occupational disease, and risk is increased for individuals who work in industries involving exposure to wood dust, tanning of leather, and nickel refining (Llorente et al., 2014).

Nasal cavity and paranasal sinus tumors are treated initially with surgery followed by postoperative external beam radiation therapy (Holliday & Frank, 2014). Conventional photon-based external beam radiation therapy, proton-based intensity-modulated radiation therapy, or three-dimensional conformal radiation therapy help to spare normal tissue yet provide an effective dose to the tumor site (Holliday & Frank, 2014).

Surgical Approaches

Total Maxillectomy With Orbital Exenteration

Total maxillectomy with orbital exenteration is an en bloc resection of the maxilla, including dental structures, ethmoid labyrinth, anterior zygoma, and the orbit and adnexal structures. The procedure is indicated for malignant tumors of the maxillary sinus or maxilla with superior extension into the orbit (Eley, Watt-Smith, Boland, Potter, & Golding, 2014). Pathways of invasion leading from the maxillary sinus to the orbit include direct bony extension, perivascular or perineural invasion through infraorbital or ethmoidal neurovascular bundles, infraorbital fissure, or nasolacrimal duct (Holliday & Frank, 2014).

Survival rates for patients who have advanced disease requiring orbital exenteration are poor despite advances over the past half century (Su et al., 2014). Total maxillectomy with orbital exenteration is associated with defects that include loss of smell (which negatively affects taste), loss of vision, cosmetic facial deformity, facial numbness, paralysis, and difficulty with swallowing and speech (Eley et al., 2014). Reconstruction and rehabilitation are accomplished with flaps, grafts, and prosthodontic devices.

Restoration of Surgical Defects

Reconstructive procedures continue to evolve to restore tissue and bone defects secondary to surgical resection of sinonasal malignancies. Reconstructive procedures include microvascular free tissue transfers, which are used for complex tissues defects, specifically in previously irradiated fields (Joseph et al., 2014). Surgical defects created by a total maxillectomy with orbital exenteration require a flap that has substantial muscle and skin to reconstruct the resected area. Bony restoration is ideal to reconstruct the orbital rim and floor but is a complex procedure (Joseph et al., 2014). Various microvascular myocutaneous free flaps, including latissimus dorsi, rectus abdominus, anterolateral thigh, or scapular fasciocutaneous flap, can be used (Joseph et al., 2014). Soft tissue flaps must include mesh to provide support for inferior and superior healing (Joseph et al., 2014).

The components to reconstruct an orbitomaxillary defect include facial bony and soft tissue contour defect, orbital socket with walls, palatal defect, skull base defect, and skin defect (Joseph et al., 2014). Ultimately, the goals include primary wound healing, cranionasal and oronasal separation, facial contour skin cover, and orbital and dental rehabilitation (Joseph et al., 2014). Flap reconstruction can facilitate speech and swallowing rehabilitation.

A split-thickness skin graft may be placed over exposed areas. Packing or a bolster is frequently inserted intraoperatively and secured over the graft to ensure adherence to the exposed areas of the undersurface of the cheek flap. The bolster temporarily fills the surgical defect, allowing the patient to speak and swallow after surgery. The bolster is removed five to seven days postoperatively (Joseph et al., 2014).

A prosthetic device known as a palatal obturator often is used. The prosthesis is prepared preoperatively and resembles an upper denture (see Figure 6-7). At the time of resection, this device is wired to any remaining dentition or to the hard palate (de Sousa & Mattos, 2014) to hold packing in place and allow for swallowing and intelligible speech during the postoperative phase. Once the packing is removed, additional denture material is applied to the obturator to fill in

Figure 6-7. Prosthetic Obturator for Patient Following Maxillectomy

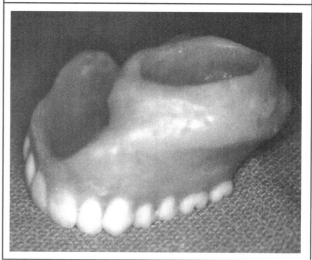

the surgical defect. Refinements are made postoperatively as healing occurs and edema subsides (de Sousa & Mattos, 2014). The obturator must fit properly to provide for swallowing and speech and should be easy to remove for daily cleaning.

Lateral Rhinotomy

A lateral rhinotomy is indicated for surgical access to the nasal cavity, paranasal sinuses, and nasopharynx. It is a useful approach for the removal of lesions limited to the anterior nasal cavity and adjacent medial third of the maxillary and ethmoid sinuses. Lateral rhinotomy is also used for en bloc resections of the ethmoid labyrinth and the wall between the antrum and nasal cavity when infiltrated by tumor (Verqez et al., 2012).

The lateral rhinotomy incision is made along the side of the nose and extends from the nostril around the alar groove, up the side of the nose, over the upper lateral cartilage, and around the frontal process of the maxilla to the medial canthus and the medial end of the eyebrow (see Figure 6-8). The incision should be made within natural creases of the skin to prevent cosmetic deformity. The incision is made to the depth of the periosteum of the bone. To provide more access to the antrum, the incision can be extended at its lower end to split the upper lip. It also can be extended further to form a full-face flap for maxillectomy or into the upper eyelid for exenteration of the orbital contents. The basic incision contains the flexibility needed for all sinus and nasal operations (Verqez et al., 2014).

Endoscopic Endonasal Surgery

Endoscopic procedures have been developed and tested over the last decade for use in sinonasal surgeries. The standard endoscopic endonasal resection begins with removal of the malignancy for identification of its origin; further resection is completed for clear margins (Su et al., 2014). Multiple anatomic sections are removed including the lamina papyracea, cribriform plate, fovea ethmoidalis, planum sphenoidale, dura, and olfactory bulbs and tracts (Su et al., 2014). Various approaches are under study, including extended transcribriform, transpterygoid, and transclival (Su et al., 2014). A combination of transnasal and transorbital approaches can be used to reach deep tumors; transfacial or transcranial approaches are recommended when skin is involved (Su et al., 2014). Transmaxillary, transethmoidal, and transsphenoidal endoscopic approaches can be used to access skull-based tumors (Grewal et al., 2014).

Potential side effects associated with the endoscopic approach include cerebrospinal fluid leaks, decrease or absence of senses, fistula development, and vascular injury (Nelson, Burke-Smith, & Kirkpatrick, 2014). Quality-of-life outcomes have been scored as favorable at one year after surgery as compared to open resection (Su et al., 2014). Endoscopic surgery has multiple advantages, including avoidance of soft tissue

Figure 6-8. Lateral Rhinotomy

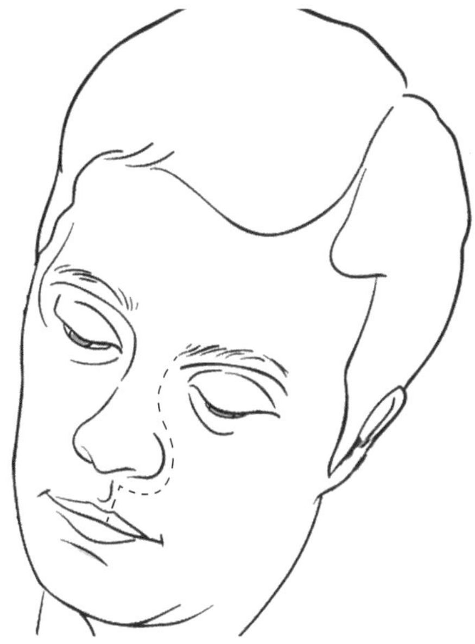

Note. LifeArt image copyright 2002 by Lippincott Williams & Wilkins. All rights reserved.

dissection, removal of skeletal segments, and brain retraction (Su et al., 2014). Multiple vascularized reconstructive options exist for restoration of removed structures.

Cancers of the Oral Cavity

The oral cavity comprises the lips, tongue, buccal mucosa, floor of the mouth, hard palate, and alveolar ridges. The area of transition to the oropharynx is the retromolar trigone (see Figure 2-5 in Chapter 2), which is located behind the third molar and anterior to the tonsillar pillar and soft palate (Belcher, Hayes, Fedewa, & Chen, 2014). The mouth is easy to examine, although some lesions deep in posterior corners may be missed or confused with premalignant changes, including leukoplakia and erythroplakia (Belcher et al., 2014). Appropriate diagnosis and treatment of such lesions are extremely important in a patient's prevention portfolio given that leukoplakia can harbor a malignancy in 20% of cases and erythroplakia up to 50% of the time (Belcher et al., 2014). These lesions can be treated with excision, cold steel, or laser treatments. Chemoprevention using retinoids or beta-carotene antioxidants may prevent a second primary (Belcher et al., 2014). Of urgency is a discussion about avoidance of tobacco products and guidance for cessation if needed.

Early oral malignant lesions can be treated with surgery or radiation therapy with the same expected outcomes. Surgery remains the primary treatment modality given relatively easy access to the oral cavity (Belcher et al., 2014). Lesions that have infiltrated bone or extend close to the mandible and disallow a clean margin require a segment of the mandible to be removed. Advanced or metastatic lesions of the oral cavity may require surgical excision, radiation therapy, chemotherapy, or a combination of these modalities. Chemotherapy and radiation therapy may be combined or concurrent and may replace surgery, depending on the location and stage of the tumor (Belcher et al., 2014).

These surgical options allow for rapid rehabilitation of the patient and avoidance of radiation side effects. However, the major disadvantages are short- or long-term functional disability or cosmetic defect, depending on the size of the resection (Cuellar et al., 2014). Radiation therapy may provide full treatment with avoidance of surgery and anesthesia and other associated risks. However, patients undergoing radiation therapy for oral cancers may suffer from symptoms, such as xerostomia, dysgeusia, and loosening of teeth (Belcher et al., 2014).

Surgery is preferred over radiation in patients who continue to smoke and drink excessive amounts of alcohol, as these individuals are at increased risk for developing additional primary tumors. Surgical resection in combination with radiation therapy is recommended for advanced tumors of the oral cavity with invasion of the mandible or the mandibular periosteum (Belcher et al., 2014).

Mandibular Resection

A segmental mandibulectomy (partial or marginal) or complete resection of the mandible (e.g., mandibulectomy) is indicated as an ablative surgery to treat primary malignant neoplasms. The extent of resection is often dependent on the anatomy of the involved areas, face, or oropharynx (Singh, Bhatnagar, Bansal, & Singh, 2014). An infected or necrotic segment of the jaw may be removed secondary to bisphosphonate-related necrosis (Spinelli et al., 2014), which can occur in women or men taking bisphosphonates as part of their cancer treatment or rehabilitation. A marginal mandibulectomy is performed when cancer cells are found near or on the alveolar ridge but without marrow involvement (Lin et al., 2014). The segmental mandibulectomy is performed when the mandibular marrow is involved by tumor (i.e., when malignant cells are found in the bone of the edentulous or irradiated mandible or with significant mandibular adherence) (Lin et al., 2014).

A tracheotomy is performed to ensure a stable airway and to provide better intraoral exposure. A lip-splitting incision or a visor flap incision is often performed with elevation of the flap to ensure integrity of the marginal mandibular nerve. The mandibular bone is resected en bloc with surrounding soft tissue to provide a clear surgical margin of 1–1.5 cm. The inferior alveolar nerve is resected and sent intraoperatively to

pathology for a frozen section. If this biopsy is positive, the entire inferior alveolar canal is resected.

Mandibular Reconstruction

Defects from a segmented or complete mandibulectomy are surgically corrected with immediate reconstruction depending on the amount of tumor invasion and resection margins. Reconstruction should be meticulously planned preoperatively with a personalized approach for bone and intraoral reconstruction, osseointegrated implants, and functional rehabilitation (Cuellar et al., 2014). The insertion of a titanium plate with soft tissue flap is useful for patients with a poor prognosis or multiple comorbid conditions that preclude extensive surgery (Fang, Wang, Chen, & Zhang, 2014). In these instances, a mandibular reconstructive plate may be used with a pectoralis major pedicle flap. This approach provides adequate reconstruction and closure to the wound; however, it has considerable bulk resulting in a prominence in the neck that can be cosmetically unappealing and restrict range of motion. Delayed reconstruction with a secondary closure using bone and soft tissue is amenable, should the patient's condition improve (Cuellar et al., 2014).

Ideally, a vascularized flap of bone and adjacent soft tissue is used and intended to match the ipsilateral jaw in length, height, and width (Cuellar et al., 2014; Lin et al., 2014). The free flap procedures require microvascular surgical expertise and a significant increased operative time. Candidates for these types of reconstructive procedures must be considered carefully, with attention to underlying medical conditions, such as cardiovascular disease, diabetes mellitus, and poor nutritional status. Continued tobacco use may compromise vascularity and jeopardize viability of the flaps. Successful outcomes depend on careful preoperative assessment and a well-coordinated multidisciplinary approach to treatment.

Bone and tissue flaps may be obtained from a variety of sources, including the fibula osteoseptocutaneous free flap or soft tissue flaps from anterolateral thigh, vastus lateralis myocutaneous, radial forearm, or nasolabial area (Cuellar et al., 2014; Lin et al., 2014). Two common osteomyocutaneous flaps are the fibular free flap and the iliac crest free flap; the scapular flap does not provide the required length of bone (Lin et al., 2014). The fibular free flap is used when bone is required and there is a minimal need for soft tissue reconstruction. The fibula is a straight bone with a rich blood supply providing a length of approximately 25 cm (Lin et al., 2014). Because of its rich blood supply, multiple osteotomies (cuts in the bone) can be made to allow the bone to be contoured as needed. Muscle, tissue, and skin that are harvested with the fibula can be used to reconstruct soft tissue defects that were created at the time of resection (Lin et al., 2014).

The iliac crest free flap is another type of osteomyocutaneous flap, as its natural shape enables conforming to the mandible with fewer osteotomies. The blood supply to the skin pedicle in this type of flap is poor, thus requiring a larger skin pedicle to provide additional blood vessels. This results in a bulky soft tissue component with little mobility. The iliac crest flap is used for reconstruction that requires a large amount of soft tissue, such as those found in large craniofacial defects.

Radiation therapy may be a planned intervention following surgery depending on the stage and pathology of the tumor. The role of radiation and its timing is imperative in surgical planning. Radiation can destruct capillaries in bone, decrease bone regeneration, and cause neorevascularization (Cuellar et al., 2014). To ensure complete osseointegration, osseous dental implants require at least three months of healing (Cuellar et al., 2014).

Any type of mandibulectomy can result in alterations of anatomic and biomedical structures in the oral cavity and face with functional and aesthetic consequences (Cuellar et al., 2014). Defects in bone and muscle result in gaps between mandibular segments, muscular imbalance, or dissymmetry of muscle movements with ptosis of the lower lip and retrusion (e.g., posterior to normal position) of the jaw (Cuellar et al., 2014; Singh et al., 2014). Functional results can include incompetence of the lower lip; salivary drooling; chewing, swallowing, or mastication difficulties; and phonation issues (Cuellar et al., 2014). With or without reconstruction, patients suffer from alterations in social relationships and quality of life (Cuellar et al., 2014).

Prosthodontic rehabilitation with osseointegrated dental implants has been shown to improve patients' contentment, happiness, physical and mental health, and quality of life (Singh et al., 2014). Endosseous implants provide support for prosthetic teeth that perform similarly to native teeth and gums, as opposed to conventional dentures that are difficult to fit because of their absence of bony support (Singh et al., 2014).

Cancer of the Tongue

Cancer of the tongue is the most common head and neck malignancy in the world with a primary pathology of squamous cell carcinoma (Shin et al., 2012; Vishak & Vinayak, 2014). Tongue cancers are prevalent worldwide as a result of the increasing epidemic of HPV in the oral cavity (Valakh, Miyamoto, Mazurenka, & Liu, 2014). With the exception of extensive disease, most malignant tumors of the tongue are confined to the body of the tongue. Surgery and radiation therapy can significantly improve patients' outcomes, but quality of life can be negatively affected with impaired basic and social activities of daily life (Canis et al., 2015).

Partial Glossectomy

Partial glossectomy is indicated for T1, T2, and limited T3 lesions confined to the anterior two-thirds of the tongue. Functional outcomes after a partial glossectomy can vary from severe swallowing and unintelligible speech to near-normal function (Lee et al., 2014). The volume of tissue loss is significantly related to swallowing and speech performance (Canis et al., 2015). When the floor of the mouth is involved, the area requires resection and repair with a split-thickness skin graft to restore mobility of the remaining tongue (Shin et al., 2012). T3 lesions that require more than primary closure or resections that communicate with structures in the neck will benefit from restoration with a free tissue flap (Canis et al., 2015). Restoring large surgical defects increases the odds that speech and swallowing will be positively affected (Shin et al., 2012). A radial forearm fasciocutaneous flap is commonly used to provide a barrier between the oral cavity and the neck to prevent wound breakdown and fistula formation. These surgeries are far more involved than a partial glossectomy and will require a tracheostomy due to postoperative edema. Therefore, careful consideration of each person is necessary to tailor the surgery based on planned resection volume, age, total operative time, presence of tracheostomy, and potential flap complications (Lee et al., 2014).

Controversy exists concerning elective neck dissection for early-stage tongue lesions without palpable lymphadenopathy, as there appears to be no survival benefit of the surgery itself (Vishak & Vinayak, 2014). A staging neck dissection is performed for all tongue lesions that are greater than 3 mm in thickness, as lymph node metastasis remains a strong prognostic predictor (Vishak & Vinayak, 2014). Therefore, the reasoning behind an elective neck dissection is to identify patients with early tongue lesions who have positive lymph node metastasis and will require further adjuvant therapy. A neck dissection should be performed on all T2, T3, and T4 lesions to identify micrometastases that will require further interventions (Vishak & Vinayak, 2014).

The use of postoperative external beam radiation therapy can negatively contribute to functional outcomes of speech and swallowing, even in early-stage tongue cancers (Shin et al., 2012). Referrals to appropriate speech rehabilitation resources are necessary to minimize permanent changes. The use of high-dose-rate brachytherapy in early oral cancers may provide fewer side effects than external beam radiation therapy and reduce the risk of dysfunctional speech and swallowing (Petera et al., 2014).

Total Glossectomy

The decision to perform a total glossectomy depends on the invasion of the tumor into the substance of the tongue as well as involvement of the neurovascular supply to the tongue. Total glossectomy is indicated for massive tumors of the tongue, tumors involving both sides of the base of the tongue, and large tumors of the floor of the mouth involving the ventral surface of the tongue or extending deeply in the submental area. A total glossectomy is associated with significant morbidity (Rihani, Lee, Lee, & Ducic, 2013) and oral disabilities (Dziegielewski et al., 2013). A tracheostomy is created for airway maintenance at the beginning of the procedure and for postoperative swelling. A bilateral neck dissection is performed for a clinically node-negative neck, whereas a modified radical neck dissection is performed on patients with palpable adenopathy.

Historically, patients who had a total glossectomy also had a total laryngectomy to prevent intractable aspiration pneumonia. With modern reconstructive techniques, retention of the larynx should be considered in medically stable patients who are motivated to relearn swallowing and airway protection (Rihani et al., 2013). The goal of reconstruction should be to optimize speech and to give patients an independent life without a tracheostomy and gastric feeding tube (Rihani et al., 2013). Free tissue transfer may provide sufficient tissue volume for a neotongue; based on body habitus, however, a pedicled flap transfer may be desired (Rihani et al., 2013).

Summary

This review provides an outline of the common types of oropharyngeal cancers and the surgeries performed for management of tumor recurrence in the head and neck. The challenges for both surgeons and patients are significant. Head and neck malignancies can inhibit the common functions of breathing, swallowing, and talking, and decrease socialization and quality of life because of their debilitating effects and visibility to the public.

Patients with head and neck cancer require optimal care that includes active, intense nursing support following the acute surgical intervention and discharge to an outpatient setting. This support includes assistance in maintaining an adequate airway and nutritional status as well as developing new ways to communicate. The quality of life and survival of these patients are directly dependent on their ability to become self-sufficient, receive supportive care, and cope with the remaining demands of their bodies. A coordinated, multidisciplinary approach that uses hospital, community, and family resources can ensure optimal care for patients with head and neck cancers, as it is a group of devastating diseases.

The authors would like to acknowledge Jose Zevallos, BA, for his contribution to this chapter that remains unchanged from the first edition of this book.

References

Al-Dhahri, S.F., Mubasher, M., Mufarji, K., Allam, O.S., & Terkawi, A.S. (2014). Factors predicting post-thyroidectomy hypoparathyroidism recovery. *World Journal of Surgery, 38*, 2304–2310. doi:10.1007/s00268-014-2571-6

Allegra, E., Ferrise, P., Trapasso, S., Trapuzzano, O., Barca, A., Tamburrini, S., & Garozzo, A. (2014). Early glottic cancer: Role of MRI in the preoperative setting. *BioMed Research International, 2014*, Article ID 890385. doi:10.1155/2014/890385

Barry, C.P., Ahmed, F., Rogers, S.N., Lowe, D., Bekiroglu, F., Brown, J.S., & Shaw, R.J. (2015). Influence of surgical margins on local recurrence in T1/T2 oral squamous cell carcinoma. *Head and Neck, 37*, 1176–1180. doi:10.1002/hed.23729

Belcher, R., Hayes, K., Fedewa, S., & Chen, A.Y. (2014). Current treatment of head and neck squamous cell cancer. *Journal of Surgical Oncology, 110*, 551–574. doi:10.1002/jso.23724

Boing, A.F., Antunes, J.L., de Carvalho, M.B., de Góis Filho, J.F., Kowalski, L.P., Michaluart, P., Jr., ... Wünsch-Filho, V. (2011). How much do smoking and alcohol consumption explain socioeconomic inequalities of head and neck cancer risk? *Journal of Epidemiology and Community Health, 65*, 709–714. doi:10.1136/jech.2009.097691

Breda, E., Catarino, R., & Monteiro, E. (2015). Transoral laser microsurgery for laryngeal carcinoma: Survival analysis in a hospital-based population. *Head and Neck, 37*, 1181–1186. doi:10.1002/hed.23728

Canis, M., Weiss, B.G., Ihler, F., Hummers-Pradier, E., Matthias, C., & Wolff, H.A. (2015). Quality of life in patients after resection of pT3 lateral tongue carcinoma: Microvascular reconstruction vs. primary closure. *Head and Neck, 38*, 89–94. doi:10.1002/hed.23862

Chang, C.C., Kao, H.K., Huang, J.J., Tsao, C.K., Cheng, M.H., & Wei, F.C. (2013). Postoperative alcohol withdrawal syndrome and neuropsychological disorder in patients after head and neck cancer ablation followed by microsurgical free tissue transfer. *Journal of Reconstructive Microsurgery, 29*, 131–136. doi:10.1055/s-0032-1329927

Checcoli, E., Bianchini, C., Ciorba, A., Candiani, M., Riberti, C., Pelucchi, S., & Pastore, A. (2013). Reconstructive head and neck surgery: Oncological and functional results. *Tumori, 99*, 493–499. doi:10.1700/1361.15100

Choi, J.W., Lee, M.Y., & Oh, T.S. (2013). The application of multilobed flap designs for anatomic and functional oropharyngeal reconstructions. *Journal of Craniofacial Surgery, 24*, 2091–2097. doi:10.1097/SCS.0b013e3182a2442c

Cohen, E.E., Karrison, T.G., Kocherginsky, M., Mueller, J., Egan, R., Huang, C.H., ... Vokes, E.E. (2014). Phase III randomized trial of induction chemotherapy in patients with N2 or N3 locally advanced head and neck cancer. *Journal of Clinical Oncology, 32*, 2735–2743. doi:10.1200/JCO.2013.54.6309

Cuellar, C.N., Caicoya, S.J.O., Sanz, J.J.A., Cuellar, I.N., Muela, C.M., & Vila, C.N. (2014). Mandibular reconstruction with iliac crest free flap, nasolabial flap, and osseointegrated implants. *Journal of Oral and Maxillofacial Surgery, 72*(6), e1–e15. doi:10.1016/j.joms.2014.02.031

Denaro, N., Russi, E.G., Adamo, V., & Merlano, M.C. (2014). State-of-the-art and emerging treatment options in the management of head and neck cancer: News from 2013. *Oncology, 86*, 212–229. doi:10.1159/000357712

Department of Veterans Affairs Laryngeal Cancer Study Group. (1991). Induction chemotherapy plus radiation compared with surgery plus radiation in patients with advanced laryngeal cancer. *New England Journal of Medicine, 324*, 1685–1690. doi:10.1056/NEJM199106133242402

de Sousa, A.A., & Mattos, B.S. (2014). Finite element analysis of stability and functional stress with implant-supported maxillary obturator prostheses. *Journal of Prosthetic Dentistry, 112*, 1578–1584. doi:10.1016/j.prosdent.2014.06.020

Dik, E.A., Willems, S.M., Ipenburg, N.A., Adriaansens, S.O., Rosenberg, A.J., & van Es, R.J. (2014). Resection of early oral squamous cell carcinoma with positive or close margins: Relevance of adjuvant treatment in relation to local recurrence: Margins of 3 mm as safe as 5 mm. *Oral Oncology, 50*, 611–615. doi:10.1016/j.oraloncology.2014.02.014

Dubner, S. (2013). Head and neck cancer—Resection and neck dissection treatment and management. Retrieved from http://emedicine.medscape.com/article/1289474-overview#a04

Duke, W.S., Chaung, K., & Terris, D.J. (2014). Contemporary surgical techniques. *Otolaryngologic Clinics of North America, 47*, 529–544. doi:10.1016/j.otc.2014.04.002

Dziegielewski, P.T., Ho, M.L., Rieger, J., Singh, P., Langille, M., Harris, J.R., & Seikaly, H. (2013). Total glossectomy with laryngeal preservation and free flap reconstruction: Objective functional outcomes and systematic review of the literature. *Laryngoscope, 123,* 140–145. doi:10.1002/lary.23505

Eley, K.A., Watt-Smith, S.R., Boland, P., Potter, M., & Golding, S.J. (2014). MRI pre-treatment tumour volume in maxillary complex squamous cell carcinoma treated with surgical resection. *Journal of Cranio-Maxillo-Facial Surgery, 42,* 119–124. doi:10.1016/j.jcms.2013.03.006

Extermann, M., & Hurria, A. (2007). Comprehensive geriatric assessment for older patients with cancer. *Journal of Clinical Oncology, 25,* 1824–1831. doi:10.1200/JCO.2007.10.6559

Fan, S., Liang, F.Y., Chen, W.L., Yang, Z.H., Huang, X.M., Wang, Y.Y., … Li, J.S. (2014). Minimally invasive selective neck dissection: A prospective study of endoscopically assisted dissection via a small submandibular approach in $cT_{1-2}N_0$ oral squamous cell carcinoma. *Annals of Surgical Oncology, 21,* 3876–3881. doi:10.1245/s10434-014-3833-0

Fang, S.L., Wang, Y.Y., Chen, W.L., & Zhang, D.M. (2014). Use of extended vertical lower trapezius island myocutaneous flaps to cover exposed reconstructive plates. *Journal of Oral and Maxillofacial Surgery, 72,* e1–e37. doi:10.1016/j.joms.2014.06.420

Fiorini, F.R., Deganello, A., Larotonda, G., Mannelli, G., & Gallo, O. (2014). Tobacco exposure and complications in conservative laryngeal surgery. *Cancers, 6,* 1727–1735. doi:10.3390/cancers6031727

Forastiere, A.A., Ang, K.K., Brizel, D., Brockstein, B.E., Burtness, B.A., Cmelak, A.J., … Worden, F. (2008). Head and neck cancers. *Journal of the National Comprehensive Cancer Network, 6,* 646–695.

Genther, D.J., & Gourin, C.G. (2012). The effect of alcohol abuse and alcohol withdrawal on short-term outcomes and cost of care after head and neck cancer surgery. *Laryngoscope, 122,* 1739–1747. doi:10.1002/lary.23348

Gill, S.S., Frew, J., Fry, A., Adam, J., Paleri, V., Dobrowsky, W., … Kelly, C.G. (2011). Priorities for the head and neck cancer patient, their companion and members of the multidisciplinary team and decision regret. *Clinical Oncology, 23,* 518–524. doi:10.1016/j.clon.2011.03.014

Goldstein, D.P., Ringash, J., Irish, J.C., Gilbert, R., Brown, D., Xu, W., … Davis, A.M. (2015). Assessment of the Disabilities of the Arm, Shoulder and Hand (DASH) questionnaire for use in patients following neck dissection for head and neck cancer. *Head and Neck, 37,* 234–242. doi:10.1002/hed.23593

Grewal, S.S., Kurbanov, A., Anaizi, A., Keller, J.T., Theodosopoulos, P.V., & Zimmer, L.A. (2014). Endoscopic endonasal approach to the maxillary strut: Anatomical review and case series. *Laryngoscope, 124,* 1739–1743. doi:10.1002/lary.24528

Guttman, D., Mizrachi, A., Hadar, T., Bachar, G., Hamzani, Y., Marx, S., & Shvero, J. (2013). Post-laryngectomy voice rehabilitation: Comparison of primary and secondary tracheoesophageal puncture. *Israel Medical Association Journal, 15,* 497–499.

Haws, L., Jr., & Haws, B.T. (2014). Aerodigestive cancers: Laryngeal cancer. *Family Practice Essentials, 424,* 26–31.

Holliday, E.B., & Frank, S.J. (2014). Proton radiation therapy for head and neck cancer: A review of the clinical experience to date. *International Journal of Radiation Oncology, Biology, Physics, 89,* 292–302. doi:10.1016/j.ijrobp.2014.02.029

Hurria, A., Wildes, T., Blair, S.L., Browner, I.S., Cohen, H.J., Deshazo, M., … Sundar, H. (2014). Senior adult oncology, version 2.2014: Clinical practice guidelines in oncology. *Journal of the National Comprehensive Cancer Network, 12,* 82–126. Retrieved from http://www.jnccn.org/content/12/1/82.full.pdf+html

Iloreta, A.M., Anderson, K., & Miles, B.A. (2014). Mandibular osteotomy for expanded transoral robotic surgery: A novel technique. *Laryngoscope, 124,* 1836–1842. doi:10.1002/lary.24579

Jessri, M., & Farah, C.S. (2014). Harnessing massively parallel sequencing in personalized head and neck oncology. *Journal of Dental Research, 93,* 437–444. doi:10.1177/0022034514524783

Joseph, S.T., Thankappan, K., Mathew, J., Vijayamohan, M., Sharma, M., & Iyer, S. (2014). Defect components and reconstructive options in composite orbitomaxillary defects with orbital exenteration. *Journal of Oral and Maxillofacial Surgery, 72,* e1–e9. doi:10.1016/j.joms.2014.04.029

Kamisetty, A., Mayland, C.R., Jack, B., Lowe, D., & Rogers, S.N. (2014). Place and time of death in patients treated with palliative intent for oral cancer. *British Journal of Oral and Maxillofacial Surgery, 52,* 458–460. doi:10.1016/j.bjoms.2014.03.003

Korc-Grodzicki, B., Downey, R.J., Shahrokni, A., Kingham, T.P., Patel, S.G., & Audisio, R.A. (2014). Surgical considerations in older adults with cancer. *Journal of Clinical Oncology, 32,* 2647–2653. doi:10.1200/JCO.2014.55.0962

Lallemant, B., Chambon, G., Garrel, R., Kacha, S., Rupp, D., Galy-Bernadoy, C., … Pham, H.T. (2013). Transoral robotic surgery for the treatment of T1–T2 carcinoma of the larynx: Preliminary study. *Laryngoscope, 123,* 2485–2490. doi:10.1002/lary.23994

Lee, D.Y., Ryu, Y.J., Hah, J.H., Kwon, T.K., Sung, M.W., & Kim, K.H. (2014). Long-term subjective tongue function after partial glossectomy. *Journal of Oral Rehabilitation, 41,* 754–758. doi:10.1111/joor.12193

Lee, J., & Chung, W.Y. (2013). Robotic thyroidectomy and neck dissection: Past, present, and future. *Cancer Journal, 19,* 151–161. doi:10.1097/PPO.0b013e31828aab61

Li, L., Vikani, A.R., Harris, G.C., & Lin, F.R. (2014). Feasibility study to quantify the auditory and social environment of older adults using a digital language processor. *Otology and Neurotology, 35,* 1301–1305. doi:10.1097/MAO.0000000000000489

Lin, C.H., Kang, C.J., Tsao, C.K., Wallace, C.G., Lee, L.Y., Lin, C.Y., … Liao, C.T. (2014). Priority of fibular reconstruction in patients with oral cavity cancer undergoing segmental mandibulectomy. *PLOS ONE, 9,* e94315. doi:10.1371/journal.pone.0094315

Llorente, J.L., López, F., Suárez, C., & Hermsen, M.A. (2014). Sinonasal carcinoma: Clinical, pathological, genetic and therapeutic advances. *Nature Reviews Clinical Oncology, 11,* 460–472. doi:10.1038/nrclinonc.2014.97

Lu, B., Li, J., Gao, Q., Yu, W., Yang, Q., & Li, X. (2014). Laryngeal cancer risk and common single nucleotide polymorphisms in nucleotide excision repair pathway genes ERCC1, ERCC2, ERCC3, ERCC4, ERCC5 and XPA. *Gene, 542,* 64–68. doi:10.1016/j.gene.2014.02.043

Lucs, A.V., Saltman, B., Chung, C.H., Steinberg, B.M., & Schwartz, D.L. (2013). Opportunities and challenges facing biomarker development for personalized head and neck cancer treatment. *Head and Neck, 35,* 294–306. doi:10.1002/hed.21975

Mannelli, G., Meccariello, G., Deganello, A., Fiorini, F.R., Paiar, F., & Gallo, O. (2014). Subtotal supracricoid laryngectomy: Changing in indications, surgical techniques and use of new surgical devices. *American Journal of Otolaryngology, 35,* 719–726. doi:10.1016/j.amjoto.2014.07.010

Mitzner, R. (2013). Neck dissection classification. Retrieved from http://emedicine.medscape.com/article/849834-overview#a30

Moubayed, S.P., Rahal, A., & Ayad, T. (2014). The submental island flap for soft-tissue head and neck reconstruction: Step-by-step video description and long-term results. *Plastic and Reconstructive Surgery, 133,* 684–686. doi:10.1097/PRS.0000000000000058

National Comprehensive Cancer Network. (2015). *NCCN Clinical Practice Guidelines in Oncology (NCCN Guidelines®): Older adult oncology* [v.1.2015]. Retrieved from http://www.nccn.org/professionals/physician_gls/pdf/senior.pdf

Nelson, L., Burke-Smith, A., & Kirkpatrick, N. (2014). A novel approach for successful closure of sinonasal fistulae. *Journal of Plastic, Reconstructive and Aesthetic Surgery, 67,* 910–915. doi:10.1016/j.bjps.2014.03.015

Nichols, A.C., Fung, K., Chapeskie, C., Dowthwaite, S.A., Basmaji, J., Dhaliwal, S., … Yoo, J. (2013). Development of a transoral robotic surgery program in Canada. *Journal of Otolaryngology—Head and Neck Surgery, 42,* 8. doi:10.1186/1916-0216-42-8

Peacock, Z.S., Aghaloo, T., Bouloux, G.F., Cillo, J.E., Jr., Hale, R.G., Le, A.D., … Kademani, D. (2014). Proceedings from the 2013 American Association of Oral and Maxillofacial Surgeons Research Summit. *Journal of Oral and Maxillofacial Surgery, 72*, 241–253. doi:10.1016/j.joms.2013.09.037

Pellini, R., Manciocco, V., Turri-Zanoni, M., Vidiri, A., Sanguineti, G., Marucci, L., … Spriano, G. (2014). Planned neck dissection after chemoradiotherapy in advanced oropharyngeal squamous cell cancer: The role of US, MRI, and FDG-PET/TC scans to assess residual neck disease. *Journal of Cranio-Maxillo-Facial Surgery, 42*, 1834–1839. doi:10.1016/j.jcms.2014.06.023

Peng, K.A., Chu, A.C., Lai, C., Grogan, T., Elashoff, D., Abemayor, E., & St. John, M.A. (2014). Is there a role for neck dissection in T1 oral tongue squamous cell carcinoma? The UCLA experience. *American Journal of Otolaryngology, 35*, 741–746. doi:10.1016/j.amjoto.2014.06.019

Petera, J., Sirák, I., Laco, J., Kašaová, L., Tuček, L., & Doležalová, H. (2014). High-dose-rate brachytherapy in early oral cancer with close or positive margins. *Brachytherapy, 14*, 77–83. doi:10.1016/j.brachy.2014.08.050

Popescu, B., Berteşteanu, S.V.G., Grigore, R., Scăunaşu, R., & Popescu, C.R. (2012). Functional implications of radical neck dissection and the impact on the quality of life for patients with head and neck neoplasia. *Journal of Medicine and Life, 5*, 410–413.

Qian, W., Zhu, G., Wang, Y., Wang, X., Ji, Q., Wang, Y., & Dou, S. (2014). Multi-modality management for loco-regionally advanced laryngeal and hypopharyngeal cancer: Balancing the benefit of efficacy and functional preservation. *Medical Oncology, 31*, 178. doi:10.1007/s12032-014-0178-2

Rihani, J., Lee, M.R., Lee, T., & Ducic, Y. (2013). Flap selection and functional outcomes in total glossectomy with laryngeal preservation. *Otolaryngology—Head and Neck Surgery, 149*, 547–553. doi:10.1177/0194599813498063

Ringash, J., Bernstein, L., Cella, D., Logemann, J., Movsas, B., Murphy, B., … Ridge, J. (2015). Outcomes toolbox for head and neck cancer research. *Head and Neck, 37*, 425–439. doi:10.1002/hed.23561

Roland, N.J., & Bradley, P.J. (2014). The role of surgery in the palliation of head and neck cancer. *Current Opinion in Otolaryngology and Head and Neck Surgery, 22*, 101–108. doi:10.1097/MOO.0000000000000031

Ruberto, M., Alicandri-Ciufelli, M., Grammatica, A., Marchioni, D., Bergamini, G., & Presutti, L. (2014). Partial laryngectomies: When the problem is the pexy. *Acta Otorhinolaryngologica Italica, 34*, 247–252.

Santi, I., Kroll, L.E., Dietz, A., Becher, H., & Ramroth, H. (2014). Occupation and educational inequalities in laryngeal cancer: The use of a job index. *BMC Public Health, 13*, 1080. doi:10.1186/1471-2458-13-1080

Scarpa, R. (2014). Surgical care of head and neck cancers. In G.W. Davidson, J.L. Lester, & M. Routt (Eds.), *Surgical oncology nursing* (pp. 65–78). Pittsburgh, PA: Oncology Nursing Society.

Sharp, L., McDevitt, J., Carsin, A.E., Brown, C., & Comber, H. (2014). Smoking at diagnosis is an independent prognostic factor for cancer-specific survival in head and neck cancer: Findings from a large, population-based study. *Cancer Epidemiology, Biomarkers and Prevention, 23*, 2579–2590. doi:10.1158/1055-9965.EPI-14-0311

Sheikh, A., Shallwani, H., & Ghaffar, S. (2014). Postoperative shoulder function after different types of neck dissection in head and neck cancer. *Ear, Nose, and Throat, 93*, E21–E26.

Shin, Y.S., Koh, Y.W., Kim, S.H., Jeong, J.H., Ahn, S., Hong, H.J., & Choi, E.C. (2012). Radiotherapy deteriorates postoperative functional outcome after partial glossectomy with free flap reconstruction. *Journal of Oral and Maxillofacial Surgery, 70*, 216–220. doi:10.1016/j.joms.2011.04.014

Shukla-Dave, A., Lee, N.Y., Jansen, J.F.A., Thaler, H.T., Stambuk, H.E., Fury, M.G., … Koutcher, J.A. (2012). Dynamic contrast-enhanced magnetic resonance imaging as a predictor of outcome in head-and-neck squamous cell carcinoma patients with nodal metastases. *International Journal of Radiation Oncology, Biology, Physics, 82*, 1837–1844. doi:10.1016/j.ijrobp.2011.03.006

Shuman, A.G., Korc-Grodzicki, B., Shklar, V., Palmer, F., Shah, J.P., & Patel, S.G. (2013). A new care paradigm in geriatric head and neck surgical oncology. *Journal of Surgical Oncology, 108*, 187–191. doi:10.1002/jso.23370

Simmons, V.N., Litvin, E.B., Jacobsen, P.B., Patel, R.D., McCaffrey, J.C., Oliver, J.A., … Brandon, T.H. (2013). Predictors of smoking relapse in patients with thoracic cancer or head and neck cancer. *Cancer, 119*, 1420–1427. doi:10.1002/cncr.27880

Singh, A., Bhatnagar, A., Bansal, R., & Singh, B.P. (2014). Oral rehabilitation of segmental mandibulectomy patient with osseointegrated dental implant. *Contemporary Clinical Dentistry, 5*, 209–212. doi:10.4103/0976-237X.132336

Spinelli, G., Torresetti, M., Lazzeri, D., Zhang, Y.X., Arcuri, F., Agostini, T., & Grassetti, L. (2014). Microsurgical reconstruction after bisphosphonate-related osteonecrosis of the jaw: Our experience with fibula free flap. *Journal of Craniofacial Surgery, 25*, 788–792. doi:10.1097/SCS.0000000000000833

Su, S.Y., Kupferman, M.E., DeMonte, F., Levine, N.B., Raza, S.M., & Hanna, E.Y. (2014). Endoscopic resection of sinonasal cancers. *Current Oncology Reports, 16*, 369. doi:10.1007/s11912-013-0369-6

Tae, K., Ji, Y.B., Song, C.M., Jeong, J.H., Cho, S.H., & Lee, S.H. (2014). Robotic selective neck dissection by a postauricular facelift approach: Comparison with conventional neck dissection. *Otolaryngology—Head and Neck Surgery, 150*, 394–400. doi:10.1177/0194599813515431

Titze, I.R. (2014). Bi-stable vocal fold adduction: A mechanism of modal-falsetto register shifts and mixed registration. *Journal of the Acoustical Society of America, 135*, 2091–2101. doi:10.1121/1.4868355

Tomifuji, M., Araki, K., Yamashita, T., Mizokami, D., Kamide, D., Suzuki, H., … Shiotani, A. (2014). Risk factors for dysphagia after transoral videolaryngoscopic surgery for laryngeal and pharyngeal cancer. *Head and Neck*. Advance online publication. doi:10.1002/hed.23866

Tubachi, J., Jainkeri, V., Gadagi, V., & Gunari, P. (2013). Surgical incisions: Balancing surgical and cosmetic outcomes in head and neck oncosurgery. *Otorhinolaryngology Clinics: An International Journal, 5*, 47–50. doi:10.5005/jp-journals-10003-1110

Valakh, V., Miyamoto, C., Mazurenka, K., & Liu, J.C. (2014). A comparison of outcomes for oropharyngeal cancers treated with single-modality surgery versus radiotherapy. *Journal of Comparative Effectiveness Research, 3*, 387–397. doi:10.2217/cer.14.26

Verqez, S., Martin-Dupont, N., Lepage, B., DeBonecaze, G., Decotte, A., & Serrano, E. (2012). Endoscopic vs. transfacial resection of sinonasal adenocarcinoma. *Otolaryngology—Head and Neck Surgery, 146*, 848–853. doi:10.1177/0194599811434903

Vicini, C., Leone, C.A., Montevecchi, F., Dinelli, E., Seccia, V., & Dallan, I. (2014). Successful application of transoral robotic surgery in failures of traditional transoral laser microsurgery: Critical considerations. *Otorhinolaryngology, 76*, 98–104. doi:10.1159/000359953

Vishak, S., & Vinayak, R. (2014). Cervical node metastasis in T1 squamous cell carcinoma of oral tongue-pattern and the predictive factors. *Indian Journal of Surgical Oncology, 5*, 104–108. doi:10.1007/s13193-014-0301-z

Walko, C.M., & McLeod, H.L. (2014). Personalizing medicine in geriatric oncology. *Journal of Clinical Oncology, 32*, 2581–2586. doi:10.1200/JCO.2014.55.9047

Weinstein, G.S., O'Malley, B.W., Magnuson, J.S., Carroll, W.R., Olsen, K.D., Daio, L., … Holsinger, F.C. (2012). Transoral robotic surgery: A multicenter study to assess feasibility, safety, and surgical margins. *Laryngoscope, 122*, 1701–1707. doi:10.1002/lary.23294

Wildiers, H., Heeren, P., Puts, M., Topinkova, E., Janssen-Heijen, M.L., Extermann, M., … Hurria, A. (2014). International Society of Geriatric Oncology consensus on geriatric assessment in older patients with cancer. *Journal of Clinical Oncology, 32,* 2595–2603. doi:10.1200/ JCO.2013.54.8347

Xue, S., Wang, P., & Chen, G. (2013). Neck dissection with cervical sensory preservation in thyroid cancer. *Gland Surgery, 2,* 212–218. doi:10.3978/ j.issn.2227-684X.2013.10.02

Yu, Y., Wang, S., Xu, Z., & Wu, Y. (2014). Laryngeal reconstruction with a sternohyoid muscle flap after supracricoid laryngec-tomy: Postoperative respiratory and swallowing evaluation. *Oto-laryngology—Head and Neck Surgery, 151,* 824–829. doi:10.1177/ 0194599814549002

Zafereo, M.E. (2013). Evaluation and staging of squamous cell carcinoma of the oral cavity and oropharynx: Limitations despite technological breakthroughs. *Otolaryngologic Clinics of North America, 46,* 599–613. doi:10.1016/j.otc.2013.04.011

CHAPTER 7

Radiation Therapy

Dorothy N. Pierce, DNP, APN-C

Introduction

Radiation therapy (RT) is an essential component in the management of head and neck cancer. Radiation may be used as a primary treatment for small tumors (stages I and II), as adjuvant treatment for larger tumors (stages III and IV), or as a palliative measure for patients with unresectable or recurrent tumors. RT may be given as a single treatment modality or in conjunction with surgery and/or systemic cytotoxic agents, delivered neoadjuvantly or concurrently to provide better local-regional tumor control. RT alone is the most common treatment for certain types and stages of head and neck cancer, such as cancers of the nasopharynx, larynx, and oropharynx (Hoffmann, 2012; Mallick & Waldron, 2009). The principal goal of RT is to slow or stop tumor cell replication while minimizing toxic effects to the surrounding normal tissues (Proud, 2014; Radvansky, Pace, & Siddiqui, 2013; Rosenstein, 2009). RT can also be given to achieve cure. In cases where cure is not possible, RT is used to control the progression of disease (Stoker et al., 2013). RT is a good option for palliative relief of pain caused by bone metastasis, obstruction caused by tumor progression, or uncontrolled bleeding resulting from tumor invasion of the vascular system.

Advances in technology combined with the effects of radiobiology have led to refined treatment approaches; however, these treatments can result in both acute and late toxicity. Patients with head and neck cancer need to receive treatment from a multidisciplinary team skilled in the provision of treatment recommendations and support services (Mallick & Waldron, 2009; Mason, DeRubeis, Foster, Taylor, & Worden, 2013).

Principles of Treatment

RT is the use of ionizing radiation (electromagnetic energy) with very short wavelengths and very high-energy intensity.

Radiation is either electromagnetic or particulate and causes ionization within the cell (Ma, 2012). Ionizing radiation has sufficient energy to eject one or more orbiting electrons from an atom, changing a stable atom to an ionized or unstable atom. Ionizing radiation interacts with tissues to create physical, chemical, and biologic changes (Khan, 2010; Proud, 2014). These biologic changes occur at the cellular level, where cell damage is both direct and indirect. Direct effects are a result of damage to critical molecules, such as DNA. When the DNA is damaged, cell death or mutation may occur. Indirectly, radiation affects the water molecules surrounding the cell, resulting in biologic damage. Cell death takes place during the mitotic phase of the cell cycle, and the damaged cell is no longer able to reproduce (Altinok, Gonze, Lévi, & Goldbeter, 2011).

Radiobiology

Radiobiology investigates the effects of ionizing radiation on living organisms. Radiobiology has four cardinal concepts: repair, repopulation, redistribution, and reoxygenation. Recent research in this area of study has identified a fifth concept, radiosensitivity (Brown, Carlson, & Brenner, 2013). Repair is the ability of normal and malignant tissue to repair damage within 4–24 hours after radiation. As treatment progresses, tumor cells become less capable of repair. Repopulation or regeneration of healthy cells continues after repair of sublethal injury, allowing mitosis to take place. Malignant cells are more likely to die during mitosis. Redistribution of tumor cells in these cycles enhances the effectiveness of each succeeding radiation dose because more cells are likely to be in mitosis at the same time and healthy cells are less likely to redistribute (Brown et al., 2013; Mitchell, 2013). Reoxygenation occurs when well-oxygenated tumor cells die between daily doses, creating an environment in which previously hypoxic cells are exposed to capillary oxygenation. This reoxygenation effectively increases the success of the radiation treatments by increasing cell kill during subsequent doses.

Emerging data show that the responsiveness of tumors to RT relates mutually with the intrinsic radiosensitivity of tumors. Radiosensitivity is the sensitivity of cells, tissues, or tumors to radiation (Brown et al., 2013). The effects of ionizing radiation on intracellular DNA, leading to cellular damage, influence radiosensitivity; the cell will die if double-strand breaks are not repaired (Fukumoto, 2014; Proud, 2014).

Fractionation

A radiation oncologist prescribes a total dose of ionized radiation to the tumor site via external beam. This total dose is divided into smaller daily doses called *fractions*. Fractionation allows for reoxygenation of tumor cells as they become exposed to improved circulation, enhancing their radiosensitivity (Brown et al., 2013). The dose of radiation is expressed in units of gray (Gy), centigray (cGy), and radiation-absorbed dose (rad) (1 Gy = 100 cGy = 100 rad). In general, 44–50 Gy of radiation, delivered in increments of 1.8–2 Gy per fraction, is administered to regions that have a risk of 15% or more of harboring microscopic disease (Khan, 2010; Ma, 2012). Typically, 66–70 Gy is prescribed for primary tumors measuring 2 cm or less. A patient with advanced disease may receive RT as primary treatment. Doses of 70 Gy or more are necessary in these cases to control the primary tumor and involved lymph nodes (Harris, 2012). The goal of fractionation is to deliver a dose of radiation sufficient to kill the tumor while allowing the nearby healthy tissue time to repair. A standard fractionation schedule is given five days a week for six to eight weeks of therapy.

Altered Fractionation

Until recently, locoregional control in advanced head and neck cancer was suboptimal when RT as a primary treatment modality was administered on a once-daily schedule. Improvements in treatment outcomes have been reported by using altered fractionation RT schedules and/or concurrent adjuvant chemotherapy for individuals with locoregional advanced stage III–IV disease (Beitler et al., 2014). The intent of altered fractionation is to improve cure rates, decrease late complications, and improve locoregional control. Conventional fractionation occurs in a continuous course of one fraction per day, five days a week, for six to eight weeks. A typical dose fractionation schedule includes 2 Gy versus 1.6 Gy per fraction for eight weeks. For radiobiologic reasons, altered fractionation schedules in which two or three doses of radiation are delivered daily (at least six hours apart to minimize toxicity) have been studied in the treatment of advanced head and neck cancers (Mendenhall, Riggs, Vaysberg, Amdur, & Werning, 2010). Altered fractionation schedules can be analyzed as *hyperfractionated* or *accelerated*. *Hyperfractionation* refers to RT delivered twice daily. Accelerated fractionation integrates the same total

dose, number of fractions, and dose per fraction given over a shorter overall treatment time of four to six weeks (e.g., 66 Gy in 33 twice-daily fractions over three weeks as compared to 66 Gy in 33 once-daily fractions over 6.5 weeks).

Accelerated fractionation uses a total dose and fraction size similar to conventional treatment but achieves a shorter overall treatment time by giving two to three doses daily. Accelerated hyperfractionation incorporates features of both accelerated fractionation and hyperfractionation. This miscegenation regimen has been studied as a way of increasing tumor kill without increasing the risk of late complications (Mendenhall et al., 2010). Concomitant boost technique is a regimen that delivers hyperfractionation (81.6 Gy at 1.2 Gy twice daily over seven weeks). Accelerated split-course RT delivers 67.2 Gy at 1.6 Gy twice daily over six weeks. Accelerated concomitant boost RT delivers 72 Gy at 1.8–1.5 Gy per fraction given over six weeks, with RT given twice daily over the last 12 treatment days (Mendenhall et al., 2010). Hyperfractionation makes use of an increased number of fractions and total dose, a lower dose per fraction, and the same overall treatment time. For example, Mendenhall et al. (2010) noted that patients were randomized to hyperfractionation schedules to receive 81.6 Gy at 1.2 Gy twice daily over seven weeks compared with conventional RT (70 Gy in 35 once-daily fractions over seven weeks).

A concluding approach to the treatment plan is hypofractionation, which is most commonly defined as administration of fewer than five fractionations per week. This program can deliver higher doses of treatment (e.g., 40 Gy in 10 fractions [equivalent dose: 49.8 Gy in conventional fractionation], with two fractions per week on Mondays and Thursdays only). Hypofractionation has been used to give RT to the head and neck region for surgically unresectable stage IVb head and neck cancer (extension to the infratemporal fossa, carotid space invasion, prevertebral fascia invasion, and fixed-fungating nodal mass) (Das, Thomas, Pal, Isiah, & John, 2013).

Chemotherapy

A number of antineoplastic agents appear to have radiosensitizing properties. The term *radiosensitizer* refers to compounds that enhance the damaging effects of ionizing radiation. Concurrent treatment to include platinum-based chemotherapy combined with RT is an accepted standard for definitive therapy for locally advanced unresectable head and neck carcinomas. Based on the findings of van der Linden et al. (2015), the standard of care for locally advanced squamous cell carcinoma of the head and neck is RT with concurrent platinum-based chemotherapy plus cetuximab, a monoclonal antibody that inhibits the epidermal growth factor receptors. Komatsu et al. (2014) reported results of a retrospective study that showed excellent survival and organ preservation rates for the patients with locally advanced squamous cell carcinoma of the head and neck who were treated with concurrent chemo-radiation therapy with docetaxel, cisplatin, and 5-fluorouracil. The acute toxicities of chemotherapy with RT can be much more severe than either therapy alone.

Radiation Therapy Delivery Techniques

External Beam

External beam RT (EBRT), or teletherapy, is the delivery of local treatment by a linear accelerator. The linear accelerator can deliver treatment by high-energy x-rays (photons), gamma rays, or electrons. High-energy x-ray beams can penetrate intermediate to deep tissue depths, depending on the energy level used. Electron beam therapy delivers a shallow treatment and spares deeper tissues. Photon and electron beams often are used together to treat head and neck cancers. The high-energy x-rays are the primary treatment, and the electrons boost (i.e., give extra radiation dose) superficial tissues at the tumor site (Ang & Garden, 2012).

Traditional radiation planning is performed in two dimensions. An external contour of the patient's treatment area is traced on paper and digitized into a computer. X-ray films are taken of the area to be treated, and the radiation oncologist draws the anatomy on the film. These data are then combined to determine the treatment plan (Ma, 2012).

Three-Dimensional Conformal

Three-dimensional conformal RT (3DCRT), which began in the late 1980s and early 1990s, provides precise delivery of the radiation dose by using three-dimensional diagnostic images and computerized treatment programs to target the tumor from several angles (Spiotto & Weichselbaum, 2014). 3DCRT has increased the accuracy of treatments; therefore, higher doses can be delivered to tumors with less damage to critical normal tissues (Spiotto & Weichselbaum, 2014). Both traditional RT and 3DCRT use custom-molded Wood's metal or lead blocks to shape the radiation beam. A different block is used for each treatment angle. These blocks are mounted on the linear accelerator by hand, which is a slow and labor-intensive process (Ang & Garden, 2012). A collimator can hold up to 120 individually controlled leaves housed inside a linear accelerator (Ang & Garden, 2012; Khan, 2010). A multileaf collimator is a computer-controlled treatment shaping system that is programmed to shape the radiation beam to an individual's treatment field automatically. This process allows 3DCRT to be given accurately and quickly.

Intensity Modulated

Intensity-modulated RT (IMRT) is considered the gold standard in the latest technologic advances in EBRT. IMRT can deliver radiation more conformally than 3DCRT. IMRT differs from 3DCRT in that each x-ray beam is broken up into many "beamlets," and the intensity of each beamlet can be adjusted individually (Khan, 2010; Ma, 2012). The adjustable leaves of the multileaf collimator control not only the shape of the beam, but also the exposure duration for each segment of the tumor, effectively modulating the dose within the treatment volume (Ang & Garden, 2012). IMRT especially is useful in treating tumors of the nasal cavity, ethmoid and sphenoid sinuses, and skull base, where the risks of optic neuropathy and retinopathy following conventional RT are high (Ang & Garden, 2012; Ma, 2012). IMRT is used in all head and neck sites to minimize xerostomia and improve side effects. It has been shown to be better than 3DCRT in improving side effects (Duarte et al., 2014). Stereotactic radiosurgery provides the precise delivery of a single large dose of radiation to a target that typically measures less than 3.5 cm in diameter. This therapy has been used to treat tumors of the base of the skull and nasopharynx (Allen, 2012).

Intraoperative

Intraoperative RT (IORT) provides a single large dose of electron beam radiation to the tumor bed during surgery while sparing healthy tissue. IORT has been investigated and is frequently combined with EBRT to provide the best combination of local and locoregional treatment. IORT has been used to treat head and neck cancers, applying both intraoperative electron RT and high-dose-rate RT. Side effects and complications from IORT in the head and neck population include carotid artery blowout, osteoradionecrosis of bones in the portal field, neuropathy, edema, and wound-healing complications (Debenham, Hu, & Harrison, 2013).

Radiogenomics

Radiogenomics is the study of the genetic link and the clinical variability observed in individual response to RT (Proud, 2014; Rosenstein et al., 2014). Researchers are investigating the genetic marker single-nucleotide polymorphisms (SNPs), a DNA sequence variation in which one of the nucleotides (i.e., adenine, cytosine, guanine, thymine) is altered. According to Proud (2014), the completion of the Human Genome Project in 2003 paved the way for genome studies that look at how SNPs influence radiation toxicity. SNPs may help predict radiation responses as well as the severity of radiation side effects, allowing clinicians and patients to make the best treatment decisions individually. This may lead to personalized treatment in radiation oncology in the future. The effects of ionizing radiation on intracellular DNA cells will lead to cellular damage or death. Radiation also triggers the release of various cytokines, proteins that are involved with the cell regulation and immune system. Approximately 5%–10% of patients who receive RT exhibit a heightened sensitivity to conventional radiation doses (Proud, 2014). Patients receiving RT are at higher risk of developing radiation-induced inflammation and subsequent fibrosis. Figure 7-1 lists the clinical toxicities related to head and neck radiation-induced inflammation and fibrosis. Multiple variants of the *XRCC2*, *XRCC3*, and *RAD-5* genes were identified in patients with head and neck cancer who were treated with RT; the genes have been associated with mucositis, dermatitis, and dysphagia (Minicucci, da Silva, & Salvadori, 2014; Proud, 2014). Proud (2014) suggested that researchers have discovered other genetic mutations that increase radiation toxicity (e.g., Nijmegen breakage syndrome, Fanconi anemia). These disorders show a generalized sensitivity to all forms of radiation (e.g., environmental, diagnostic, cosmic). For now, genome studies have identified several SNPs that might cause radiation toxicity. Current research has shown conflicting data; therefore, radiogenomic research is warranted to accurately determine treatment-related toxicity in patients with cancer (Proud, 2014).

Neutron and Proton Beam

Neutron and proton (particle) beam RTs have been used since the 1950s. In the past few years, an increasing interest in this form of treatment has greatly affected both the number of patients and the variety of tumors being treated with proton therapy. Proton beam therapy is a modality of EBRT in which a particle accelerator is used to create a focused beam of protons that can be used therapeutically. Like EBRT with photons, proton therapy acts by damaging the DNA of cells. Proton therapy is useful for treating

---

Figure 7-1. Acute Toxicities by System Attributed to Radiation-Induced Inflammation and Fibrosis

Head and Neck
- Dysphagia
- Loss of taste
- Mucositis
- Voice changes
- Xerostomia

Skin
- Altered cosmesis
- Decreased elasticity
- Dermatitis
- Desquamation
- Edema
- Erythema
- Retraction
- Telangiectasia
- Thickening

Note. Based on information from Proud, 2014.

---

head and neck cancers near the spinal cord, at the base of the skull, and in the paranasal sinus region. Proton therapy can spare surrounding healthy tissues from unintended irradiation. Multiple researchers are investigating the potential use of proton therapy for tumors of the head and neck to collect data on efficacy, toxicity, and quality of life (Holliday & Frank, 2014). Randomized controlled trials are being done that directly compare proton therapy to the better-established IMRT treatment modality. According to Holliday and Frank (2014), phase II and III randomized trials are currently accruing at the University of Texas MD Anderson Cancer Center for patients with oropharyngeal cancer. Its findings should provide valuable insight into the potential benefits and liabilities for both modalities.

Brachytherapy

Brachytherapy is the temporary or permanent placement of a radioactive source either on or within the tumor. Brachytherapy is also called *internal radiation* or *implant therapy*. This therapy offers the advantage of delivering a high dose of radiation to a specific tumor volume with a rapid falloff in dose to adjacent normal tissues (Ang & Garden, 2012). Brachytherapy can be classified as low dose rate (LDR) (4–20 Gy/hr), medium dose rate (20–120 Gy/hr), or high dose rate (HDR) (doses greater than 120 Gy/hr) (Rudžianskas et al., 2012).

Brachytherapy is used in the treatment of head and neck malignancies. The radiation oncologist and head and neck surgeon work together in the operating room to place hollow brachytherapy catheters directly into the tumor. One or two days following surgery, the patient is taken to the radiation oncology department for loading of the catheters with iridium-192 radioactive seeds (Khan, 2010; Wiegand et al., 2013). The treatment area then is x-rayed to verify the placement of the seeds. The patient returns to the inpatient room. The radiation oncologist and medical physicist determine the dosage and time needed to treat the cancer safely and adequately by placing nonradioactive seed sources into the catheters. A process similar to the simulation is conducted to determine dosage and time of treatment. After treatment is completed, the catheters and seeds are removed. Brachytherapy also may be given in combination with EBRT using LDR and/or HDR. An average LDR brachytherapy treatment varies from 48–66 Gy with a median treatment duration of 87 hours. HDR brachytherapy treatment is usually performed using nine fractions with 4 Gy, delivering 36 Gy in five days and occasionally two fractions delivered per day. Minimal time interval between fractions is six hours (Ghadjar et al., 2012). Brachytherapy techniques usually are temporary interstitial or intracavitary implants, but permanent interstitial implants also have been used for treatment of tumor extending into the base of the skull (Rudžianskas et al., 2012).

Radiation Therapy Process

Consultation

The primary care provider, medical oncologist, or surgeon refers the patient with head and neck cancer to a radiation facility. The radiation oncologist or another member of the team performs an in-depth history and physical examination. Previous staging workup, including pathology and surgical reports, along with studies (i.e., computed tomography [CT], magnetic resonance imaging, and positron-emission tomography) are reviewed. Additional studies may be needed to complete the process. The patient is counseled regarding the goals of RT and expected acute and chronic treatment side effects and consent is obtained. When salivary glands and tissue are part of the radiation field, loss of saliva causes xerostomia, or dry mouth, and results in the development of dental caries following treatment. Dental care and oral health are essential components of the treatment planning process. Patients with head and neck cancer need to undergo a pretreatment prophylactic dental evaluation. Dental work, such as extractions, fillings, or gum surgery, must be done prior to RT. Patients are instructed in the use of custom-made fluoride trays molded for daily dental prophylaxis (Ang & Garden, 2012; Lambertz et al., 2010).

Prior to starting RT, patients who have concurrent chemotherapy often will have a venous access device placed to allow for reliable IV access for chemotherapy. Because acute dysphagia makes it difficult to get the necessary caloric intake by mouth during treatment, patients receiving RT to the head and neck may require a gastrostomy tube for nutritional support. Ideally, the gastrostomy tube should be placed prior to starting treatment to allow the insertion site time to heal so that the patient may lie flat during treatment without discomfort (Lambertz et al., 2010).

Simulation: Treatment Planning

Simulation is the planning session that enables the radiation oncologist to simulate a patient's treatment prior to starting actual therapy. The simulation process uses CT scan, fluoroscopy, or radiographs to establish a target volume and parameters for treatment delivery on digitally reconstructed images. The simulation process can take several hours to complete. During this time, the patient is positioned lying on an x-ray table with an immobilization device in place. The nurse may start an IV line to administer a contrast agent or x-ray dye while scanning (Tantiwongkosi, Yu, Kanard, & Miller, 2014). The contrast allows the radiation oncologist to assess the tumor as well as the lymph nodes of the area being treated (Ang & Garden, 2012). The immobilization device (see Figure 7-2) typically is a soft, thermoplastic mesh mask that is placed over the patient's face and molded to adhere firmly.

Figure 7-2. Head and Neck Immobilization Device

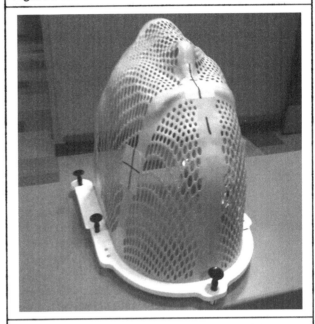

Note. Image courtesy of Dorothy N. Pierce. Used with permission.

The patient can see and breathe normally through holes in the plastic mask. Some patients may experience increased anxiety related to the immobilization mask and may require medication prior to simulation. A custom-made bite block to maintain head position may be placed in the patient's mouth. Depending on the treatment area, the patient's shoulders also may be immobilized and pulled away from the treatment field by using handles similar to jump rope handles. These handles connect to the board at the patient's feet. Pressure from the patient's feet helps to hold tension on the ropes, thus pulling the shoulders down and out of the field. Tracheal and oral suctioning should be done before immobilization and during simulation as needed. Tattoos are placed under the skin via pinpricks with black ink; this procedure permanently records the radiation field. Tattoos also may be placed on the neck and supraclavicular region. To avoid placing tattoos on the patient's face, marks are made directly on the mask using a permanent felt marker to note treatment areas (Ang & Garden, 2012).

Templates of blocking, defining the treatment areas, and shielding of normal structures are drawn on the simulation x-ray planning films. CT simulation allows the physician to outline the tumor area and identify normal structures on each CT slice. Following simulation, the medical physicist and dosimetrist determine an optimal dose distribution to the area. The radiation oncologist reviews and approves various generated treatment areas identified on the scan and prescribes the fractionation schedule, dose, and treatment type (IMRT, 3DCRT, or traditional two-dimensional fields) (Ang & Garden, 2012).

Treatment

RT is delivered using a team approach (Vichare et al., 2013). Each RT team member (see Figure 7-3) plays an important role in a patient's care. Prior to starting RT, the patient must have treatment verification films accepted and approved by the radiation oncologist. This process ensures that the prescribed treatment area is correct and that vital, nonmalignant tissue is spared from toxic doses of radiation. Often, minor improvements are made to the treatment plan at this time, and the process can take 30–60 minutes. The first treatment is given after the verification has been approved and completed. Daily treatment times range from 10–20 minutes, depending on the number of treatment areas. Patients will undergo treatment Monday through Friday, five days a week, until the prescribed dose is reached. Port verification films are taken weekly for quality assurance to document the accuracy of the radiation treatment. The radiation oncologist sees patients once a week and as necessary for assessment of tumor response and severity of side effects. The nurse provides regular monitoring of treatment effects and nutritional stability and provides recommendations and referrals to pain management or a registered dietitian for symptom control during treatment. Most radiation side effects are site specific and usually develop during the third week of treatment, lasting several weeks after treatment completion. The nursing staff and radiation oncologist advise patients, family members, and other support personnel about side effects from treatment. They continue to monitor the severity and will intervene by prescribing medications to help minimize or relieve the symptoms, along with determining the need to withhold treatment.

Follow-Up Care

After the prescribed radiation treatments have been completed, patients will enter the next phase, surveillance follow-up care. It is during follow-up care that patients are monitored for resolution of acute side effects and surveillance of chronic side effects. The radiation oncologist monitors the frequency of follow-up visits, which may occur as often as weekly or extended to months between visits. The frequency of follow-up visits is dependent on resolution of toxic side effects and response to treatment. In addition, close follow-up with the multidisciplinary team is essential for optimum outcomes. A multidisciplinary team is a group of healthcare clinicians from different disciplines who each provide specific services to patients with the aim of ensuring that they receive optimum care and support (El Saghir, Keating, Carlson, Khoury, & Fallowfield, 2014; Naugler, Alsina, Frenette, Rossaro, & Sellers, 2015). The team may include a speech-language pathologist, dietitian, nurse, surgeon, oncologist, physiotherapist, and social worker. This multidisciplinary team has the potential to improve quality of life and clinical outcomes as well as increase survival for patients with cancer (Thewes, Butow, Davis, Turner, & Mason, 2014).

Side Effects

Side effects of RT are divided into three groups: acute, subacute, and chronic. Acute side effects occur during treatment or up to two weeks after treatment and are caused by edema and inflammation in the normal tissues. The side effects occur in most rapidly dividing cells, such as mucosal surfaces, gastrointestinal cells, hair follicles, bone marrow, and the urinary bladder. Subacute side effects occur within three weeks to three months after treatment completion and are in the more slowly dividing cells of the liver, bone, and endocrine tissues. Chronic side effects occur between four months and two years after RT. They occur in the most slowly dividing cells of the nerve, cartilage, and muscle tissue (Servagi-Vervat et al., 2014). Figure 7-4 lists specific side effects of RT to the head and neck area, which vary according to treatment fields. Each of these side effects will be examined at length along with the appropriate nursing care and patient education needed to care for a patient receiving RT to the head and neck.

Patient Education

The Oncology Nursing Society's (ONS's) *Standards of Oncology Education: Patient/Significant Other and Public* (Blecher, Ireland, & Watson, 2016) described education as integral segments of in-depth nursing care for patients, significant others, and the public experiencing cancer. Patient education is designed to increase knowledge, improve attitudes and behaviors, and promote coping (Sobecki-Ryniak & Krouse, 2013). Patients need information about their treatment, general emotional support, and practical help with side

---

Figure 7-3. Radiation Therapy Team

- Managers/administrators
- Medical dosimetrists
- Medical physicist
- Medical secretaries
- Nurse practitioners or physician assistants
- Primary radiation oncology nurse
- Radiation oncologist
- Radiation technologist/therapist
- Residents
- Treatment assistant staff

Figure 7-4. Side Effects of Treatment

Acute Side Effects
• Dysphagia, odynophagia
• Esophagitis, pharyngitis
• Fatigue, depression
• Mucositis, oral infection, oral pain
• Nasal dryness
• Pain
• Taste alterations, nutritional changes
• Xerostomia, secretion changes

Chronic Side Effects
• Dental caries, osteoradionecrosis
• Laryngeal edema
• Ocular and otologic changes
• Radiation dermatitis, alopecia
• Spinal cord injury
• Thyroid dysfunction
• Tissue fibrosis
• Xerostomia

effects of treatment. The information should include presentation, prevalence, and duration of side effects to reduce anxiety and enhance self-care (O'Gorman, Sasiadek, Denieffe, & Gooney, 2014). Patients receiving RT need ongoing education throughout their course of treatment. The nurse, radiation oncologist, or radiation therapist may initiate teaching and must discuss signs and symptoms, as well as duration and management of treatment side effects. Multidisciplinary patient and family education is an important aspect of patient care because RT is a frightening concept for the public to grasp. Most information regarding radiation is thought to be negative, and turning these thoughts into a positive experience is challenging for the RT team.

Teaching may be performed in a group setting or one-on-one using a variety of resources, such as verbal and written information, video, or demonstration (Lambertz et al., 2010). Patient pathways about the RT experience are useful for educating patients with head and neck cancer. A patient pathway is a written patient education tool that maps or charts the expected course of treatment from the pretreatment phase through the recovery period (Kinsman, Rotter, James, Snow, & Willis, 2010). Communication for patients with head and neck cancer often is impaired by tumor invasion or anatomic changes resulting from surgery. Patients may be in the early stages of speech therapy and unable to speak clearly. In these situations, patience and consideration need to be implemented (Lambertz et al., 2010). Staff should encourage patients to write their questions and concerns and provide adequate time for them to do so. Family members often are useful as interpreters for patients with impaired communication. Patients and families must be assessed for their level of understanding of the education being delivered. Reinforcement of teaching must be offered throughout therapy.

Symptom Management

RT to the head and neck results in both acute and chronic side effects. Nursing interventions are aimed at symptom management and patient education.

Mucositis, Oral Infection, and Oral Pain

Mucositis is inflammation of the mucous membrane. Stomatitis refers specifically to inflamed erosive or ulcerative lesions of the oral cavity (Lalla, Saunders, & Peterson, 2014). See Figure 7-5 for the National Cancer Institute Cancer Therapy Evaluation Program (NCI CTEP) mucositis toxicity criteria. Mucositis typically occurs during the first two weeks of RT because of epithelial cells' impaired ability to replicate and replenish (Macann et al., 2014). An abundance of papers have been published in the medical literature documenting the clinical investigations aimed at the prevention, palliation, or reduction of RT-induced oral mucositis in patients with head and neck cancer. The most effective measure to treat RT-induced mucositis is frequent oral rinsing with a bland mouthwash, such as saline or sodium bicarbonate rinse, to reduce the amount of microbial flora (Gu et al., 2014). Patients with severe stomatitis should not use hydrogen peroxide rinses because new tissue is easily broken down by hydrogen peroxide. Cryotherapy and keratinocyte growth factor (palifermin) have been recommended for adult and pediatric patients with head and neck cancer who receive radiation or chemotherapy to prevent oral mucositis (Lalla et al., 2014; Lang, 2013).

Infection of the oral mucosa is often seen in patients receiving head and neck RT. Oral infections may be caused by bacteria (e.g., *Pseudomonas*, *Klebsiella*, *Staphylococcus*, *Streptococcus*) or fungus (e.g., *Candida*). Culture and sensitivity studies are necessary to treat bacterial infections appropriately. Fungal infections usually present as a burning sensation of the tongue and mucous membranes and the appearance of small, white "cottage cheese–like" patches in the oral cavity. Antifungal therapy may be necessary throughout RT (Bensadoun, Patton, Lalla, & Epstein, 2011; Deng et al., 2010).

Figure 7-5. Grading of Mucositis Caused by Radiation

0—None
1—Erythema of the mucosa
2—Patchy pseudomembranous reaction (noncontiguous patches usually < 1.5 cm in diameter)
3—Confluent pseudomembranous reaction (contiguous patches generally > 1.5 cm in diameter)
4—Necrosis or deep ulceration; may include bleeding not induced by minor trauma or abrasion

Note. Based on information from Bensinger et al., 2008; National Cancer Institute Cancer Therapy Evaluation Program, 2010.

Oral pain from mucositis or oral infection must be treated promptly and effectively. Topical oral rinses may coat or numb areas of discomfort temporarily. Nonsteroidal anti-inflammatory drugs or narcotics may be indicated for moderate to severe pain. Liquid, intranasal, or transdermal routes of administration may be a better alternative to pills for patients with head and neck cancer. See Figure 7-6 for nursing interventions useful for patients with mucositis.

Bell and Butler (2013) highlighted five case reports in which patients receiving RT were treated with fentanyl pectin nasal spray (FPNS) for predictable breakthrough pain in cancer (BTPc). The authors noted that BTPc might be associated with RT processes, such as mucositis-associated pain and dysphagia. The authors noted that in a radiation oncology department survey, more than half of the patients who were treated experienced pain. Of these patients, 39% indicated that their pain was inadequately treated, which could affect their ability to complete their treatment.

Bell and Butler (2013) noted that in RT, more than half of the patients treated experienced pain, and 39% indicated that their pain was inadequately treated, which could affect their ability to complete their treatment.

Dysphagia, Odynophagia, and Esophagitis

Dysphagia is defined as the inability to swallow or difficulty swallowing, odynophagia is painful swallowing, and esophagitis is inflammation of the esophagus (Brockbank, Miller, Owen, & Patterson, 2014). The severity of dysphagia depends on many factors, including fraction size and sched-

> **Figure 7-6. Nursing Interventions for Mucositis**
>
> - Encourage frequent mouth care, every 2–4 hours, especially after meals and at bedtime.
> - Provide frequent nonalcohol mouth rinses with salt water or sodium bicarbonate solution.
> - Recommend avoiding commercial mouth care products and lemon/glycerine swabs.
> - Recommend avoiding irritating substances such as cigarettes, alcohol, and spicy or acidic foods.
> - Recommend a soft toothbrush or foam swabs for oral care.
> - Instruct the patient to remove dentures between meals and at bedtime.
> - Treat dentures with antifungal prescription medication if a fungal infection is present.
> - Encourage the completion of antifungal or antibiotic therapy as prescribed.
> - Recommend eating foods that are cold or room temperature; hot foods may be more irritating.
> - Encourage the use of topical/systemic measures prescribed to ease pain.
> - Assess the patient's pain level as often as necessary to maintain comfort.
> - Assess oral mucosa weekly and as needed for infection.
> - Educate the patient to perform oral inspection daily and to report changes immediately.

ule, treatment delivery techniques, target volumes, total radiation dose, and concurrent chemoradiotherapy (Balusik, 2014). These acute side effects may occur when a patient is receiving radiation to the throat and upper chest, usually starting within two weeks of treatment and subsiding two or more weeks after treatment completion. See Figure 7-7 for the most appropriate nursing interventions.

> **Figure 7-7. Nursing Interventions for Dysphagia, Odynophagia, and Esophagitis**
>
> - Suggest that the patient consume soft, moist foods that have minimal irritation to the esophagus.
> - Suggest that the patient avoid hot or cold extremes in temperature; room-temperature foods may be more soothing.
> - Provide straws for drinks and a cup or glass instead of a bowl and spoon for soups.
> - Encourage topical/systemic pain medication prior to meals.
> - Weigh the patient at least once weekly.

Taste Alterations and Nutritional Changes

Dysgeusia is the perversion of the gustatory sense where ordinary tastes are interpreted as unpleasant or different from the characteristic taste of a particular food or chemical compound. Ageusia is the absence, partial loss, or impairment of the sense of taste (Lambertz et al., 2010). Prolonged alteration in taste sensation is an anticipated and unpleasant side effect of head and neck RT. Taste alterations may appear subtle and more pronounced as treatment continues. Taste alterations may take six or more months to return to normal. Some patients report permanent taste alterations (Baharvand, ShoalehSaadi, Barakian, & Moghaddam, 2013; Hovan et al., 2010). Patients with head and neck cancer who are treated with various modalities are at high risk for nutritional changes to occur for multiple reasons, such as taste alterations, anorexia, mucositis, and fatigue. It is important to educate patients and families on the importance of good nutrition during RT. See Figure 7-8 for nursing interventions for nutrition.

Xerostomia and Secretion Changes

Xerostomia is dryness of the mouth caused by a reduction in produced saliva. Xerostomia occurs when the salivary glands (parotid, submandibular, and sublingual) receive significant exposure in the radiation treatment field. Patients may experience xerostomia during the first week of treatment, and it is thought to be permanent once the RT exceeds 40–50 Gy (Koukourakis et al., 2009). Xerostomia is both an acute and a chronic side effect of RT. As an acute side effect, the patient's saliva may become thick, ropy, and tenacious. Salivary fibrosis leads to the chronic state of xerostomia. Xerostomia may result in tenderness; burning and pain in the oral cavity; difficulty wearing dentures; and difficulty eating, speaking, and sleeping. These side effects significantly affect patients' quality of life and affect up to 90% of patients undergoing RT (Beech, Robinson, Porceddu, & Batstone, 2014). Figure 7-9 lists nursing interventions for patients with xerostomia.

Two medications have been developed to reduce the chronic side effects of radiation-induced xerostomia. Oral pilocarpine is a sialogogic agent and salivary stimulant that can be used during and after RT. If effective, pilocarpine can be taken daily for the patient's lifetime. The U.S. Food and Drug Administration (FDA) has approved pilocarpine for radiation-induced salivary hypofunction

---

Figure 7-8. Nursing Interventions for Improved Nutrition

- Encourage small, frequent meals (five to six per day).
- Choose and prepare foods that look and smell good.
- Marinate meat, chicken, or fish with mild seasoning or sweet fruit juice.
- Use bacon, ham, or onion to flavor bland foods.
- Instruct the patient to rinse his or her mouth with baking soda solution prior to meals to moisten mucosa and stimulate taste buds.
- Recommend high-calorie liquids or nutritional supplements.
- Instruct the patient on ways to increase the calorie content of food.
- Suggest eating foods at room temperature, which may be more palatable.
- Recommend the use of plastic utensils and plates to decrease metallic taste.
- Encourage the patient to eat with others or while watching TV.
- Weigh the patient frequently.
- Consult with a dietitian as needed.

Figure 7-9. Nursing Interventions for Xerostomia

- Confirm that a dental evaluation has been done prior to therapy.
- Encourage the patient to follow the mouth care regimen provided by his or her dentist.
- Suggest the patient moisten his or her mouth frequently with water, artificial saliva, or sugar-free liquids.
- Suggest frequent oral rinses with salt water and/or sodium bicarbonate solution.
- Suggest the use of a humidifier to decrease mucosal dryness.
- Order home suction equipment as needed.
- Increase the patient's intake of fluids to at least 8–10 glasses a day.
- Encourage the use of the oral rinse Biotène®, a product that relieves dry mouth symptoms.
- Suggest foods with sauces, gravies, and salad dressing to make them moist and easier to swallow.
- Encourage the use of lip balm to relieve lip dryness (do not use petroleum jelly–based products while receiving radiation).
- Suggest the use of sugar-free candy or gum to moisten the mouth.

(Kałużny, Wierzbicka, Nogala, Milecki, & Kopeć, 2014; Lovelace, Fox, Sood, Nguyen, & Day, 2014). Pilocarpine tablets are prescribed at an initial dose of 5 mg three times daily. Depending on therapeutic response, the dose can be adjusted up to 30 mg per day. The most common side effect of pilocarpine is sweating. Additionally, chills, flushing, headache, rhinitis, frequent urination, diarrhea, dyspepsia, nausea, and dizziness may occur. The authors stated that the pilocarpine is a muscarinic agonist; its use is contraindicated in individuals with asthma, acute iritis, glaucoma, and cardiovascular or pulmonary conditions (Lovelace et al., 2014). Amifostine is a cytoprotectant that selectively protects normal tissues from the effects of chemotherapy and radiation. Amifostine accumulates in many epithelial tissues with the highest concentrations found in the salivary glands and kidneys (Gu et al., 2014). FDA has approved amifostine for use in patients who are undergoing postoperative radiation for head and neck cancer when the radiation port includes a substantial portion of the parotid gland (Gu et al., 2014). Although amifostine is well tolerated, nausea, vomiting, and hypotension are the most commonly reported side effects (Gu et al., 2014). Antiemetics and prehydration are essential for patients to tolerate amifostine treatment. Amifostine is given daily, 30 minutes prior to RT. To date, amifostine is the only approved cytoprotective agent; cytoprotectives are the latest agents developed and approved for the treatment of radiation-induced xerostomia.

Multiple studies have identified different therapeutic applications, some of which have already been mentioned for the management of xerostomia. Lovelace et al. (2014) suggested other preventive strategies to minimize xerostomia that have been under investigation, including muscarinic acetylcholine agonists such as cevimeline, salivary substitutes, bethanechol, acupuncture, and hyperbaric oxygen therapy (HBOT). Cevimeline is a muscarinic acetylcholine receptor agonist with a high affinity for muscarinic M3 receptors found in salivary gland cells. It may prove to be a better agent than pilocarpine to treat xerostomia, as it has been shown to have a longer half-life and action and with fewer respiratory and cardiac side effects (Lovelace et al., 2014). Cevimeline has been approved in the United States for the treatment of xerostomia associated with Sjögren syndrome; however, cevimeline has not yet been approved for radiation-induced xerostomia (Lovelace et al., 2014). In their study, Lovelace et al. (2014) found that the tolerable dosage for cevimeline was 30–45 mg three times daily with only mild to moderate side effects. Bethanechol is a cholinergic choline carbamate with mostly M3 muscarinic activity, muscarinic adverse effects, and a longer half-life. However, limited studies have been conducted on the use of bethanechol for the treatment of radiation-induced hyposalivation (Kałużny et al., 2014; Lovelace et al., 2014). Lovelace and colleagues (2014) illuminated that acupuncture, HBOT, and electrical stimulation may provide potential relief for radiation-induced xerostomia without serious complications; however, research is needed to substantiate this finding. These authors also highlighted the potential for gene transfer and stem cell transplant therapy in the management of radiation-induced xerostomia. These interventions are still in the early stage of research.

Nasal Dryness

Cancers of the sinus and nasopharynx may require the administration of RT to the nasal passages. Su et al. (2014) highlighted that when radiation dose to the nasopharynx reaches 40 Gy, patients experience acute mucosal reaction that is similar to toxicity of the oral mucosa. The nasal mucosa may become parched and irritated, leading to cracking and bleeding. Mucus secretions become dry, hard, and crusty, making them hard to remove with nose blowing (Remenschneider, Sadow, Lin, & Gray, 2013). See Figure 7-10 for nursing interventions for nasal dryness.

Laryngeal Edema

Laryngeal edema, or swelling of the larynx, can be caused by RT. Symptoms of edema of the larynx include hoarseness, dyspnea, and stridor, which require intubation or tracheostomy. Voice changes usually will progress during radiation and improve slowly after therapy is completed (Deng, Ridner, & Murphy, 2011). Figure 7-11 lists nursing interventions for laryngeal edema.

Radiation Dermatitis and Alopecia

Radiation dermatitis is an expected side effect of RT. Most patients receiving RT to the head and neck will have some degree of skin reaction because of normal tissue breakdown from ionizing radiation (Bensadoun et al., 2011; Ryan, 2012). Skin reactions may include mild to brisk erythema, dry or moist desquamation, or skin necrosis and ulceration of the dermis (NCI CTEP, 2010). Nursing interventions for dermatitis are listed in Figure 7-12. Moist desquamation results from the inability of the basal layer to proliferate sufficiently to replace the epidermal surface (Bergstrom, 2011; Dendaas, 2012; McQuestion, 2011). Moist desquamation may be painful for the patient. Like many radiation side effects, skin reaction usually will begin two to three weeks after the start of treatment and continue for two to four weeks after treatment is completed.

For patients with head and neck cancer undergoing RT, alopecia, or hair loss caused by follicular death, results in loss of facial hair in addition to the loss of scalp hair, depending on the treatment field. During RT, alopecia begins with an exposure of more than 3 Gy, and total hair loss may occur within weeks of exposure to 6 Gy (Nanashima, Ito, Ishikawa, Nakano, & Nakamura, 2012). Hair growth usually will resume six to eight weeks after RT, but the growth may be patchy and thin. Nanashima and colleagues noted that blood

---

Figure 7-10. Nursing Interventions for Nasal Dryness

- Encourage fluid intake of 8–10 glasses throughout the day.
- Suggest the use of a humidifier, especially at night in the bedroom.
- Administer saline nasal spray to moisten nasal passages.
- Apply petroleum jelly or hydrocortisone ointment intranasally to moisten the membrane and provide comfort. (Do not use petroleum jelly during radiation treatment.)
- Consult with the otorhinolaryngology department for nasal lavage for obstructive secretions.

Figure 7-11. Nursing Interventions for Laryngeal Edema

- Assess the patient's voice quality weekly.
- Monitor for symptoms of breathing difficulty (i.e., stridor/dyspnea).
- Encourage frequent gargling with salt water or sodium bicarbonate solution.
- Encourage the patient to rest voice.
- Explain voice quality changes to the patient and family.
- Administer steroids, as ordered, to decrease swelling.

Figure 7-12. Nursing Interventions for Dermatitis

- Teach the patient and family proper skin care during radiation therapy, including
  - Use mild soap.
  - Avoid friction when washing and rinse completely with water.
  - Use an electric razor for shaving.
  - Avoid the use of shaving creams or aftershave lotion.
  - Avoid the use of perfume and makeup.
  - Avoid sun exposure to treatment areas; wear a hat and clothing to protect skin.
- Moisturize skin three times a day with recommended gels or creams.
- Use hydrocortisone cream for itchy skin.
- Do not apply skin care products for two to four hours before the radiation treatment, depending on the product(s) used.
- Advise patient to avoid tight-fitting clothing that may cause irritation of the treatment area.
- When treating a patient with moist desquamation,
  - Avoid gauze dressings that stick and may cause bleeding.
  - Do not apply tape to the skin in the radiation treatment area.
  - Nonstick dressings may be useful.
  - Antibiotic ointment combined with lidocaine may provide comfort to the reaction area.
  - Give pain medication as prescribed.

stem cells are sensitive to radiation; hair loss is considered to be caused by irradiation-induced stem cell damage. Patients must be prepared for the cosmetic changes that may appear.

Skin care products used to treat radiation dermatitis vary among institutions. Nurses should be aware that some patients might be predisposed to skin problems and should stay abreast of newly developed products and research regarding these products so that effective treatment can be instituted. Recent research done by Haddad, Amouzgar-Hashemi, Samsami, Chinichian, and Oghabian (2013) concluded that adding aloe vera gel to patients' skin care regimens may offer a protective effect and reduce the intensity of radiation-induced dermatitis. Aloe vera gel is low cost and usually easy to find, unlike many other skin care products.

Dental Caries and Osteoradionecrosis

Patients receiving ionizing radiation to the parotid glands usually develop xerostomia. Even with recent advances in medication, it is not known if saliva has the same chemical composition after RT. Saliva is composed of electrolytes, minerals, small organic molecules, and essential proteins that continuously coat the oral mucosa. Patients with xerostomia are at increased risk for dental decay (dental caries) because of the inability of saliva to lubricate and cleanse the mouth and act as a buffer to acid (Ede et al., 2011). Osteoradionecrosis and chondronecrosis are radiation damage to the bone and cartilage, respectively. Irradiation can adversely affect cellular elements of bone, which can limit the potential for wound maintenance and ability to heal after a traumatic event. Elective oral surgical procedures are contraindicated within an irradiated field. If surgical intervention (e.g., extractions, endodontic or periodontal surgery) is required after RT, pre- and postoperative HBOT treatments may increase the potential for healing and minimize the risk for osteoradionecrosis (Ede et al., 2011). See Figure 7-13 for nursing interventions.

Tissue Fibrosis and Trismus

Soft tissue fibrosis is the development of soft tissue firmness of the neck. Trismus is the tightening of the mastication muscles in the jaw, which, if not prevented or treated, can significantly hinder patients' ability to chew (Ede et al., 2011). Additionally, trismus is viewed as the result of fibrosis, leading to a loss of flexibility and extension; an oral opening less than 20 mm can be considered trismus (Ede et al., 2011). The prevalence of trismus ranges from 5%–38% (Kamstra, Roodenburg, Beurskens, Reintsema, & Dijkstra, 2013). According to Kamstra et al. (2013), mouth opening improved an average of 5.4 mm after jaw-stretching exercises using the Thera-Bite® device. Nursing interventions include

---

Figure 7-13. Nursing Interventions for Dental Care

- Confirm that the patient has had a prophylactic dental evaluation.
- Encourage compliance with prescribed treatments, such as
  - Applying fluoride daily for life
  - Brushing and flossing regularly (use soft toothbrush)
  - Avoiding candy, gum, and drinks high in sugar
  - Rinsing often.

- Encourage frequent exercises such as chewing.
- Refer patient to physical therapy for a dynamic bite opener.
- Make dietary changes as needed.
- Assess mouth opening measurement periodically.

Ocular and Otologic Changes

Radiation can cause long-term injury to the structures of the eyes, particularly when the retina receives doses greater than 45 Gy (Higginson et al., 2013). Careful planning is performed to avoid treating these structures whenever possible. If the area surrounding the eye must be treated, a lead shield may be placed under the eyelid to block the radiation from injuring the eye. Radiation-induced optic neuropathy presents with sudden, painless, and irreversible vision loss in one or both eyes and can develop three months to nine years following RT (Zhao et al., 2013). Serous otitis media is the development of sterile fluid within the middle ear. In some situations, patients have drainage tubes surgically placed in the ear. Cerumen (earwax) can harden in the ear canal, which an ear, nose, and throat specialist must lavage and remove. If these patients develop subtle changes in hearing, immediate evaluation with an otolaryngologist or audiologist is warranted (Harris, 2012). Nurses should assess patients for hearing changes. Pretreatment and post-treatment ototoxic assessment is essential to preserve hearing for patients who receive cytotoxic agents along with RT to the head and neck. Hearing preservation must be assessed using formal audiograms at six-month follow-ups for two years and annually thereafter (Brown et al., 2011).

Hypothyroidism

Hypothyroidism is the decreased function of the thyroid gland; this is a subacute side effect of RT to the neck. According to Kim, Yu, and Wu (2014), approximately 10%–15% of patients develop hypothyroidism after RT to the head and neck using fields that include all or part of the thyroid gland. Because of the frequency of hypothyroidism, the National Comprehensive Cancer Network® recommends that thyroid function tests should be monitored and repeated every 6–12 months after RT to the neck (Kim et al., 2014), and levothyroxine should be prescribed to treat this problem. Once patients are diagnosed with hypothyroidism, they will need to take levothyroxine for life and may require many dose adjustments to restore the quality of life and decrease morbidity and mortality (Rønjom et al., 2013). Hypothyroidism left untreated could cause weight problems, fatigue, and hair changes (Carter, Sippel, & Chen, 2014). Research shows that prompt referral to an endocrinologist for thyroid monitoring and intervention with hormonal replacement is indicated for all patients diagnosed with clinical, symptomatic, and subclinical hypothyroidism after head and neck RT (Ma, Li, Zou, & Zhou, 2013).

Spinal Cord Injury

Radiation-induced myelopathy is injury to the spinal cord that could result in paralysis. Lhermitte sign is characterized by shock-like sensations that radiate down the back and extremities when the neck is flexed. Often, these symptoms pass with time; a neck collar is sometimes prescribed to help with the discomfort. Fortunately, with today's knowledge of radiobiology and availability of advanced treatment planning techniques, radiation injury to the spinal cord is avoidable in most situations (Mul et al., 2012).

Fatigue and Depression

Patients who commonly receive head and neck radiation also experience fatigue to some degree. The actual mechanism of fatigue is not clearly defined and appears to be related to excess toxic metabolite and waste products, causing cell destruction (Erickson, Spurlock, Kramer, & Davis, 2013; Gulliford et al., 2012). Nutrition, sleep patterns, mucosal discomfort, secretion management, and daily activity all can affect fatigue. Depression often is seen in patients with head and neck cancer. Mo et al. (2014) reported a moderate level of perceived depression in patients receiving RT for cancers of the head and neck. Patients need monitoring and professional intervention for depression. See Figure 7-14 for nursing interventions for fatigue and depression.

Summary

RT is an essential treatment modality in the management of head and neck cancer. Advanced technologies have dramatically changed the delivery of RT to the head and neck area. Patients with head and neck cancer require complex patient management that is guided by a dedicated healthcare team. Nursing care has become highly specialized within the realm of radiation oncology nursing practice. In particular, the role of the nurse is inherent in providing patients and their families with the information necessary to understand the anticipated treatment course and to manage the side effects of their treatment.

Figure 7-14. Nursing Interventions for Fatigue and Depression

- Teach the patient to reduce activity levels when tired.
- Encourage frequent naps or rest periods throughout the day.
- Limit the patient's naps to one to two hours so that the patient can sleep at night.
- Increase the patient's hours of sleep at night with earlier bedtimes or sleeping in.
- Encourage the use of sleep medication as prescribed.
- Recommend short periods of light exercise to decrease fatigue.
- Encourage the use of pain medication as prescribed so the patient may be more comfortable at sleep times.
- Encourage the patient to maintain high-calorie and high-protein intake to improve energy level.
- Refer the patient to a social worker for emotional, spiritual, and financial support, as needed.

The author would like to acknowledge Lisa L. Blevins, RN, BSN, OCN®, for her contribution to this chapter that remains unchanged from the first edition of this book.

References

Allen, K.J. (2012). Stereotactic radiosurgery. In R.R. Iwamoto, M.L. Haas, & T.K. Gosselin (Eds.), *Manual for radiation oncology nursing practice and education* (4th ed., pp. 274–281). Pittsburgh, PA: Oncology Nursing Society.

Altinok, A., Gonze, D., Lévi, F., & Goldbeter, A. (2011). An automaton model for the cell cycle. *Interface Focus, 1,* 36–47. doi:10.1098/rsfs.2010.0009

Ang, K.K., & Garden, A.S. (2012). *Radiotherapy for head and neck cancers: Indications and techniques* (4th ed.). Philadelphia, PA: Lippincott Williams & Wilkins.

Baharvand, M., ShoalehSaadi, N., Barakian, R., & Moghaddam, E.J. (2013). Taste alteration and impact on quality of life after head and neck radiotherapy. *Journal of Oral Pathology and Medicine, 42,* 106–112. doi:10.1111/j.1600-0714.2012.01200.x

Balusik, B. (2014). Management of dysphagia in patients with head and neck cancer. *Clinical Journal of Oncology Nursing, 18,* 149–150. doi:10.1188/14.CJON.149-150

Beech, N., Robinson, S., Porceddu, S., & Batstone, M. (2014). Dental management of patients irradiated for head and neck cancer. *Australian Dental Journal, 59,* 20–28. doi:10.1111/adj.12134

Beitler, J.J., Zhang, Q., Fu, K.K., Trotti, A., Spencer, S.A., Jones, C.U., ... Ang, K.K. (2014). Final results of local-randomized trial of altered fractionation radiation for locally advanced head and neck cancer. *International Journal of Radiation Oncology, Biology, Physics, 89,* 13–20. doi:10.1016/j.ijrobp.2013.12.027

Bell, B.C., & Butler, E.B. (2013). Management of predictable pain using fentanyl pectin nasal spray in patients undergoing radiotherapy. *Journal of Pain Research, 6,* 843–848. doi:10.2147/JPR.S54788

Bensinger, W., Schubert, M., Ang, K.K., Brizel, D., Brown, E., Eilers, J.G., ... Trotti, A.M., III. (2008). NCCN Task Force report: Prevention and management of mucositis in cancer care. *Journal of the National Comprehensive Cancer Network, 6*(Suppl. 1), S1–S21. Retrieved from http://www.nccn.org/JNCCN/PDF/mucositis_2008.pdf

Bergstrom, K. (2011). Development of a radiation skin care protocol and algorithm using the Iowa Model of Evidence-Based Practice. *Clinical Journal of Oncology Nursing, 15,* 593–595. doi:10.1188/11.CJON.593-595

Blecher, C.S., Ireland, A.M., & Watson, J.L. (2016). *Standards of oncology education: Patient/significant other and public* (4th ed.). Pittsburgh, PA: Oncology Nursing Society.

Brockbank, S., Miller, N., Owen, S., & Patterson, J.M. (2014). Pretreatment information on dysphagia exploring the views of head and neck cancer patients. *Journal of Pain and Symptom Management, 49*, 89–97. doi:10.1016/j.jpainsymman.2014.04.014

Brown, J.M., Carlson, D.J., & Brenner, D.J. (2013). The tumor radiobiology of SRS and SBRT: Are more than the 5 Rs involved? *International Journal of Radiation Oncology, Biology, Physics, 88*, 254–262. doi:10.1016/j.ijrobp.2013.07.022

Brown, M., Ruckenstein, M., Bigelow, D., Judy, K., Wilson, V., Alonso-Basanta, M., & Lee, J.Y. (2011). Predictors of hearing loss after gamma knife radiosurgery for vestibular schwannomas: Age, cochlear dose, and tumor coverage. *Neurosurgery, 69*, 605–613. doi:10.1227/NEU.0b013e31821a42f3

Carter, Y., Sippel, R.S., & Chen, H. (2014). Hypothyroidism after a cancer diagnosis; etiology, diagnosis, complications, and management. *Oncologist, 19*, 34–43. doi:10.1634/theoncologist.2013-0237

Das, S., Thomas, S., Pal, S.K., Isiah, R., & John, S. (2013). Hypofractionated palliative radiotherapy in locally advanced inoperable head and neck cancer: CMC Vellore experience. *Indian Journal of Palliative Care, 19*, 93–98. doi:10.4103/0973-1075.116709

Debenham, B.J., Hu, K.S., & Harrison, L.B. (2013). Present status and future directions of intraoperative radiotherapy. *Lancet Oncology, 14*, e457–e464. doi:10.1016/S1470-2045(13)70270-5

Dendaas, N. (2012). Toward evidence and theory-based skin care in radiation oncology. *Clinical Journal of Oncology Nursing, 16*, 520–525. doi:10.1188/12.CJON.520-525

Deng, J., Ridner, S.H., & Murphy, B.A. (2011). Lymphedema in patients with head and neck cancer [Online exclusive]. *Oncology Nursing Forum, 38*, E1–E10. doi:10.1188/11.ONF.E1-E10

Deng, Z., Kiyuna, A., Hasegawa, M., Nakasone, I., Hosokawa, A., & Suzuki, M. (2010). Oral candidiasis in patients receiving radiation therapy for head and neck cancer. *Otolaryngology—Head and Neck Surgery, 143*, 242–247. doi:10.1016/j.otohns.2010.02.003

Duarte, V.M., Liu, Y.F., Rafizadeh, S., Tajima, T., Nabili, V., & Wang, M.B. (2014). Comparison of dental health of patients with head and neck cancer receiving IMRT versus conventional radiation. *Otolaryngology—Head and Neck Surgery, 150*, 81–86. doi:10.1177/0194599813509586

Ede, S.T., Centurion, B., Ferreira, L.H., Souza, A.P., Damante, J.H., & Rubira-Bullen, I.R. (2011). Oral adverse effects of head and neck radiotherapy: Literature review and suggestion of a clinical oral care guideline for irradiated patients. *Journal of Applied Oral Science, 19*, 448–454. doi:10.1590/S1678-77572011000500003

El Saghir, N.S., Keating, N.L., Carlson, R.W., Khoury, K.E., & Fallowfield, L. (2014). Tumor board: Optimizing the structure and improving efficiency of multidisciplinary management of patients with cancer worldwide. *American Society of Clinical Oncology, 2014*, e461–e466. doi:10.14694/EdBook_AM.2014.34.e461

Erickson, J.M., Spurlock, L.K., Kramer, J.C., & Davis, M.A. (2013). Self-care strategies to relieve fatigue in patients receiving radiation therapy. *Clinical Journal of Oncology Nursing, 17*, 319–324. doi:10.1188/13.CJON.319-324

Fukumoto, M. (2014). Radiation pathology: From thorotrast to the future beyond radioresistance. *Pathology International, 64*, 251–262. doi:10.1111/pin.12170

Ghadjar, P., Bojaxhiu, B., Simcock, M., Terribilini, D., Isaak, B., Gut, P., ... Aebersold, D.M. (2012). High dose-rate versus low dose-rate brachytherapy for lip cancer. *International Journal of Radiation Oncology, Biology, Physics, 83*, 1205–1212. doi:10.1016/j.ijrobp.2011.09.038

Gu, J., Zhu, S., Li, X., Wu, H., Li, Y., & Hua, F. (2014). Effect of amifostine in head and neck cancer patients treated with radiotherapy: A sys-tematic review and meta-analysis based on randomized controlled trials. *PLOS ONE, 9*, e5968. doi:10.1371/journal.pone.0095968

Gulliford, S.L., Miah, A.B., Brennan, S., McQuaid, D., Clark, C.H., Partridge, M., ... Nutting, C.M. (2012). Dosimetric explanations of fatigue in head and neck radiotherapy: An analysis from PARSPORT phase III trial. *Radiotherapy and Oncology, 104*, 205–212. doi:10.1016/j.radonc.2012.07.005

Haddad, P., Amouzgar-Hashemi, F., Samsami, S., Chinichian, S., & Oghabian, M.A. (2013). Aloe vera for prevention of radiation-induced dermatitis: A self-controlled clinical trial. *Current Oncology, 20*, E345–E348. doi:10.3747/co.20.1356

Harris, D. (2012). Head and neck. In R.R. Iwamoto, M.L. Haas, & T.K. Gosselin (Eds.), *Manual for radiation oncology nursing practice and education* (4th ed., pp. 122–145). Pittsburgh, PA: Oncology Nursing Society.

Higginson, D.S., Sahgal, A., Lawrence, M.V., Moyer, S., Stefanescu, M., Wilson, A.K., ... Chera, B. (2013). External beam radiotherapy for head and neck cancers is associated with increased variability in retinal vascular oxygenation. *PLOS ONE, 8*, e69657. doi:10.1371/journal.pone.0069657.t001

Hoffmann, T.K. (2012). Systemic therapy strategies for head-neck carcinomas: Current status. *Head and Neck Surgery, 11*, 1–25. doi:10.1055/s-0031-1297244

Holliday, E.B., & Frank, S.J. (2014). Proton radiation therapy for head and neck cancer: A review of clinical experience to date. *International Journal of Radiation Oncology, Biology, Physics, 89*, 292–302. doi:10.1016/j.ijrobp.2014.02.029

Hovan, A.J., Williams, P.M., Stevenson-Moore, P., Wahlin, Y.B., Ohrn, K.E.O., Elting, L.S., ... Brennan, M.T. (2010). A systematic review of dysgeusia induced by cancer therapies. *Supportive Care in Cancer, 18*, 1081–1087. doi:10.1007/s00520-010-0902-1

Kałużny, J., Wierzbicka, M., Nogala, H., Milecki, P., & Kopeć, T. (2014). Radiotherapy induced xerostomia: Mechanisms, diagnostics, prevention and treatment—Evidence based up to 2013. *Otolaryngologia Polska, 68*, 1–14. doi:10.1016/j.otpol.2013.09.002

Kamstra, J.I., Roodenburg, J., Beurskens, C., Reintsema, H., & Dijkstra, P. (2013). TheraBite exercises to treat trismus secondary to head and neck cancer. *Supportive Care in Cancer, 21*, 951–957. doi:10.1007/s00520-012-1610-9

Khan, F. (2010). *The physics of radiation therapy* (4th ed.). Philadelphia, PA: Lippincott Williams & Wilkins.

Kim, M.Y., Yu, T., & Wu, H.G. (2014). Dose-volumetric parameters for predicting hypothyroidism after radiotherapy for head and neck cancer. *Japanese Journal of Clinical Oncology, 44*, 331–337. doi:10.1093/jjco/hyt235

Kinsman, L., Rotter, T., James, E., Snow, P., & Willis, J. (2010). What is a clinical pathway? Development of a definition to inform the debate. *BMC Medicine, 8*, 31. doi:10.1186/1741-7015-8-31

Komatsu, M., Shiono, O., Taguchi, T., Sakuma, Y., Nishimura, G., Sano, D., & Oridate, N. (2014). Concurrent chemoradiotherapy with docetaxel, cisplatin and 5-fluorouracil (TPF) in patients with locally advanced squamous cell carcinoma of the head and neck. *Japanese Journal of Clinical Oncology, 44*, 416–421. doi:10.1093/jjco/hyu026

Koukourakis, M.I., Tsoutsou, P.G., Karpouzis, A., Tsiarkatsi, M., Karapantzos, I., Danilidis, V., & Kouskoukis, C. (2009). Radiochemotherapy with cetuximab, cisplatin, and amifostine for locally advanced head and neck cancer: A feasibility study. *International Journal of Radiation Oncology, Biology, Physics, 77*, 9–15. doi:10.1016/j.ijrobp.2009.04.060

Lalla, R.V., Saunders, D.P., & Peterson, D.E. (2014). Chemotherapy or radiation-induced oral mucositis. *Dental Clinics of North America, 58*, 341–349. doi:10.1016/j.cden.2013.12.005

Lambertz, C.K., Gruell, J., Robenstein, V., Mueller-Funaiole, V., Cummings, K., & Knapp, V. (2010). NO SToPS: Reducing treatment breaks during chemoradiation for head and neck cancer. *Clinical Journal of Oncology Nursing, 14*, 585–593. doi:10.1188/10.CJON.585-593

Lang, D. (2013). Interventions for preventing oral mucositis for patients with cancer receiving treatment. *Clinical Journal of Oncology Nursing, 17,* 340. doi:10.1188/13.CJON.340

Lovelace, T.L., Fox, N.F., Sood, A.J., Nguyen, S.A., & Day, T.A. (2014). Management of radiotherapy-induced salivary hypofunction and consequent xerostomia in patients with oral or head and neck cancer: Meta-analysis and literature review. *Oral Surgery, Oral Medicine, Oral Pathology, and Oral Radiology, 117,* 595–607. doi:10.1016/j.oooo.2014.01.229

Ma, C. (2012). The practice of radiation oncology. In R.R. Iwamoto, M.L. Haas, & T.K. Gosselin (Eds.), *Manual for radiation oncology nursing practice and education* (4th ed., pp. 17–27). Pittsburgh, PA: Oncology Nursing Society.

Ma, J.A., Li, X., Zou, W., & Zhou, Y. (2013). Grave's disease induced by radiotherapy for nasopharyngeal carcinoma: A case report and review of the literature. *Oncology Letters, 6,* 144–146. doi:10.3892/ol.2013.1332

Macann, A., Fua, T., Milross, C.G., Porceddu, S.V., Penniment, M., Wratten, C., ... Hockey, P. (2014). Phase 3 trial of domiciliary humidification to mitigate acute mucosal toxicity during radiation therapy for head-and-neck cancer: First report of Tran Tasman Radiation Oncology Group (TROG) 07.03 RadioHUM study. *International Journal of Radiation Oncology, Biology, Physics, 88,* 572–579. doi:10.1016/j.ijrobp.2013.11.226

Mallick, I., & Waldron, J. (2009). Radiation therapy for head and neck cancers. *Seminars in Oncology Nursing, 25,* 193–202. doi:10.1016/j.soncn.2009.05.002

Mason, H., DeRubeis, M.B., Foster, J.C., Taylor, J.M., & Worden, F.P. (2013). Outcomes evaluation of a weekly nurse practitioner–managed symptom management clinic for patients with head and neck cancer treated with chemoradiotherapy. *Oncology Nursing Forum, 40,* 581–586. doi:10.1188/13.ONF.40-06AP

McQuestion, M. (2011). Evidence-based skin care management in radiation therapy: Clinical update. *Seminars in Oncology Nursing, 27,* e1–17. doi:10.1016/j.soncn.2011.02.009

Mendenhall, W.M., Riggs, C.E., Vaysberg, M., Amdur, R.J., & Werning, J.W. (2010). Altered fractionation and adjuvant chemotherapy for head and neck squamous cell carcinoma. *Head and Neck, 32,* 939–945. doi:10.1002/hed.21261

Minicucci, E.M., da Silva, G.N., & Salvadori, D.M. (2014). Relationship between head and neck cancer therapy and some genetic endpoints. *World Journal of Clinical Oncology, 5,* 93–102. doi:10.5306/wjco.v5.i2.93

Mitchell, G. (2013). The rationale for fractionation in radiotherapy. *Clinical Journal of Oncology Nursing, 17,* 412–417. doi:10.1188/13.CJON.412-417

Mo, Y., Li, L., Qin, L., Zhu, X.D., Qu, S., Liang, X., & Wei, Z.J. (2014). Cognitive function, mood, and sleep quality in patients treated with intensity-modulated radiation therapy for nasopharyngeal cancer: A prospective study. *Psycho-Oncology, 23,* 1185–1191. doi:10.1002/pon.3542

Mul, V.E.M., de Jong, J.M.A., Murrer, L.H.P., van den Ende, P.L.A., Houben, R.M.A., Lacko, M., ... Baumert, B.G. (2012). Lhermitte sign and myelopathy after irradiation of cervical spinal cord in radiotherapy treatment of head and neck cancer. *Strahlentherapie und Onkologie, 188,* 71–76. doi:10.1007/s00066-011-0010-2

Nanashima, N., Ito, K., Ishikawa, T., Nakano, M., & Nakamura, T. (2012). Damage of hair follicle stem cells and alteration of keratin expression in external radiation-induced acute alopecia. *International Journal of Molecular Medicine, 30,* 579–584. doi:10.3892/ijmm.2012.1018

National Cancer Institute Cancer Therapy Evaluation Program. (2010). *Common terminology criteria for adverse events* [v.4.03]. Retrieved from http://evs.nci.nih.gov/ftp1/CTCAE/CTCAE_4.03_2010-06-14_QuickReference_5x7.pdf

Naugler, W.E., Alsina, A.E., Frenette, C.T., Rossaro, L., & Sellers, M.T. (2015). Building the multidisciplinary team for management of patients with hepatocellular carcinoma. *Clinical Gastroenterology and Hepatology, 13,* 827–835. doi:10.1016/j.cgh.2014.03.038

O'Gorman, C., Sasiadek, W., Denieffe, S., & Gooney, M. (2014). Predicting radiotherapy-related clinical toxicities in cancer: A literature review [Online exclusive]. *Clinical Journal of Oncology Nursing, 18,* E37–E44. doi:10.1188/14.CJON.E37-E44

Proud, C. (2014). Radiogenomics: The promise of personalized treatment in radiation oncology. *Clinical Journal of Oncology Nursing, 18,* 185–189. doi:10.1188/14.CJON.185-189

Radvansky, L.J., Pace, M.B., & Siddiqui, A. (2013). Prevention and management of radiation-induced dermatitis, mucositis, and xerostomia. *American Journal of Health-System Pharmacy, 70,* 1025–1032. doi:10.2146/ajhp120467

Remenschneider, A.K., Sadow, P.M., Lin, D.T., & Gray, S.T. (2013). Metastatic renal cell carcinoma to the sinonasal cavity: A case series. *Journal of Neurological Surgery Reports, 74,* 67–72. doi:10.1055/s-0033-1346972

Rønjom, M.F., Brink, C., Bentzen, S.M., Hegedüs, L., Overgaard, J., & Johansen, J. (2013). Hypothyroidism after radiotherapy for head and neck squamous cell carcinoma: Normal tissue complication probability modeling with latent time correction. *Radiotherapy and Oncology, 109,* 317–322. doi:10.1016/j.radonc.2013.06.029

Rosenstein, B.S. (2009). Molecular radiobiology. In B.G. Haffty & L.D. Wilson (Eds.), *Handbook of radiation oncology: Basic principles and clinical protocols* (pp. 73–88). Burlington, MA: Jones & Bartlett Learning.

Rosenstein, B.S., West, C.M., Bentzen, S.M., Alsner, J., Andreassen, C.N., Azria, D., ... Zenhausern, F., for the Radiogenomics Consortium. (2014). Radiogenomics: Radiobiology enters the era of Big Data and Team Science. *International Journal of Radiation Oncology, Biology, Physics, 89,* 709–713. doi:10.1016/j.ijrobp.2014.03.009

Rudžianskas, V., Inčiūra, A., Juozaitytė, E., Rudžianskienė, M., Kubilius, R., Vaitkus, S., ... Adliene, D. (2012). Reirradiation of recurrent head and neck cancer using high-dose-rate brachytherapy. *Acta Otorhinolaryngologica Italica, 32,* 297–303. Retrieved from http://www.ncbi.nlm.nih.gov/pmc/articles/PMC3546407

Ryan, J.L. (2012). Ionizing radiation: The good, the bad, and the ugly. *Journal of Investigative Dermatology, 132,* 985–993. doi:10.1038/jid.2011.411

Servagi-Vervat, S., Ali, D., Roubieu, C., Durdux, C., Laccourreye, O., & Giraud, P. (2014). Dysphagia after radiotherapy: State of the art and prevention. *European Annals of Otorhinolaryngology, Head and Neck Diseases, 14,* 25–29. doi:10.1016/j.anorl.2013.09.006

Sobecki-Ryniak, D., & Krouse, H.J. (2013). Head and neck cancer: Historical evolution of treatment and patient self-care requirements. *Clinical Journal of Oncology Nursing, 17,* 659–663. doi:10.1188/13.CJON.659-663

Spiotto, M.T., & Weichselbaum, R.R. (2014). Comparison of 3D conformal radiotherapy and intensity modulated radiotherapy with or without simultaneous integrated boost during concurrent chemoradiation for locally advanced head and neck cancers. *PLOS ONE, 9,* e94496. doi:10.1371/journal.pone.0094456

Stoker, S.D., van Diessen, J.N., de Boer, J.P., Karakullukcu, B., Leemans, C.R., & Tan, I.B. (2013). Current treatment options for residual nasopharyngeal carcinoma. *Current Treatment Options in Oncology, 14,* 475–491. doi:10.1007/s11864-013-0261-5

Su, Y.X., Liu, L.P., Li, L., Li, X., Cao, X., Dong, W., ... Hao, J.F. (2014). Factors influencing the incidence of sinusitis in nasopharyngeal carcinoma patients after intensity-modulated radiation therapy. *European Archives of Otorhinolaryngology, 271,* 3195–3201. doi:10.1007/s00405-014-3004-8

Tantiwongkosi, B., Yu, F., Kanard, A., & Miller, F.R. (2014). Role of F-FDG PET/CT in pre- and post-treatment evaluation in head and neck carcinoma. *World Journal of Radiology, 6,* 177–191. doi:10.4329/wjr.v6.i5.177

Thewes, B., Butow, P., Davis, E., Turner, J., & Mason, C. (2014). Psychologists' views of inter-disciplinary psychosocial communication within the cancer care team. *Supportive Care in Cancer, 22,* 3193–3200. doi:10.1007/s00520-014-2299-8

van der Linden, N., van Gils, C.W., Pescott, C.P., Buter, J., Vergeer, M.R., & Groot, C.A. (2015). Real-world cost-effectiveness of cetuximab in locally advanced squamous cell carcinoma of the head and neck. *European Archives of Oto-Rhino-Laryngology, 272*, 2007–2016. doi:10.1007/s00405-014-3106-3

Vichare, A., Washington, R., Patton, C., Arnone, A., Olsen, C., Fung, C.Y., … Pohar, S. (2013). An assessment of the current U.S. radiation oncology workforce: Methodology and global results of the American Society for Radiation Oncology 2012 Workforce Study. *International Journal of Radiation Oncology, Biology, Physics, 87*, 1129–1134. doi:10.1016/j.ijrobp.2013.08.050

Wiegand, S., Sesterhenn, A.M., Zimmermann, A.P., Strassmann, G., Wihelm, T., & Werner, J.A. (2013). Interstitial HDR brachytherapy for advanced recurrent squamous cell carcinoma of the head and neck. *Anticancer Research, 33*, 249–252.

Zhao, Z., Lan, Y., Bai, S., Shen, J., Xiao, S., Lv, R., … Liu, J. (2013). Late-onset radiation-induced optic neuropathy after radiotherapy for nasopharyngeal carcinoma. *Journal of Clinical Neuroscience, 20*, 702–706. doi:10.1016/j.jocn.2012.05.034

CHAPTER 8

Chemotherapy

Catherine Jansen, PhD, RN, CNS, AOCNS®

Introduction

The head and neck region is composed of the paranasal sinuses, larynx, pharynx, and oral cavity. Chemotherapy is very effective against squamous cell carcinoma of the head and neck, and some regimens can elicit response rates up to 80% (Benasso, 2013). Chemotherapy differs from other treatment modalities used for this population (e.g., surgery, radiation therapy), as antineoplastic agents have a systemic effect because of their ability to circulate throughout the body via the bloodstream. The primary purpose of chemotherapy, therefore, is to treat disease that is no longer confined to one site or has metastasized to other areas. Chemotherapy is also used as a radiosensitizer to improve the effect of radiation therapy on locoregional control of microscopic diseases. Chemotherapy has been integrated into the standard of care for locally advanced, recurrent, and metastatic disease with the goal of improving survival outcomes as well as minimizing functional and cosmetic morbidity (Denaro, Russi, Lefebvre, & Merlano, 2014).

Despite the expanded role of chemotherapy for head and neck cancers over the past three decades, its influence on overall survival rates remains limited and is associated with acute and chronic toxicities. Numerous chemotherapy approaches have been studied in the head and neck cancer population, including evaluating efficacy of individual antineoplastic agents or combination regimens, as well as varied dosing or timing in relation to other modalities (e.g., radiation therapy, biologics). Cetuximab, a monoclonal antibody (mAb), has been approved for use in patients with head and neck cancer and incorporated into treatment plans for locally advanced, metastatic, and recurrent disease. Research in this area, including the investigation of additional novel agents, is ongoing. Further clinical trials are needed to determine their impact on prognosis and toxicity profile.

Principles of Treatment

Neoadjuvant therapy, otherwise known as *induction*, refers to the use of a treatment modality prior to the principal therapy. For instance, chemotherapy can be given before surgery to decrease tumor bulk and consequently improve surgical outcome. Induction chemotherapy can be used in patients with disease that may be surgically removed, with unresectable disease that will be treated with radiation therapy, or for the goal of larynx preservation (Murphy, 2011).

Adjuvant therapy refers to cancer treatments that are given after primary treatment (e.g., surgery) to minimize disease recurrence. Radiation therapy, chemotherapy, mAbs, and a combination of these modalities have been used as adjuvant treatment for patients with head and neck cancer. *Sequential chemotherapy* describes the administration of a predetermined number of induction chemotherapy cycles, followed by evaluation for response prior to proceeding with another treatment (e.g., chemoradiotherapy). *Concomitant*, or *concurrent*, chemotherapy refers to chemotherapy cycles that are administered according to a specific protocol at the same time the patient is receiving radiation therapy (Fury, 2012).

In general, the treatment plan and the goals of care (i.e., cure, control, palliation) are based on the extent of disease at presentation. The utility of chemotherapy is related to the tumor burden and rate of tumor growth. Several cancer characteristics can influence tumor response (e.g., location of tumor, blood supply), and various factors unique to the patient and to the antineoplastic agent being considered need to be evaluated when developing the treatment plan (see Figure 8-1). Disease-related factors influence which treatment options are feasible. For example, surgery is generally limited to patients with early-stage disease who are deemed good surgical candidates. Chemotherapy is most often utilized in patients with advanced or metastatic disease.

Figure 8-1. Factors to Consider When Determining the Treatment Plan for Patients With Head and Neck Cancer

Tumor (Versus Disease-Related) Factors
- Anatomic location and extent of disease (including size and involvement of adjacent normal structures)
- Stage
- Histology
- Grade
- Vascularity of the tumor

Individual Patient Characteristics
- Age
- Health status (e.g., comorbidities that affect pulmonary, cardiac, renal, or hepatic function)
- Performance status
- Weight loss
- Human papillomavirus status
- Symptom burden
- Social support system
- Extent of prior treatment
- Compliance

Antineoplastic Agent or Targeted Therapy Factors
- Type and dose of drug
- Route of administration
- Single agent versus combination therapy
- Combination with definitive locoregional therapy
- Timing of administration (e.g., neoadjuvant, concomitant, sequential)
- Therapeutic index: toxicity and side effects (all modalities combined)

Note. Based on information from Choong & Vokes, 2012; Fury, 2012; Murphy, 2011.

Chemotherapy administration is based on the principles of pharmacokinetics, including bioavailability, distribution, metabolism, and excretion (Tortorice, 2011). Chemotherapy may not be an option for patients who have comorbidities that may influence the metabolism or excretion of antineoplastic agents, such as impaired renal or hepatic function. Key patient characteristics that can limit the use of chemotherapy include weight loss, extensive prior treatment, increased symptom burden, and poor performance status. Older adult patients are even more at risk for chemotherapy-related toxicities and are less likely to have survival benefits from treatment (Sarris, Harrington, Saif, & Syrigos, 2014).

Chemotherapy consists of several different classes of drugs that exert their effect through various mechanisms of action, are given by various routes for specific indications, and have a variety of side effects and nursing implications. Although cisplatin has been the most widely used, several antineoplastic agents have been used in variable schedules and combinations (see Figures 8-2 and 8-3). Many of the same chemotherapy drugs and regimens used in squamous cell carcinomas are also active in nasopharyngeal cancers. When determining the treatment plan, it is critical to con-

sider the therapeutic index and potential impact on the individual's symptom burden and quality of life for all proposed modalities.

Organ Preservation

In the past, advanced squamous cell carcinomas of the larynx were usually treated with extensive surgery and post-

Figure 8-2. Medications Active in Patients With Head and Neck Cancer

Chemotherapeutic Agents	Monoclonal Antibody
• Bleomycin	• Cetuximab*
• Capecitabine	
• Carboplatin	
• Cisplatin	
• Docetaxel	
• Doxorubicin	
• 5-Fluorouracil	
• Gemcitabine	
• Hydroxyurea	
• Ifosfamide	
• Methotrexate	
• Paclitaxel	
• Vincristine	
• Vinorelbine	

* Not effective for nasopharyngeal cancer

Note. Based on information from Choong & Vokes, 2012; Fury, 2012; Murphy, 2011; National Comprehensive Cancer Network®, 2015.

Figure 8-3. Chemotherapy and Targeted Therapy Regimens Used in Patients With Head and Neck Cancer

- Cisplatin + 5-fluorouracil (5-FU)
- Cisplatin + docetaxel
- Paclitaxel + cisplatin + 5-FU
- Docetaxel + cisplatin + 5-FU
- Cisplatin + paclitaxel
- Cisplatin + gemcitabine
- Cisplatin + 5-FU + cetuximab
- Cisplatin + methotrexate + 5-FU
- Cisplatin + methotrexate + bleomycin + vincristine
- Cisplatin + 5-FU + interferon
- Cisplatin + epirubicin + paclitaxel
- Cisplatin + bevacizumab
- Carboplatin + paclitaxel
- Carboplatin + 5-FU
- Carboplatin + docetaxel
- Docetaxel + carboplatin + 5-FU
- Carboplatin + 5-FU + cetuximab
- Carboplatin + gemcitabine
- Carboplatin + paclitaxel
- 5-FU + hydroxyurea
- Gemcitabine + vinorelbine

Note. Based on information from Choong & Vokes, 2012; Fury, 2012; Murphy, 2011, 2013; National Comprehensive Cancer Network®, 2015.

operative radiation therapy. In the 1980s, a pivotal trial evaluated the efficacy of induction chemotherapy with cisplatin and 5-fluorouracil (5-FU) followed by radiation therapy, with the goal of larynx preservation, improved quality of life, and comparable response rates (Department of Veterans Affairs Laryngeal Cancer Study Group, 1991). The larynx was preserved through neoadjuvant chemotherapy, and overall survival was comparable to that with surgery prior to radiation therapy. Subsequent clinical trials have evaluated various chemotherapy combinations to treat advanced cancers of the larynx, nasopharynx, and oropharynx, with the strategy to downstage locally advanced tumors to preserve organs and structures essential for speech and swallowing (Fury, 2012). Recently, three meta-analyses were published that evaluated the growing number of randomized clinical trials that have incorporated induction chemotherapy (Blanchard et al., 2013; Ma et al., 2012; OuYang et al., 2013).

Ma et al. (2012) evaluated 40 randomized trials between 1965 and 2011 to determine the specific effect of induction chemotherapy in patients with squamous cell head and neck cancers on locoregional control, rate of distant metastasis, toxicity, response to induction chemotherapy, and survival. In general, the results of their meta-analysis did not show any benefit for induction chemotherapy prior to either locoregional treatment or radiation therapy. However, a significant advantage in overall survival ($p = 0.01$) was found when the analysis was limited to studies that used cisplatin with 5-FU for induction chemotherapy.

Blanchard et al. (2013) evaluated five randomized trials to determine differences in efficacy and toxicity profiles of induction chemotherapy regimens (cisplatin with 5-FU compared with or without a taxane) in patients with locally advanced squamous cell head and neck cancers. Their meta-analysis found that the addition of a taxane to the cisplatin with 5-FU regimen resulted in a significant decrease in locoregional failures ($p = 0.007$), as well as improvement in progression-free ($p < 0.001$) and overall survival ($p < 0.001$). Based on these results, the National Comprehensive Cancer Network® (NCCN®) has recommended that the combination of docetaxel, cisplatin, and 5-FU be administered when induction chemotherapy is utilized for most squamous cell carcinomas of the head and neck (NCCN, 2015). Although this meta-analysis supported the established superiority of a taxane-based regimen for induction chemotherapy, it did not compare the efficacy of this neoadjuvant regimen with locoregional treatment or concurrent radiation therapy.

OuYang et al. (2013) compared 11 randomized trials—five neoadjuvant and six adjuvant chemotherapy—to determine differences in efficacy in patients with nasopharyngeal cancer. This meta-analysis found improved overall survival ($p = 0.03$) and decreased distant metastases ($p = 0.0002$) in patients who received neoadjuvant or induction chemotherapy. In contrast, those who received adjuvant chemotherapy

had decreased locoregional recurrence rates ($p = 0.03$) but did not have any improvement in distant metastases or overall survival.

Studies that were published after the aforementioned meta-analyses were completed have consistent findings confirming the benefit of induction chemotherapy compared to radiation therapy alone in locoregional control. These benefits do not extend to overall survival between patients who receive induction chemotherapy followed by concurrent chemoradiotherapy versus those who receive only concomitant chemoradiotherapy alone (Forastiere et al., 2013; Haddad et al., 2013; Herman et al., 2014; Hitt et al., 2014). Lefebvre et al. (2013) found similar outcomes when comparing induction chemotherapy followed either by concurrent chemoradiotherapy or radiation therapy combined with cetuximab. Although induction chemotherapy has shown a benefit in regard to organ preservation, it comes at the cost of longer treatment duration and additional toxicity. In addition, studies have not shown it to be superior to chemoradiotherapy (Cmelak, 2013). Further studies need to be done to determine whether taxane-based induction chemotherapy regimens improve progression-free and overall survival over chemoradiotherapy.

Concomitant Versus Sequential Chemotherapy

Pignon, le Maître, Maillard, Bourhis, and the MACH-NC Collaborative Group (2009) evaluated 87 randomized trials between 1994 and 2000 to determine the benefit of induction, concomitant, or adjuvant chemotherapy in patients with cancers of the oral cavity, oropharynx, hypopharynx, and larynx. Results of their meta-analysis confirmed a significant benefit of chemotherapy for overall survival ($p < 0.0001$). Moreover, there was a significantly greater benefit from concomitant chemotherapy over induction chemotherapy in overall survival ($p < 0.0001$). Of note, although platinum drugs (e.g., cisplatin, carboplatin) had a significantly higher effect on survival ($p < 0.006$) compared to other single agents, when monotherapy was compared to combination chemotherapy regimens, there were no significant differences in overall survival.

The benefit of concurrent chemoradiotherapy over induction chemotherapy has also been found in patients with nasopharyngeal cancer (Chen et al., 2013; Wu et al., 2013). Although nasopharyngeal cancers are acutely sensitive to radiation, concurrent chemoradiotherapy has been found to be superior to radiation therapy alone (Lee et al., 2010; Murphy, 2011). This benefit of combined modality is consistent with other locally advanced squamous cell carcinomas of the head and neck (Chitapanarux, Tharavichitkul, Kamnerdsupaphon, Pukanhapan, & Vongtama, 2013). Concomitant or concurrent chemotherapy with radiation therapy has therefore become the standard of care for locally advanced squamous cell carcinoma of the head and neck (NCCN, 2015).

As stated earlier, sequential chemotherapy describes the administration of a predetermined number of induction chemotherapy cycles after evaluating for response and prior to proceeding with another treatment (e.g., chemoradiotherapy). Because the role of induction chemotherapy is unclear at this time, the use of sequential chemotherapy does not appear to be a viable option, as it prolongs treatment duration with increased toxicity (Baxi, Sher, & Pfister, 2014). However, direct comparisons between taxane-based induction regimens and chemoradiotherapy have yet to be evaluated. As different chemotherapy, targeted agents, and combination regimens that have efficacy in head and neck cancer regimens are introduced, survival and toxicity outcomes will need to be reevaluated.

Several methods have been evaluated to determine the best approach for improving outcomes while minimizing toxicities with concomitant chemoradiotherapy. These have included variations in the use of chemotherapy (e.g., single-agent versus combination regimens, dosing, timing), radiation therapy (e.g., fraction size, total dose, schedule), and cetuximab (Fury, 2012). Although combination chemotherapeutic agents have proved to be more effective than single-agent therapy, they may be associated with a higher toxicity profile. For this reason, the evaluation of less-toxic chemotherapeutic agents with equivalent efficacy, such as carboplatin compared to cisplatin (Wilkins et al., 2013) and capecitabine compared to 5-FU (Gupta, Khan, Barik, & Negi, 2013), may improve patient tolerance and compliance to treatment.

In summary, the clinical evidence to date continues to demonstrate that concomitant chemoradiotherapy is the most effective approach associated with improved overall survival in locally advanced head and neck cancers. However, the combined use of chemotherapy with radiation therapy results in increased side effects. Several studies are ongoing to evaluate the ideal combinations and schedules in terms of overall survival, toxicities, and quality of life.

Systemic Treatment for Recurrent or Metastatic Disease

Treatment of recurrent or metastatic disease is more challenging than that of locally advanced squamous cell head and neck carcinomas. This is because of the aggressiveness of the disease with corresponding increased symptom burden, poorer patient performance, and residual toxicities from prior treatments. The goal of chemotherapy becomes palliative in an effort to control the disease and related symptoms. Several single-agent and combination chemotherapy regimens have been used, but response rates are limited (Denaro et al., 2014; Murphy, 2013; Xu et al.,

2013). Careful consideration should therefore be given to patients' performance status. Cetuximab may be useful in this setting, either as a single agent or in combination with chemotherapy, because it has been found to improve survival (Murphy, 2013).

Ongoing Clinical Research

In general, studies are ongoing to determine which chemotherapeutic agents and combined modalities are most effective in treating patients with squamous cell carcinoma of the head and neck. Further research is needed to determine which antineoplastic or targeted agents are the most effective in achieving locoregional control, organ preservation, and overall survival while minimizing toxicity and long-term side effects (Fury, 2012).

Studies evaluating several alternative chemotherapeutic agents (e.g., pemetrexed, nedaplatin, albumin-bound paclitaxel) are ongoing (Denaro et al., 2014). Pemetrexed is an antimetabolite, similar to 5-FU, and therefore has been considered a novel chemotherapeutic agent for squamous cell carcinomas of the head and neck (Argiris, Pennella, Koustenis, Hossain, & Obasaju, 2013). Early trials demonstrated activity in this population, but the only phase III clinical trial published to date compared pemetrexed and cisplatin to cisplatin alone and did not find any benefit in overall survival (Urba et al., 2013). Further studies with other chemotherapeutic agents or cetuximab may be warranted (Argiris, 2013).

Alternative routes of chemotherapy administration are also being examined. Although intra-arterial chemotherapy has been most widely studied in head and neck cancer, findings are limited by small, early-phase studies (Damascelli, Patelli, & Ticha, 2014). Similar to current chemoradiotherapy protocols, cisplatin has been the most common antineoplastic agent used and has been given in combination with fractionated or hyperfractionated radiation therapy. Rasch et al. (2010) compared intra-arterial versus IV cisplatin in combination with radiation therapy and found significantly less renal toxicity with the intra-arterial route (p < 0.0001). However, no benefit in disease-free or overall survival was found. Ackerstaff et al. (2012) reviewed quality-of-life measures and found no differences between patients who received intra-arterial versus IV chemotherapy.

Approximately 90% of head and neck squamous cell carcinomas express epidermal growth factor receptors (EGFRs), and it is overexpressed in 20%–43% of patients (Bauman & Ferris, 2014; Cohen, 2014). Therefore, EGFR is currently one of the most extensively studied targets, with cetuximab being the first mAb approved for treatment. Other antibodies currently in clinical trials include bevacizumab, panitumumab, zalutumumab, and nimotuzumab. Several small-molecule inhibitors of EGFR include gefitinib, erlotinib, lapatinib, afatinib, and dacomitinib; these are also being evaluated for potential efficacy in head and neck cancers.

In a recent meta-analysis, Zhang, Chen, Jiang, Ma, and Yang (2012) found that anti-EGFR mAbs were effective in improving progression-free and overall survival for locally advanced, as well as recurrent and metastatic, head and neck cancers. Tyrosine kinase inhibitors (TKIs), however, were not found to provide any benefit for either locally advanced or metastatic disease (Zhang et al., 2012). In contrast, a meta-analysis by Petrelli and Barni (2012) found significantly increased response rates in patients who were receiving anti-EGFR therapies. Recently published studies involving the use of TKIs have been disappointing, however, and sufficient data are not yet available for many ongoing trials (Cohen, 2014; Hsu et al., 2014; Limaye et al., 2013). More than 90% of squamous cell head and neck carcinomas also express angiogenic factors, such as vascular endothelial growth factor (VEGF). Studies currently evaluating bevacizumab, vandetanib, sorafenib, and sunitinib are underway (Agulnik, 2012; Hsu et al., 2014).

Another avenue for research is tailoring treatment for human papillomavirus (HPV) infection associated with carcinomas of the oropharynx. Because HPV is a viral infection, immunotherapy has been proposed as a potential treatment (Gildener-Leapman, Lee, & Ferris, 2014). HPV has been found to be a favorable prognostic factor in recurrent or metastatic disease, and patients who are HPV-positive tend to respond well to multimodal therapy (Argiris et al., 2014). In one retrospective study, however, HPV status did not predict response to cetuximab (Vermorken et al., 2014).

In summary, several opportunities exist for exploring novel chemotherapeutic or targeted agents, as well as different combinations or schedules of administering current antineoplastics. The use of biomarkers, such as HPV status, may be useful in the future to further tailor treatments to individuals.

The Nursing Role

Nurses have a responsibility to be aware of their patients' diagnosis, stage of disease, and goals of care, as these factors direct the treatment plan. The administration of chemotherapy requires specialized training and knowledge in order to ensure that it is given safely. The Oncology Nursing Society (ONS) has published a position statement that provides recommendations for this training. It incorporates an understanding of the principles of chemotherapeutic agents, pharmacology, administration procedures, safe handling, patient assessments (including monitoring and symptom management), and patient education (ONS, 2015). Nursing responsibilities continue throughout the treatment plan and include evaluation of the patient prior to, during, and after chemotherapy administration.

The individualized treatment plan is based on cancer and patient characteristics. Prior to the initiation of chemotherapy or any other treatment modality, it is important to review and document patients' diagnosis, current treatment history, pertinent medical history, current medication regimen, and allergies. It is crucial to obtain patients' current weight, as chemotherapy doses are based on their body surface area and are calculated using their height and weight (Polovich, Olsen, & LeFebvre, 2014).

Nursing assessment prior to chemotherapy administration for patients with head and neck cancer should include a baseline physical assessment that examines condition of the lips, tongue, buccal mucosa, gums and teeth, hard and soft palates, and oropharynx (Ellis, 2014). At the time of diagnosis, it has been found that as many as 60% of patients are malnourished, increasing to as high as 88% during chemoradiotherapy (Alshadwi et al., 2013; Langius et al., 2013). For this reason, a referral to a dietitian for a nutritional evaluation should be completed prior to starting therapy. This is warranted because individualized dietary counseling has been shown to significantly benefit nutritional status and quality of life. The use of prophylactic feeding tubes, however, remains controversial. Romesser et al. (2012) found that the placement of percutaneous gastrostomy in patients receiving chemoradiotherapy did not improve albumin levels or decrease acute toxicity such as dysphagia or mucositis (Romesser et al., 2012).

Patients' veins should be evaluated to determine whether they have adequate venous access or if a central line will need to be placed (Camp-Sorrell, 2011). A careful review of the regimen for antineoplastic agents with vesicant or irritant properties and how they will be given may also indicate whether a venous access device may be indicated. 5-FU, a known irritant, can be given either as an IV push or by continuous infusion. However, when it is administered as a continuous infusion, a central venous catheter is preferable because of the potential for severe phlebitis when given peripherally.

Nurses must be familiar with the specific agent(s) being administered, particularly pertinent recent laboratory parameters to review prior to treatment (e.g., complete blood count [CBC] with differential, liver function tests [LFTs], renal function), potential side effects (especially dose-limiting toxicities), and any relevant requirements for adequate hydration, premedications (including, but not limited to, antiemetics), and monitoring recommendations. For example, the most commonly used chemotherapy drug for the head and neck cancer population, cisplatin, has been known to cause acute and delayed nausea and vomiting. The emetogenic potential of individual agents or combinations needs to be assessed to ensure that appropriate antiemetics are prescribed for the entire duration of expected nausea and vomiting (Tipton, 2014). The American Society of Clinical Oncology (ASCO), Multinational Association of Supportive Care in Cancer, and NCCN have developed guidelines regarding the use of antiemetics (Basch et al., 2011; Ettinger et al., 2012; Jordan, Gralla, Jahn, & Molassiotis, 2014). When chemotherapy is combined with radiation therapy, antiemetics should be geared toward the specific antineoplastic agents being used (Basch et al., 2011). Based on these guidelines, when cisplatin is given as monotherapy or in a combination regimen, a three-drug antiemetic regimen would be indicated that would include a serotonin antagonist, a neurokinin-1 (NK_1) antagonist, and a corticosteroid. Because nausea and vomiting can occur soon after the administration of chemotherapy, it is essential that patients be given prophylactic antiemetics.

Finally, prior to starting chemotherapy, patients should be queried for their understanding of the treatment plan and their willingness to proceed. Patient and caregiver education regarding the prevention and management of treatment side effects is crucial. Of equal importance is informing patients to promptly report changes, such as nausea and vomiting not controlled by antiemetics, inability to maintain adequate fluids, difficulty swallowing or talking, or pain.

During administration of chemotherapy, nurses must be careful to follow safe handling recommendations (Polovich, 2011). Care must be given to promote safe medication administration by double-checking each individual antineoplastic agent with another chemotherapy-competent licensed person at the chair- or bedside. Nurses should follow the guidelines that were jointly developed by ONS and ASCO (Neuss et al., 2013).

Throughout the treatment continuum, focal assessments of the head and neck region, particularly the oral cavity, are critical. Each area should be critically inspected for color, moisture, swelling, lesions, or any signs of inflammation (Ellis, 2014). Changes may indicate that the patient is dehydrated or malnourished or has an infection. Examination of the nose and sinuses with particular attention to color, swelling, and discharge is similarly important in patients being treated for cancer of the nasopharynx (Ellis, 2014).

Approximately 50% of patients receiving concurrent chemoradiotherapy will experience severe dysphagia and significant mucositis throughout treatment (Romesser, Riaz, Ho, Wong, & Yee, 2014). Mucositis may be accompanied by pain and can significantly decrease quality of life, depending on level of morbidity (Lewis, Brody, Touger-Decker, Parrott, & Epstein, 2014; Wujcik, 2014). Although the prophylactic placement of feeding tubes prior to treatment is controversial, it often becomes necessary, and early placement can ensure greater ability to complete all chemotherapy cycles, as well as maintain nutritional requirements and avoid weight loss (Lewis et al., 2014). Several guidelines exist for the management of mucositis (Lalla et al., 2014; Saunders et al., 2013; Wujcik, 2014).

Fatigue is the most commonly reported problem in patients with cancer; it is multifactorial and can occur throughout the cancer continuum. Chemotherapy and its treatment-related toxicities may intensify the degree of fatigue. Nurses should discuss evidence-based interventions with patients, including exercise, energy-conservation techniques, behavioral approaches to ensuring improved sleep quality, and management of concurrent symptoms (Mitchell, 2014).

Finally, several treatment-related toxicities that patients experience may put them at a significant risk for neutropenic complications (e.g., mucositis that interferes with swallowing, nausea/vomiting, diarrhea, potential for renal insufficiency). It is also important to monitor patients carefully for neutropenia, altered skin integrity, and alterations in the mucosal barrier (Zitella, 2014). Of note, tube feeding and the comorbidity of diabetes mellitus have been found to be independent predictors of febrile neutropenia in patients with head and neck cancer undergoing chemotherapy (Takenaka et al., 2013).

Treatment of head and neck cancers can be challenging for nurses, patients, and caregivers. Nurses need to be aware of the potential toxicities that coincide with the antineoplastic regimens being administered so that they can complete a comprehensive assessment and provide appropriate teaching. Active communication with patients, caregivers, and all members of the treatment team is crucial when determining if patients are experiencing any signs of toxicities from chemotherapy. Nurses should reinforce patient education and manage symptoms as they occur.

Chemotherapeutic and Targeted Agents Used to Treat Head and Neck Cancers

Although several chemotherapy drugs have shown activity against squamous head and neck carcinomas, some are more commonly used. The following section describes many of these agents in detail, including the dose most often used for this population. Agents are listed in the order of most commonly administered.

Cisplatin

Cisplatin is the most commonly used antineoplastic agent for head and neck cancers (Murphy, 2011). It also has the most data to support its use as a radiosensitizer (Choong & Vokes, 2011; Fury, 2012). Therefore, it may be used as a single agent in combination with radiation therapy for locally advanced head and neck cancers, as well as in several combination regimens (as described in Figure 8-3) for locally advanced, metastatic, or recurrent head and neck (including nasopharyngeal) cancers (Murphy, 2011; NCCN, 2015).

Classification
Alkylating agent

Route
IV

Usual Dose
100 mg/m^2 (when given with radiation or in combination regimens, dose may be decreased to 60–75 mg/m^2)

Mechanism of Action
Causes breakage of the double helix, thereby preventing protein, DNA, and RNA synthesis. It is cell cycle nonspecific.

Dose-Limiting Side Effects
• Severe nephrotoxicity
• Myelosuppression, transient (Fury, 2012)

Other Side Effects
• Nausea and vomiting (acute and/or delayed)
• Ototoxicity (e.g., high-frequency hearing loss or tinnitus)
• Peripheral neuropathy
• Hyperuremia
• Hypersensitivity reaction
• Electrolyte abnormalities (e.g., hypomagnesemia, hypokalemia, hypophosphatemia, hypocalcemia)

Nursing Considerations and Management
• A baseline audiogram should be obtained prior to treatment (Polovich et al., 2014).
• Prior to administration, the following laboratory values should be reviewed.
  – CBC with differential
  – Serum creatinine, creatinine clearance (CrCl)
  – Electrolytes (especially potassium and magnesium)
• Verify that patient's labs meet parameters for cisplatin administration and notify physician if white blood cell (WBC) count < 3,000/mm^3; absolute neutrophil count (ANC) < 1,500/mm^3; platelets < 100,000/mm^3; serum creatinine > 1.5 mg/dl; CrCl > 60 ml/min; or for any electrolyte abnormalities prior to administration.
• The drug should be held if serum creatinine is > 1.5 mg/dl to prevent irreversible renal tubular damage (Polovich et al., 2014).
• Amifostine may be used as a chemoprotectant because it selectively protects normal tissue from the effects of chemotherapy and radiation therapy (Wilkes & Barton-Burke, 2014).
  – When used to prevent nephrotoxicity, amifostine is dosed at 740 mg/m^2 in 50 ml of normal saline to be given over five minutes, 30 minutes prior to chemotherapy.
  – It can help prevent or minimize xerostomia for patients with head and neck cancer undergoing radiation treatment.

– Of note, toxicities related to amifostine include hypotension and severe nausea and vomiting. The transient and profound hypotension found with amifostine may occur during or soon after administration. Therefore, it is essential to withhold hypertensive medications the day prior to treatment, encourage adequate hydration prior to administration, and maintain the patient in a supine position. The potential for nausea/vomiting requires premedications that include a serotonin antagonist and corticosteroid.
• Review the orders for completeness.
  – Hydration
  – Antiemetics for acute nausea/vomiting prophylaxis should include a serotonin antagonist, corticosteroid, and NK$_1$ antagonist.
  – Electrolyte replacement and diuretics, if ordered
• Vigorous hydration (e.g., one to two liters of fluid prior to and after administration) is needed to prevent nephrotoxicity. Ensure that patients void prior to and during cisplatin infusion.
• Cisplatin is an irritant that has a vesicant potential if > 20 ml of 0.5 mg/ml is extravasated (Polovich et al., 2014). If extravasation occurs, attempt to aspirate residual cisplatin and apply cold compresses.

Patient Education
• Immediate side effects (within 24 hours)
  – Nausea or vomiting can begin within one to two hours after receiving cisplatin and can last for 24–48 hours (Polovich et al., 2014). Nausea may continue or recur for several days.
  – Loss of appetite may occur 24–48 hours after treatment.
  – Allergic reactions can occur but are rare.
• Early side effects (within one week)
  – Diarrhea may occur but usually subsides within a day.
  – Kidney damage may occur unless cisplatin is given with large amounts of IV and oral fluids.
• Late side effects (after one week post-treatment)
  – A temporary decrease in red blood cell (RBC), WBC, and platelet counts may occur 7–14 days after treatment. This usually is mild and does not warrant any intervention or alteration in dosage or treatment plan.
  – Tinnitus or difficulty hearing may occur after the initial treatment and may persist or worsen after subsequent doses.
  – Temporary thinning or loss of hair may occur several weeks after treatment.
  – Numbness, tingling, or burning in the hands and feet may occur after several treatments but is uncommon.
• During cisplatin infusion, report any signs of
  – An allergic reaction (e.g., hives, itching, tightness in the chest or throat, trouble breathing)
  – Irritation or extravasation (e.g., redness, burning, pain, swelling, leaking of fluids in area of IV infusion).

• Take antiemetics as instructed. Doses should not be skipped, even if no nausea is noted. Call if experiencing nausea or vomiting that is not controlled with current antiemetic regimen or if unable to maintain hydration.
• Drink at least two liters of fluid a day for 72 hours and report any potential signs of kidney problems (e.g., difficulty urinating, blood in urine, increasing weight).
• Report any potential signs or symptoms of electrolyte problems (e.g., muscle pain or weakness, abnormal heartbeats, confusion).
• Report any signs or symptoms of infection (e.g., fever of 100.4°F [38°C] or higher, chills).
• Notify physician of any changes in hearing or unusual feelings of numbness or tingling in hands or feet.

Carboplatin

Carboplatin has a mechanism of action similar to cisplatin but is less nephrotoxic and exhibits more myelosuppression (Fury, 2012). Therefore, it is often substituted for cisplatin in several combination regimens. Cisplatin has a higher response rate than carboplatin when used as a single agent for recurrent disease (Murphy, 2011). Similar to cisplatin, it is also a radiosensitizer (Choong & Vokes, 2011).

Classification
Alkylating agent

Route
IV

Usual Dose
Target area under the curve (AUC) of 5

Mechanism of Action
Breaks the DNA helix strand, thereby interfering with DNA replication. It is cell cycle nonspecific.

Dose-Limiting Side Effect
• Thrombocytopenia

Other Side Effects
• Neutropenia (Myelosuppression is more pronounced with renal impairment.)
• Nausea and vomiting (acute and/or delayed)
• Hypersensitivity can occur after several cycles (approximately fifth or sixth cycle).
• Renal and hepatic toxicity
• Hyperuremia
• Electrolyte abnormalities (e.g., hyponatremia, hypomagnesemia, hypokalemia, hypocalcemia)
• Peripheral neuropathy (Schwartz, Rockey, Surati, & Gullatte, 2014)

Nursing Considerations and Management
• Prior to administration, the following laboratory values should be reviewed.
  – CBC with differential
  – Serum creatinine
  – LFTs
• Verify that patient's labs meet parameters for carboplatin administration and notify physician if WBC < 3,000/mm³; ANC < 1,500/mm³; platelets < 100,000/mm³; serum creatinine > 1.5 mg/dl; or abnormal LFTs prior to administration.
• Double-check carboplatin dose based on AUC, calculation of glomerular filtration rate, and Calvert formula (Polovich et al., 2014).
• Review the orders for completeness.
  – Antiemetics for acute nausea/vomiting prophylaxis should include a serotonin antagonist and a corticosteroid.
  – Hydration is usually not necessary because carboplatin is less nephrotoxic and doses are based on renal function.
• Carboplatin is considered an irritant (Polovich et al., 2014).
• If given in combination with a taxane, carboplatin is generally given first to decrease myelosuppression (Polovich et al., 2014).

Patient Education
• Immediate side effects (within 24 hours)
  – Nausea or vomiting can begin within hours after receiving carboplatin and can last for 72 hours (Polovich et al., 2014).
  – Allergic reactions (e.g., flushing, shortness of breath, low blood pressure, hives, itching) can occur but are more common with the fifth or sixth cycles of administration rather than the initial dose.
• Late side effects (after one week post-treatment)
  – A temporary decrease in RBC, WBC, and platelet counts may occur 7–14 days after treatment. This usually is mild and does not warrant any intervention or alteration in dosage or treatment plan.
  – Temporary elevations in LFTs may occur but usually do not warrant any intervention or alteration in dosage or treatment plan.
  – Temporary thinning or loss of hair may occur several weeks after treatment.
  – Numbness, tingling, or burning in the hands and feet may occur after several treatments but are uncommon.
• During carboplatin infusion, report any signs of
  – An allergic reaction (e.g., hives, itching, tightness in the chest or throat, trouble breathing)
  – Irritation (e.g., redness, aching, or pain in area of IV infusion).
• Antiemetics should be taken as instructed. Doses should not be skipped, even if no nausea is noted. Notify physician if

experiencing nausea or vomiting that is not controlled with current antiemetic regimen or if unable to maintain fluids.
- Report any potential signs or symptoms of electrolyte problems (e.g., muscle pain or weakness, abnormal heartbeats, confusion).
- Report any signs or symptoms of infection (e.g., fever of 100.4°F [38°C] or higher, chills) or bleeding (e.g., dark or tarry stool, unusual bruising).
- Notify physician of any changes in hearing or unusual feelings of numbness or tingling in hands or feet.

5-Fluorouracil

5-FU has efficacy as a single agent but is generally given in conjunction with other chemotherapeutic agents in treating squamous cell carcinoma of the head and neck (Murphy, 2011). Of note, patients with a genetic dihydropyrimidine dehydrogenase deficiency will have increased toxicity because of prolonged clearance of the drug (Schwartz et al., 2014).

Classification
Antimetabolite

Route
IV

Usual Dose
1,000 mg/m² per day for 4–5 days

Mechanism of Action
Acts in S phase and inhibits enzyme production for DNA synthesis, leading to strand breaks or premature chain termination. It is considered cell cycle specific.

Dose-Limiting Side Effects
- Mucositis
- Myelosuppression

Other Side Effects
- Nausea
- Vomiting
- Anorexia
- Diarrhea
- Alopecia
- Photosensitivity
- Darkening of the veins
- Dry skin
- Ocular toxicity
- Cardiac toxicity (rare)

Nursing Considerations and Management
- Prior to administration, the following laboratory values should be reviewed.
  - CBC with differential
  - Serum creatinine
  - LFTs
- Verify that patient's labs meet parameters for 5-FU administration and notify physician if WBC < 3,000/mm³; ANC < 1,500/mm³; platelets < 100,000/mm³; serum creatinine > 1.5 mg/dl; or for any LFT abnormalities prior to administration.
- Review the orders for completeness.
- 5-FU is an irritant that can cause severe phlebitis and therefore should be administered through a central line when given by continuous infusion (Polovich et al., 2014).

Patient Education
- Immediate side effects (within 24 hours)
  - Discomfort at IV site as a result of irritant properties of the drug
  - Increased darkening along the vein
- Early side effects (within one week)
  - Mucositis
  - Diarrhea
  - Skin reactions
- Late side effects (after one week post-treatment)
  - A temporary decrease in RBC, WBC, and platelet counts may occur 7–14 days after treatment. This usually is mild and does not warrant any intervention or alteration in dosage or treatment plan.
  - Darkening of the nail beds, skin, and veins in which the drug was given may begin four to six weeks after treatment and may persist.
  - Temporary thinning or loss of hair may occur several weeks after treatment.
  - Photophobia, conjunctivitis, and watering of the eyes may occur three to four weeks after treatment.
- During the 5-FU infusion, report any signs of irritation (e.g., redness, aching, or pain in area of IV infusion).
- Perform oral care after meals and prior to bedtime and observe mouth for any redness, swelling, or sores. Report any mouth sores or difficulty maintaining hydration or nutrition.
- Report any diarrhea.
- Report any signs or symptoms of infection (e.g., fever of 100.4°F [38°C] or higher, chills).
- Sun exposure increases skin reactions. Follow photosensitivity precautions (e.g., wear protective clothing and use sunscreen [SPF 15 or greater] when in the sun).

Capecitabine

Capecitabine has efficacy as a single agent for metastatic or recurrent squamous cell (including nasopharyngeal) cancers (Murphy, 2011; NCCN, 2015). Its toxicity profile is similar to 5-FU but with some exceptions. Of note, ongoing studies are evaluating the substitution of capecitabine for 5-FU in regimens where locally advanced disease is warranted (Ahn, Kim, Sohn, Sin, & Lee, 2013; Gupta et al., 2013).

Classification
Antimetabolite

Route
Oral

Mechanism of Action
Acts in S phase and inhibits enzyme production for DNA synthesis, leading to strand breaks or premature chain termination and therefore is cell-cycle specific.

Dose-Limiting Side Effects
• Palmar-plantar erythrodysesthesia
• Diarrhea

Other Side Effects
• Myelosuppression (especially anemia)
• Nausea
• Vomiting
• Mucositis
• Fatigue
• Elevated LFTs
• Photosensitivity
• Skin rashes and/or itching
• Nail changes
• Cardiac toxicity (rare)

Nursing Considerations and Management
• Prior to administration, the following laboratory values should be reviewed.
  – CBC with differential
  – LFTs
• Verify that patient's labs meet parameters for capecitabine administration and notify physician if WBC < 3,000/mm³; ANC < 1,500/mm³; platelets < 100,000/mm³; or for any LFT abnormalities prior to administration.
• Review the orders for completeness.
• Multiple drug interactions can occur (e.g., warfarin).

Patient Education
• Immediate side effects (within 24 hours)
  – Nausea and vomiting
• Early side effects (within one week)
  – Mucositis
  – Diarrhea
  – Skin reactions
• Late side effects (after one week post-treatment)
  – A temporary decrease in RBC, WBC, and platelet counts may occur 7–14 days after treatment.
  – Redness, swelling, blistering, peeling, and discomfort in the palms of the hands and/or soles of the feet may occur.

– Changes in the nails may develop and persist.
• Take medication within 30 minutes after eating with plenty of water.
• Monitor skin for any changes and notify physician of any redness or discomfort.
• Perform oral care after meals and prior to bedtime and observe mouth for any redness, swelling, or sores. Report any mouth sores or difficulty maintaining hydration or nutrition.
• Report any diarrhea.
• Report any signs or symptoms of infection (e.g., fever of 100.4°F [38°C] or higher, chills).
• Sun exposure increases skin reactions. Follow photosensitivity precautions (e.g., wear protective clothing and use sunscreen [SPF 15 or greater] when in the sun).

Paclitaxel

Paclitaxel is a radiosensitizer, but compared to other chemotherapeutic agents, it causes increased mucositis (Fury, 2012). It is used in combination regimens for locally advanced, metastatic, and recurrent squamous cell (including nasopharyngeal) carcinomas (Murphy, 2011; NCCN, 2015).

Classification
Plant alkaloid, taxane

Route
IV

Usual Dose
175–250 mg/m² every three weeks, or 60–120 mg/m² if given weekly

Mechanism of Action
Stabilizes microtubules to inhibit cell division. Effective in G_2 and M phases and therefore is cell cycle specific.

Dose-Limiting Side Effects
• Hypersensitivity reaction
• Peripheral neuropathy (Polovich et al., 2014)

Other Side Effects
• Myelosuppression (dose dependent) (Schwartz et al., 2014)
• Alopecia
• Myalgia
• Fatigue
• Bradycardia

Nursing Considerations and Management
• Consider a baseline multigated acquisition (MUGA) scan or echocardiogram to evaluate left ventricular ejection fraction (LVEF) in patients with cardiac risk factors prior to treatment (Schwartz et al., 2014).

- Prior to administration, the following laboratory values should be reviewed.
  - CBC with differential
  - Serum creatinine
  - LFTs
- Verify that patient's labs meet parameters for paclitaxel administration and notify physician if WBC < 3,000/mm³; ANC < 1,500/mm³; platelets < 100,000/mm³; or for any LFT abnormalities prior to administration.
- Review the orders for completeness.
  - Premedications to prevent hypersensitivity reactions are prescribed, including
    * Corticosteroids (e.g., dexamethasone 20 mg IV)
    * H₂ receptor antagonist (e.g., cimetidine 300 mg, famotidine 20 mg IV)
    * H₁ receptor antagonist (e.g., diphenhydramine 50 mg IV).
- Administer paclitaxel using non–polyvinyl chloride (PVC) bags and tubing with a 0.2 micron in-line filter.
- When combined with a platinum drug, paclitaxel is generally given first to lessen the severity of myelosuppression (Polovich et al., 2014).
- Paclitaxel is an irritant that has vesicant potential if extravasated. If extravasation occurs, attempt to aspirate residual paclitaxel and apply cold compresses (Polovich et al., 2014).
- Monitor vital signs frequently during infusion and at least one hour after infusion, especially with first infusion.

Patient Education
- Immediate side effects (within 24 hours)
  - Allergic reactions (e.g., urticaria, facial flushing, trouble breathing) can occur within the initial 15–60 minutes of the administration. Premedications are given prior to paclitaxel; however, reactions can still occur, so the nurse will monitor frequently (especially with the first cycle).
  - Fatigue
  - Mild nausea and vomiting
- Early side effects (within one week)
  - Mucositis and/or diarrhea
  - Joint pain and body aches
- Late side effects (after one week post-treatment)
  - A temporary decrease in RBC, WBC, and platelet counts may occur 7–10 days after treatment.
  - Temporary partial or complete loss of hair may occur.
  - Numbness, tingling, or burning in the hands and feet may occur and worsen with subsequent treatments.
- During the paclitaxel infusion, report any signs of
  - An allergic reaction (e.g., hives, itching, tightness in the chest or throat, trouble breathing)
  - Irritation or extravasation (e.g., redness, burning, pain, swelling, leaking of fluids in area of IV infusion).
- Acetaminophen may be helpful to relieve any joint pain or body aches. Notify physician if pain or aches are not relieved with acetaminophen.

- Report any signs or symptoms of infection (e.g., fever of 100.4°F [38°C] or higher, chills).
- Notify physician of any changes or unusual feelings of numbness or tingling in hands or feet.

Docetaxel

Docetaxel is similar to paclitaxel but with a slightly different toxicity profile. It is also considered a radiosensitizer and is used in combination regimens for locally advanced, metastatic, and recurrent squamous cell (including nasopharyngeal) carcinomas (Murphy, 2011; NCCN, 2015).

Classification
Plant alkaloid, taxane

Route
IV

Usual Dose
75–100 mg/m² every three weeks, or 30–40 mg/m² if given weekly (Murphy, 2011)

Mechanism of Action
Stabilizes microtubules to inhibit cell division. Effective in G_2 and M phases and therefore is cell cycle specific.

Dose-Limiting Side Effect
- Myelosuppression (Schwartz et al., 2014)

Other Side Effects
- Fluid retention, which can lead to weight gain and pulmonary edema
- Hypersensitivity reaction
- Peripheral neuropathy
- Alopecia
- Skin and nail changes
- Stomatitis
- Myalgia
- Fatigue (Polovich et al., 2014)

Nursing Considerations and Management
- Prior to administration, the following laboratory values should be reviewed.
  - CBC with differential
  - Serum creatinine
  - LFTs
- Verify that patient's labs meet parameters for docetaxel administration and notify physician if WBC < 3,000/mm³; ANC < 1,500/mm³; platelets < 100,000/mm³; or for any LFT abnormalities prior to administration.
- Review the orders for completeness, in particular that premedications to prevent fluid retention and hypersensitivity reactions are prescribed, including corticosteroids (i.e.,

dexamethasone 8 mg BID starting the day before treatment for a total of three days).
- Administer docetaxel using non-PVC bags and tubing with a 0.2 micron in-line filter.
- When combined with a platinum drug, docetaxel is generally given first to lessen the severity of myelosuppression (Polovich et al., 2014).
- Docetaxel is an irritant that has vesicant potential if extravasated. If extravasation occurs, attempt to aspirate residual docetaxel and apply cold compresses (Polovich et al., 2014).

Patient Education
- Immediate side effects (within 24 hours)
  - Allergic reactions (e.g., urticaria, facial flushing, trouble breathing) can occur within the initial 15–60 minutes of the administration. Premedications are given prior to docetaxel; however, reactions can still occur, so the nurse will monitor the infusion frequently (especially with the first cycle).
  - Fatigue
  - Mild nausea and vomiting
- Early side effects (within one week)
  - Mucositis and/or diarrhea
  - Joint pain and body aches
- Late side effects (after one week post-treatment)
  - A temporary decrease in RBC, WBC, and platelet counts may occur 7–10 days after treatment.
  - Temporary partial or complete loss of hair may occur.
- During the docetaxel infusion, report any signs of
  - An allergic reaction (e.g., hives, itching, tightness in the chest or throat, trouble breathing)
  - Irritation or extravasation (e.g., redness, burning, pain, swelling, leaking of fluids in area of IV infusion).
- Acetaminophen may be helpful to relieve any joint pain or body aches. Notify physician if pain or aches are not relieved with acetaminophen.
- Report any signs or symptoms of infection (e.g., fever of 100.4°F [38°C] or higher, chills).
- Notify physician of weight gain and/or shortness of breath.

Doxorubicin

Doxorubicin has shown activity in salivary gland (NCCN, 2015) and nasopharyngeal (Murphy, 2011) cancers but is not widely used.

Classification
Antitumor antibiotic

Route
IV

Mechanism of Action
Binds with DNA, thereby inhibiting DNA and RNA synthesis. It is cell cycle nonspecific.

Dose-Limiting Side Effects
- Myelosuppression
- Cardiotoxicity (lifetime dose of 550 mg/m^2)
- Hepatotoxicity (Polovich et al., 2014)

Other Side Effects
- Nausea and vomiting
- Alopecia
- Mucositis
- Photosensitivity
- Radiation recall (acute inflammatory reaction confined to radiation areas)
- Drug may turn urine red.

Nursing Considerations and Management
- A baseline MUGA or echocardiogram must be done to evaluate LVEF prior to treatment.
- Prior to administration, the following laboratory values should be reviewed.
  - CBC with differential
  - Serum creatinine
  - Electrolytes (especially potassium and magnesium)
- Verify that patient's labs meet parameters for doxorubicin administration and notify physician if WBC < 3,000/mm^3; ANC < 1,500/mm^3; platelets < 100,000/mm^3; serum creatinine > 1.5 mg/dl; or for any LFT abnormalities prior to administration.
- Calculate current total dose and notify physician if approaching lifetime dose limit.
- Review the orders for completeness; antiemetics for acute nausea/vomiting prophylaxis should include a serotonin antagonist and corticosteroid.
- Doxorubicin may cause flare reaction.
- Monitor IV site prior to, during (every 2–5 ml), and after completion of doxorubicin administration for signs and symptoms of extravasation (Polovich et al., 2014). If extravasation occurs, attempt to aspirate residual doxorubicin, administer antidote (i.e., dexrazoxane), and apply cold compresses for 15–20 minutes at least four times within the first 24 hours. Remove at least 15 minutes prior to dexrazoxane (Polovich et al., 2014).
  - Dexrazoxane hydrochloride, when used for anthracycline extravasations, is dosed at 1,000 mg/m^2 on days 1 and 2, then 500 mg/m^2 on day 3 and infused over one to two hours in a large vein that is in a different area than where the extravasation occurred.
  - The first infusion should be initiated as soon as possible and no later than within six hours of the extravasation.

Patient Education
- Immediate side effects (within 24 hours)
  - Flare reaction (localized allergic reaction) evidenced by itching, blotches, or streaking along vein may occur during doxorubicin administration.

- Extravasation evidenced by redness, swelling, loss of blood return, and pain may occur during or shortly after doxorubicin administration.
- Nausea or vomiting can begin within one to three hours after receiving doxorubicin and can last for 24–48 hours (Polovich et al., 2014).
- Urine may appear pink or red in color and persist up to 48 hours after treatment.
• Early side effect (within one week)
  - Mucositis
• Late side effects (after one week post-treatment)
  - A temporary decrease in RBC, WBC, and platelet counts may occur 10–14 days after treatment.
  - Temporary thinning or loss of hair may occur two to four weeks after treatment.
  - Redness of the skin can develop in areas where the patient previously received radiation therapy.
  - Damage to the heart muscle can occur (especially when nearing cumulative dose limits). MUGA scans, electrocardiograms, and echocardiograms are performed at periodic intervals to monitor patient's status.
• During the doxorubicin administration, report any signs of
  - A local allergic reaction (e.g., hives, itching)
  - Extravasation (e.g., redness, burning, pain, swelling, leaking of fluids in area of IV infusion).
• Antiemetics should be taken as instructed. Doses should not be skipped, even in the absence of nausea. Call physician if experiencing nausea or vomiting that is not controlled with current antiemetic regimen or if unable to maintain fluids.
• Report any signs or symptoms of infection (e.g., fever of 100.4°F [38°C] or higher, chills).
• Sun exposure increases skin reactions. Follow photosensitivity precautions (e.g., wear protective clothing and use sunscreen [SPF 15 or greater] when in the sun).
• Report any potential signs or symptoms of cardiotoxicity (e.g., weight gain, ankle swelling, abnormal heartbeats, shortness of breath).

Methotrexate

Methotrexate has efficacy as a single agent against squamous cell carcinomas of the head and neck (Murphy, 2011) and is used mainly for palliation.

Classification
Antimetabolite

Route
IV

Usual Dose
40–60 mg/m^2

Mechanism of Action
Acts in S phase; inhibits enzyme production for DNA synthesis, leading to strand breaks or premature chain termination. It is cell cycle specific.

Dose-Limiting Side Effects
• Hepatotoxicity
• Renal toxicity (Polovich et al., 2014)

Other Side Effects
• Mucositis
• Nausea
• Myelosuppression
• Photosensitivity
• Fatigue

Nursing Considerations and Management
• Prior to administration, the following laboratory values should be reviewed.
  - CBC with differential
  - Serum creatinine
  - LFTs
• Verify that patient's labs meet parameters for methotrexate administration and notify physician if WBC < 3,000/mm^3; ANC < 1,500/mm^3; platelets < 100,000/mm^3; serum creatinine > 1.5 mg/dl; or any LFT abnormalities prior to administration.
• Review the orders for completeness, including antiemetics for acute nausea/vomiting.
• Multiple drug interactions can occur (e.g., warfarin).

Patient Education
• Immediate side effects (within 24 hours)
  - Nausea or vomiting can occur after receiving methotrexate. However, it is dose-related and therefore not generally problematic with doses used for head and neck carcinomas.
• Early side effects (within one week)
  - Diarrhea may occur but usually subsides within a day.
  - Kidney damage can occur but generally is more associated with higher doses of methotrexate.
  - Photosensitivity
• Late side effects (after one week post-treatment)
  - A temporary decrease in RBC, WBC, and platelet counts may occur five to seven days after treatment (Schwartz et al., 2014).
  - Temporary thinning or loss of hair may occur several weeks after treatment.
• Antiemetics should be taken as instructed. Call physician if experiencing nausea or vomiting that is not controlled with current antiemetic regimen or if unable to maintain fluids.
• Perform oral care after meals and prior to bedtime and observe mouth for any redness, swelling, or sores. Report

any mouth sores or difficulty maintaining hydration or nutrition.
• Avoid taking multivitamins with folic acid.
• Report any signs or symptoms of infection (e.g., fever of 100.4°F [38°C] or higher, chills) or bleeding (e.g., dark or tarry stool, unusual bruising).

Gemcitabine

Gemcitabine binds to DNA, interfering with synthesis of DNA and, to a lesser extent, RNA and protein synthesis. Gemcitabine is a radiosensitizer and is highly effective in nasopharyngeal cancers that are refractory to platinum agents (Choong & Vokes, 2011).

Classification
Antimetabolite

Route
IV

Usual Dose
1,000 mg/m² weekly

Mechanism of Action
Binds with DNA, thereby inhibiting DNA and RNA synthesis. It is cell cycle specific.

Dose-Limiting Side Effect
• Myelosuppression (especially thrombocytopenia) (Polovich et al., 2014)

Other Side Effects
• Fever and flulike symptoms
• Nausea and vomiting
• Pulmonary toxicity
• Fatigue

Nursing Considerations and Management
• Prior to administration, the following laboratory values should be reviewed.
  – CBC with differential
  – Serum creatinine
  – Electrolytes (especially potassium and magnesium)
• Verify that patient's labs meet parameters for gemcitabine administration and notify physician if WBC < 3,000/mm³; ANC < 1,500/mm³; platelets < 100,000/mm³; serum creatinine > 1.5 mg/dl; or any LFT abnormalities prior to administration.
• Review the orders for completeness.

Patient Education
• Immediate side effects (within 24 hours)
  – Nausea or vomiting

• Early side effects (within one week)
  – Diarrhea
  – Generalized edema
• Late side effects (after one week post-treatment)
  – A temporary decrease in RBC, WBC, and platelet counts may occur 7–14 days after treatment.
• Antiemetics should be taken as instructed. Doses should not be skipped, even if no nausea is noted. Call physician if experiencing nausea or vomiting that is not controlled with current antiemetic regimen or if unable to maintain fluids.
• Report any signs or symptoms of infection (e.g., fever of 100.4°F [38°C] or higher, chills) or bleeding (e.g., dark or tarry stool, unusual bruising).

Bleomycin

Bleomycin has limited and short-lived efficacy against nasopharyngeal cancer (Murphy, 2011).

Classification
Antitumor antibiotic

Route
IV or intramuscular

Usual Dose
10–20 mg/m² weekly

Mechanism of Action
Binds with DNA, thereby inhibiting DNA and RNA synthesis and is cell cycle specific.

Dose-Limiting Side Effects
• Pulmonary fibrosis
• Hypersensitivity (rare) (Polovich et al., 2014)

Other Side Effects
• Fever and chills
• Mucositis
• Alopecia
• Photosensitivity
• Renal toxicity
• Hepatotoxicity

Nursing Considerations and Management
• A baseline pulmonary function test should be obtained prior to treatment (Polovich et al., 2014).
• Prior to administration, the following laboratory values should be reviewed.
  – CBC with differential
  – Serum creatinine
• Verify that patient's labs meet parameters for bleomycin administration and notify physician if WBC < 3,000/mm³; ANC < 1,500/mm³; platelets < 100,000/mm³; serum cre-

atinine > 1.5 mg/dl; or CrCl > 60 ml/min prior to administration.
- Review the orders for completeness.
- Bleomycin is an irritant.
- Bleomycin often causes flulike symptoms.
- Cumulative lifetime dose of bleomycin should not exceed 400 units. Higher doses can result in pulmonary fibrosis.
- Calculate current total dose and notify physician if approaching lifetime dose limit.

Patient Education
- Immediate side effects (within 24 hours)
  - Fever and/or chills can begin within 4–6 hours after receiving bleomycin and can last for approximately 12 hours (Schwartz et al., 2014).
- Early side effect (within one week)
  - Hyperpigmentation
- Late side effect (after one week post-treatment)
  - Pulmonary toxicity
- During the bleomycin infusion, report any signs of
  - An allergic reaction (e.g., hives, itching, tightness in the chest or throat, trouble breathing)
  - Irritation (e.g., redness, burning, pain or discomfort in area of IV infusion).
- Acetaminophen should be taken as instructed.
- History of bleomycin must be disclosed if anesthesia is required for any surgical intervention (Polovich et al., 2014).
- Report any potential signs or symptoms of respiratory problems (e.g., cough, shortness of breath).
- Report any signs or symptoms of infection (e.g., fever of 100.4°F [38°C] or higher, chills).

Hydroxyurea

Hydroxyurea has been used in combination with other chemotherapeutic agents for induction therapy for organ preservation, as well as with concurrent radiation therapy for squamous cell carcinomas (NCCN, 2015).

Classification
Miscellaneous

Route
Oral

Mechanism of Action
Interferes with DNA synthesis phase similar to antimetabolites and is therefore cell cycle specific.

Dose-Limiting Side Effect
- Myelosuppression (Polovich et al., 2014)

Other Side Effects
- Nausea

- Vomiting
- Mucositis
- Diarrhea
- Renal toxicity
- Fever
- Hyperuricemia
- Hepatotoxicity

Nursing Considerations and Management
- Prior to administration, the following laboratory values should be reviewed.
  - CBC with differential
  - Serum creatinine
  - LFTs
- Verify that patient's labs meet parameters for hydroxyurea administration and notify physician if WBC < 3,000/mm^3; ANC < 1,500/mm^3; platelets < 100,000/mm^3; serum creatinine > 1.5 mg/dl; or abnormal LFTs prior to administration.
- Review the orders for completeness.

Patient Education
- Immediate side effects (within 24 hours)
  - Nausea and vomiting
- Early side effects (within one week)
  - Mucositis
  - Diarrhea
  - Rashes
- Late side effect (after one week post-treatment)
  - Myelosuppression
- Report any nausea or vomiting that is not controlled with antiemetics or if unable to maintain fluids.
- Report any signs or symptoms of infection (e.g., fever of 100.4°F [38°C] or higher, chills).

Ifosfamide

Ifosfamide has activity against head and neck squamous cell carcinomas and has been utilized in combination regimens for metastatic or recurrent disease (Murphy, 2011).

Classification
Alkylating agent

Route
IV

Usual Dose
1,000 mg/m^2/day

Mechanism of Action
Breaks the DNA helix strand, thereby interfering with DNA replication. It is cell cycle nonspecific.

Dose-Limiting Side Effects
- Hemorrhagic cystitis
- Myelosuppression (Polovich et al., 2014)

Other Side Effects
- Nausea and vomiting
- Alopecia
- Neurotoxicity

Nursing Considerations and Management
- Prior to administration, the following laboratory values should be reviewed.
  - CBC with differential
  - Serum creatinine
  - LFTs
  - Urine to assess for blood
- Verify that patient's labs meet parameters for ifosfamide administration and notify physician if WBC < 3,000/mm³; ANC < 1,500/mm³; platelets < 100,000/mm³; serum creatinine > 1.5 mg/dl; CrCl > 60 ml/min prior to administration; any LFT abnormalities; or blood in urine.
- Review the orders for completeness.
  - Antiemetics for acute and delayed nausea/vomiting
  - Mesna (equivalent to 60%–100% of ifosfamide dose) to prevent hemorrhagic cystitis
- Ifosfamide is an irritant.

Patient Education
- Immediate side effects (within 24 hours)
  - Hemorrhagic cystitis
  - Nausea and vomiting
  - Neurotoxicity
- Early side effect (within one week)
  - Myelosuppression
- Late side effect (after one week post-treatment)
  - Alopecia
- During the ifosfamide infusion, report any signs of irritation (e.g., redness, burning, pain, or discomfort in area of IV infusion).
- Report any nausea or vomiting that is not controlled with antiemetics or if unable to maintain fluids.
- Report any signs or symptoms of infection (e.g., fever of 100.4°F [38°C] or higher, chills).
- Report any signs or symptoms of difficulty with urination, including pain or bleeding.

Vincristine

Vincristine has been utilized in combination regimens for metastatic or recurrent squamous cell carcinomas of the head and neck (NCCN, 2015).

Classification
Plant alkaloid

Route
IV

Mechanism of Action
Blocks DNA production in the G_2 phase and prevents cell division during mitosis. It is cell cycle specific.

Dose-Limiting Side Effect
- Neurotoxicity (Polovich et al., 2014)

Other Side Effects
- Peripheral neuropathy
- Constipation
- Foot drop
- Alopecia
- Renal toxicity
- Hepatotoxicity
- Extravasation

Nursing Considerations and Management
- Intrathecal administration is fatal (Polovich et al., 2014).
- Prior to administration, review the following laboratory values.
  - Serum creatinine
  - LFTs
- Verify that patient's labs meet parameters for vincristine administration and notify physician if serum creatinine > 1.5 mg/dl or any LFT abnormalities prior to administration.
- Assess patient for any peripheral neuropathy.
- Review the orders for completeness.
- Vincristine is a vesicant.
- Monitor IV site prior to, during (every 5–10 ml if given by IV piggyback), and after completion of vincristine administration for signs/symptoms of extravasation (Polovich et al., 2014). If extravasation occurs, attempt to aspirate residual vincristine, administer antidote (i.e., hyaluronidase), and apply warm compresses for 15–20 minutes four times a day for the first 24 hours.
- Hyaluronidase, when used for vinca alkaloid extravasations, is drawn up as 1 ml (equivalent to 150 units) and administered as five separate injections of 0.2 ml each subcutaneously around the area of infiltration, using a 25-gauge or smaller needle, which is changed with each injection (Polovich et al., 2014).

Patient Education
- Immediate side effect (within 24 hours)
  - Extravasation evidenced by redness, swelling, loss of blood return, and pain may occur during or shortly after vincristine administration.
- Late side effects (after one week post-treatment)
  - Neurotoxicity
  - Peripheral neuropathy
  - Constipation

- During vincristine infusion, report any signs of extravasation (e.g., redness, burning, pain, or discomfort in area of IV infusion).
- Report any peripheral neuropathy (e.g., feeling of numbness or tingling in hands or feet).
- Report any difficulty with constipation or abdominal pain.

Vinorelbine

Vinorelbine has shown activity against squamous cell head and neck (including nasopharyngeal) carcinomas (NCCN, 2015).

Classification
Plant alkaloid

Route
IV

Mechanism of Action
Blocks DNA production in the G_2 phase and prevents cell division during mitosis. It is cell cycle specific.

Dose-Limiting Side Effect
- Myelosuppression (Polovich et al., 2014)

Other Side Effects
- Nausea
- Vomiting
- Peripheral neuropathy
- Constipation
- Alopecia
- Hepatotoxicity
- Extravasation

Nursing Considerations and Management
- Intrathecal administration is fatal (Polovich et al., 2014).
- Prior to administration, the following laboratory values should be reviewed.
  - CBC with differential
  - Serum creatinine
  - LFTs
- Verify that patient's labs meet parameters for vinorelbine administration and notify physician if WBC < 3,000/mm³; ANC < 1,500/mm³; platelets < 100,000/mm³; serum creatinine > 1.5 mg/dl; CrCl > 60 ml/min prior to administration; or any LFT abnormalities.
- Assess patient for any peripheral neuropathy.
- Review the orders for completeness.
- Vinorelbine is a vesicant.
- Monitor IV site prior to, during (every 5–10 ml), and after completion if given by IV infusion for signs/symptoms of extravasation (Polovich et al., 2014). If extrav-

asation occurs, attempt to aspirate residual vinorelbine, administer antidote (i.e., hyaluronidase), and apply warm compresses for 15–20 minutes four times a day for the first 24 hours.
- Hyaluronidase, when used for vinca alkaloid extravasations, is drawn up as 1 ml (equivalent to 150 units) and administered as five separate injections of 0.2 ml each subcutaneously around the area of infiltration, using a 25-gauge or smaller needle (Polovich et al., 2014).

Patient Education
- Immediate side effect (within 24 hours)
  - Extravasation evidenced by redness, swelling, loss of blood return, and pain may occur during or shortly after vinorelbine administration.
- Late side effects (after one week post-treatment)
  - Neurotoxicity
  - Peripheral neuropathy
  - Constipation
- During the vinorelbine infusion, report any signs of extravasation (e.g., redness, burning, pain, or discomfort in area of IV infusion).
- Report any nausea or vomiting that is not controlled with antiemetics or if unable to maintain fluids.
- Report any signs or symptoms of infection (e.g., fever of 100.4°F [38°C] or higher, chills).
- Report any peripheral neuropathy (e.g., feeling of numbness or tingling in hands or feet).
- Report any difficulty with constipation or abdominal pain.

Cetuximab

Cetuximab is a mAb and EGFR inhibitor (Schwartz et al., 2014) that is used alone or in combination with radiation therapy for locally advanced squamous cell carcinoma. It is also combined with chemotherapy for recurrent or metastatic disease (NCCN, 2015).

Classification
EGFR inhibitor and mAb

Route
IV

Usual Dose
Initial dose of 400 mg/m² over two hours, followed by weekly doses of 250 mg/m² over one hour

Mechanism of Action
Binds to the extracellular domain of EGFR, thereby blocking phosphorylation and activation of receptor-associated kinases, resulting in growth inhibition, apoptosis, and decreased VEGF production.

Common Side Effects
- Acne-like rash
- Generalized weakness, malaise
- Fever with or without infusion reaction
- Electrolyte abnormalities, especially hypomagnesemia, hypokalemia, and hypocalcemia

Other Side Effects
- Nausea and vomiting
- Anorexia
- Stomatitis
- Diarrhea
- Nail changes
- Infusion reactions
- Elevated LFTs

Nursing Considerations and Management
- Prior to administration, the following laboratory values should be reviewed.
  - CBC with differential
  - Serum creatinine
  - Electrolytes (especially magnesium)
  - LFTs
- Verify that patient's labs meet parameters for cetuximab administration and notify physician if WBC < 3,000/mm³; ANC < 1,500/mm³; platelets < 100,000/mm³; serum creatinine > 1.5 mg/dl; or for any electrolyte or LFT abnormalities prior to administration.
- Review the orders for completeness, including premedications to prevent hypersensitivity reactions.
- Premedicate with an H₁ antagonist.
- Monitor vital signs frequently during infusion and at least one hour after infusion, especially with first infusion.
- Administer oral or topical antibiotics for rash.
- Monitor magnesium, calcium, and potassium levels for eight weeks after last dose.

Patient Education
- Immediate side effects (within 24 hours)
  - Hypersensitivity reactions can occur.
  - Fever is possible irrespective of whether a hypersensitivity reaction occurs.
- Early to late side effects (within one week)
  - Low magnesium levels (may occur up to eight weeks after the completion of treatment)
  - Nail changes
- During the cetuximab infusion, patients should report any signs of an allergic reaction (e.g., hives, itching, tightness in the chest or throat, trouble breathing).
- Report any potential signs or symptoms of electrolyte problems (e.g., muscle pain or weakness, abnormal heartbeats, confusion).

Summary

Although chemotherapy used alone is not effective for overall survival, it has been integrated into the standard of care for locally advanced, recurrent, and metastatic disease. The combination of chemotherapy with radiation therapy has been proved to be effective in minimizing functional and cosmetic morbidities in patients with laryngeal cancer.

Prospective clinical trials are ongoing to examine chemotherapy drugs, targeted agents, and combined modalities, as well as varied dosing and/or timing approaches, for their effectiveness in achieving locoregional control, organ preservation, and overall survival, while minimizing toxicity and long-term side effects.

Nurses play a major role in caring for this patient population throughout the continuum of care. It is essential to perform a comprehensive physical assessment, paying particular attention to the head and neck region, as well as evaluating for any comorbidities that may influence the patient's overall well-being. This assessment should be started prior to the initiation of therapy and continue during and after completion.

Nursing assessment should also include patient support systems and coping strategies. Additionally, nurses need to stay on the front line for educating patients and their caregivers regarding their cancer treatment plan and potential toxicities. Finally, nurses are patient advocates, communicating pertinent findings with other members of the healthcare team and assisting with referrals to other disciplines, as warranted.

The author would like to acknowledge Jill Solan, RN, MS, ANP, OCN®, and Mary Jo Dropkin, PhD, RN, for their contributions to this chapter that remain unchanged from the first edition of this book.

References

Ackerstaff, A.H., Rasch, C.R.N., Balm, A.J.M., de Boer, J.P., Wiggenraad, R., Rietveld, D.H., … Hilgers, F.J. (2012). Five-year quality of life results of the randomized clinical phase III (RADPLAT) trial, comparing concomitant intra-arterial versus intravenous chemoradiotherapy in locally advanced head and neck cancer. *Head and Neck, 34,* 974–980. doi:10.1002/hed.21851

Agulnik, M. (2012). New approaches to EGFR inhibition for locally advanced metastatic squamous cell carcinoma of the head and neck (SCCHN). *Medical Oncology, 29,* 2481–2491. doi:10.1007/s12032-012-0159-2

Ahn, D., Kim, J.H., Sohn, J.H., Sin, C.M., & Lee, J.E. (2013). Laryngeal preservation in stage III/IV resectable laryngo-hypopharyngeal squamous cell carcinoma following concurrent chemoradiotherapy with capecitabine/cisplatin. *Molecular and Clinical Oncology, 1,* 685–691. doi:10.3892/mco.2013.113

Alshadwi, A., Nadershah, M., Carlson, E.R., Young, L.S., Burke, P.A., & Daley, B.J. (2013). Nutritional considerations for head and neck cancer patients: A review of the literature. *Journal of Oral and Maxillofacial Surgery, 71,* 1853–1860. doi:10.1016/j.joms.2013.04.028

Argiris, A. (2013). Current status and future directions in induction chemotherapy for head and neck cancer. *Critical Reviews in Oncology/Hematology, 88*, 57–74. doi:10.1016/j.critrevonc.2013.03.001

Argiris, A., Li, S., Ghebremichael, M., Egloff, A.M., Wang, L., Forastiere, A.A., ... Mehra, R. (2014). Prognostic significance of human papillomavirus in recurrent or metastatic head and neck cancer: An analysis of Eastern Cooperative Oncology Group trials. *Annals of Oncology, 25*, 1410–1416. doi:10.1093/annonc/mdu167

Argiris, A., Pennella, E., Koustenis, A., Hossain, A.M., & Obasaju, C.K. (2013). Pemetrexed in head and neck cancer: A systematic review. *Oral Oncology, 49*, 492–501. doi:10.1016/j.oraloncology.2013.01.007

Basch, E., Prestrud, A.A., Hesketh, P.J., Kris, M.G., Feyer, P.C., Somerfield, M.R., ... Lyman, G.H. (2011). Antiemetics: American Society of Clinical Oncology clinical practice guideline update. *Journal of Clinical Oncology, 29*, 4189–4198. doi:10.1200/JCO.2010.34.4614

Bauman, J.E., & Ferris, R.L. (2014). Integrating novel therapeutic monoclonal antibodies into the management of head and neck cancer. *Cancer, 120*, 624–632. doi:10.1002/cncr.28380

Baxi, S.S., Sher, D.J., & Pfister, D.G. (2014). Value considerations in the treatment of head and neck cancer: Radiation, chemotherapy, and supportive care. *American Society of Clinical Oncology Educational Book, 2014*. Retrieved from http://meetinglibrary.asco.org/content/11400296-144

Benasso, M. (2013). Induction chemotherapy for squamous cell head and neck cancer: A neverending story? *Oral Oncology, 49*, 747–752. doi:10.1016/j.oraloncology.2013.04.007

Blanchard, P., Bourhis, J., Lacas, B., Posner, M.R., Vermorken, J.B., Hernandez, J.J., ... Pignon, J.P. (2013). Taxane-cisplatin-fluorouracil as induction chemotherapy in locally advanced head and neck cancers: An individual patient data meta-analysis of chemotherapy in head and neck cancer group. *Journal of Clinical Oncology, 31*, 2854–2860. doi:10.1200/JCO.2012.47.7802

Camp-Sorrell, D. (Ed.). (2011). *Access device guidelines: Recommendations for nursing practice and education* (3rd ed.). Pittsburgh, PA: Oncology Nursing Society.

Chen, Y., Sun, Y., Liang, S.B., Zong, J.F., Li, W.F., Chen, M., ... Ma, J. (2013). Progress report of a randomized trial comparing long-term survival and late toxicity of concurrent chemoradiotherapy with adjuvant chemotherapy versus radiotherapy alone in patients with stage III to IVB nasopharyngeal carcinoma from endemic regions of China. *Cancer, 119*, 2230–2238. doi:10.1002/cncr.28049

Chitapanarux, I., Tharavichitkul, E., Kamnerdsupaphon, P., Pukanhapan, N., & Vongtama, R. (2013). Randomized phase III trial of concurrent chemoradiotherapy vs accelerated hyperfractionation radiotherapy in locally advanced head and neck cancer. *Journal of Radiation Research, 54*, 1110–1117. doi:10.1093/jrr/rrt054

Choong, N.W., & Vokes, E.E. (2012). Chemotherapy for head and neck cancer. In M.C. Perry, D.C. Doll, & C.E. Freter (Eds.), *Perry's the chemotherapy source book* (5th ed., pp. 366–384). Philadelphia, PA: Lippincott Williams & Wilkins.

Cmelak, A.J. (2012). Current issues in combined modality therapy in locally advanced head and neck cancer. *Critical Reviews in Oncology/Hematology, 84*, 261–273. doi:10.1016/j.critrevonc.2012.04.004

Cohen, R.B. (2014). Current challenges and clinical investigations of epidermal growth factor receptor (EGFR)- and ErbB family-targeted agents in the treatment of head and neck squamous cell carcinoma (HNSCC). *Cancer Treatment Reviews, 40*, 567–577. doi:10.1016/j.ctrv.2013.10.002

Damascelli, B., Patelli, G., & Ticha, V. (2014). Transcatheter chemotherapy for malignancies in the brain, head, and neck. In S.T. Kee, R. Murthy, & D.C. Madoff (Eds.), *Clinical interventional oncology* (pp. 227–233). Philadelphia, PA: Elsevier.

Denaro, N., Russi, E.G., Lefebvre, J.L., & Merlano, M.C. (2014). A systematic review of current and emerging approaches in the field of larynx preservation. *Radiotherapy and Oncology, 110*, 16–24. doi:10.1016/j.radonc.2013.08.016

Department of Veterans Affairs Laryngeal Cancer Study Group. (1991). Induction chemotherapy plus radiation compared with surgery plus radiation in patients with advanced laryngeal cancer. *New England Journal of Medicine, 324*, 1685–1690. doi:10.1056/NEJM199106133242402

Ellis, K.K. (2014). Ears, nose, mouth, and throat. In M.E. Estes (Ed.), *Health assessment and physical examination* (5th ed., pp. 407–446). Clifton Park, NY: Delmar Cengage Learning.

Ettinger, D.S., Armstrong, D.K., Barbour, S., Berger, M.J., Bierman, P.J., Bradbury, B., ... Urba, S.G. (2012). Antiemesis. *Journal of the National Comprehensive Cancer Network, 10*, 456–485. Retrieved from http://www.jnccn.org/content/10/4/456.full

Forastiere, A.A., Zhang, Q., Weber, R.S., Maor, M.H., Goepfert, H., Pajak, T.F., ... Cooper, J.S. (2013). Long-term results of RTOG 91-11: A comparison of three nonsurgical treatment strategies to preserve the larynx in patients with locally advanced larynx cancer. *Journal of Clinical Oncology, 31*, 845–852. doi:10.1200/JCO.2012.43.6097

Fury, M. (2012). Chemotherapy. In J.P. Shah, S.G. Patel, & B. Singh (Eds.), *Jatin Shah's head and neck surgery and oncology* (4th ed., pp. 788–799). Philadelphia, PA: Elsevier.

Gildener-Leapman, N., Lee, J., & Ferris, R.L. (2014). Tailored immunotherapy for HPV positive head and neck squamous cell cancer. *Oral Oncology, 50*, 780–784. doi:10.1016/j.oraloncology.2013.09.010

Gupta, S., Khan, H., Barik, S., & Negi, M.P.S. (2013). Clinical benefits of concurrent capecitabine and cisplatin versus concurrent cisplatin and 5-fluorouracil in locally advanced squamous cell head and neck cancer. *Drug Discoveries and Therapeutics, 7*, 36–42. doi:10.5582/ddt.2013.v7.1.36

Haddad, R.I., O'Neill, A., Rabinowits, G.S., Tishler, R., Khuri, F., Adkins, D., ... Posner, M. (2013). Induction chemotherapy followed by concurrent chemoradiotherapy (sequential chemoradiotherapy) versus chemoradiotherapy alone in locally advanced head and neck cancer (PARADIGM): A randomised phase 3 trial. *Lancet Oncology, 14*, 257–264. doi:10.1016/S1470-2045(13)70011-1

Herman, L.C., Chen, L., Garnett, A., Feldman, L.E., Smith, B., Weichselbaum, R.R., & Spiotto, M.T. (2014). Comparison of carboplatin-paclitaxel to docetaxel-cisplatin-5-flurouracil induction chemotherapy followed by concurrent chemoradiation for locally advanced head and neck cancer. *Oral Oncology, 50*, 52–58. doi:10.1016/j.oraloncology.2013.08.007

Hitt, R., Grau, J.J., López-Pousa, A., Berrocal, A., García-Girón, C., Irgoyen, A., ... Cruz-Hernández, J.J. (2014). A randomized phase III trial comparing induction chemotherapy followed by chemoradiotherapy versus chemoradiotherapy alone as treatment of unresectable head and neck cancer. *Annals of Oncology, 25*, 216–225. doi:10.1093/annonc/mdt461

Hsu, H.W., Wall, N.R., Hsueh, C.T., Kim, S., Ferris, R.L., Chen, C.S., & Mirshahidi, S. (2014). Combination antiangiogenic therapy and radiation in head and neck cancers. *Oral Oncology, 50*, 19–26. doi:10.1016/j.oraloncology.2013.10.003

Jordan, K., Gralla, R., Jahn, F., & Molassiotis, M. (2014). International antiemetic guidelines on chemotherapy induced nausea and vomiting: Content and implementation in daily routine practice. *European Journal of Pharmacology, 722*, 197–202. doi:10.1016/j.ejphar.2013.09.073

Lalla, R.V., Bowen, J., Barasch, A., Elting, L., Epstein, J., Keefe, D.M., ... The Mucositis Guidelines Leadership Group of the Multinational Association of Supportive Care in Cancer and the International Society of Oral Oncology (MASCC/ISOO). (2014). MASCC/ISOO clinical practice guidelines for the management of mucositis secondary to cancer therapy. *Cancer, 120*, 1453–1461. doi:10.1002/cncr.28592

Langius, J.A., Zandbergern, M.C., Eerenstein, S.E., van Tulder, M.W., Leemans, C.R., Kramer, M.H., & Weijs, P.J. (2013). Effect of nutritional interventions on nutritional status, quality of life, and mortality in patients with head and neck cancer receiving (chemo)radiotherapy: A systematic review. *Clinical Nutrition, 32*, 671–678. doi:10.1016/j.clnu.2013.06.012

Lee, A.W., Tung, S.Y., Chua, D.T., Ngan, R.K., Chappell, R., Tung, R., ... Lau, W.H. (2010). Randomized trial of radiotherapy plus concurrent-adjuvant chemotherapy vs radiotherapy alone for regionally advanced nasopharyngeal carcinoma. *Journal of the National Cancer Institute, 102*, 1188–1198. doi:10.1093/jnci/djq258

Lefebvre, J.L., Pointreau, Y., Rolland, F., Alfonsi, M., Baudoux, A., Sire, C., ... Bardet, E. (2013). Induction chemotherapy followed by either chemoradiotherapy or bioradiotherapy for larynx preservation: The TREMPLIN randomized phase II study. *Journal of Clinical Oncology, 31*, 853–859. doi:10.1200/JCO.2012.42.3988

Lewis, S.L., Brody, R., Touger-Decker, R., Parrott, J.S., & Epstein, J. (2014). Feeding tube use in patients with head and neck cancer. *Head and Neck, 36*, 1789–1795. doi:10.1002/hed.23538

Limaye, S., Riley, S., Zhao, S., O'Neill, A., Posner, M., Adkins, D., ... Haddad, R. (2013). A randomized phase II study of docetaxel with or without vandetanib in recurrent or metastatic squamous cell carcinoma of head and neck (SCCHN). *Oral Oncology, 49*, 835–841. doi:10.1016/j.oraloncology.2013.04.010

Ma, J., Liu, Y., Huang, X.L., Zhang, Z.Y., Myers, J.N., Neskey, D.M., & Zhong, L.P. (2012). Induction chemotherapy decreases the rate of distant metastasis in patients with head and neck squamous cell carcinoma but does not improve survival or locoregional control: A meta-analysis. *Oral Oncology, 48*, 1076–1084. doi:10.1016/j.oraloncology.2012.06.014

Mitchell, S.A. (2014). Cancer-related fatigue. In C.H. Yarbro, D. Wujcik, & B.H. Gobel (Eds.), *Cancer symptom management* (4th ed., pp. 27–43). Burlington, MA: Jones & Bartlett Learning.

Murphy, B.A. (2011). Carcinomas of the head and neck. In R.T. Skeel & S.N. Khlief (Eds.), *Handbook of cancer chemotherapy* (8th ed., pp. 69–93). Philadelphia, PA: Lippincott Williams & Wilkins.

Murphy, B.A. (2013). To treat or not to treat: Balancing therapeutic outcomes, toxicity, and quality of life in patients with recurrent and/or metastatic head and neck cancer. *Journal of Supportive Oncology, 11*, 149–159. Retrieved from http://www.oncologypractice.com/fileadmin/content_images/jso/SUPONC_11-4_Enhanced.pdf

National Comprehensive Cancer Network. (2015). *NCCN Clinical Practice Guidelines in Oncology (NCCN Guidelines®): Head and neck cancers* [v.1.2015]. Retrieved from http://www.nccn.org/professionals/physician_gls/pdf/head-and-neck.pdf

Neuss, M.N., Polovich, M., McNiff, K., Esper, P., Gilmore, T.R., LeFebvre, K.B., ... Jacobson, J.O. (2013). 2013 updated American Society of Clinical Oncology/Oncology Nursing Society chemotherapy administration safety standards including standards for the safe administration and management of oral chemotherapy. *Journal of Oncology Practice, 9*(Suppl. 2), 5s–13s. doi:10.1200/JOP.2013.000874

Oncology Nursing Society. (2015). Education of the nurse who administers and cares for the individual receiving chemotherapy and biotherapy. Retrieved from https://www.ons.org/advocacy-policy/positions/education/chemotherapy-biotherapy

OuYang, P.Y., Xie, C., Mao, Y.P., Zhang, Y., Liang, X.X., Su, Z., ... Xie, F.Y. (2013). Significant efficacies of neoadjuvant and adjuvant chemotherapy for nasopharyngeal carcinoma by meta-analysis of published literature-based randomized, controlled trials. *Annals of Oncology, 24*, 2136–2146. doi:10.1093/annonc/mdt146

Petrelli, F., & Barni, S. (2012). Anti-EGFR-targeting agents in recurrent or metastatic head and neck cancer: A meta-analysis. *Head and Neck, 34*, 1657–1664. doi:10.1002/hed.21858

Pignon, J.P., le Maître, A., Maillard, E., Bourhis, J., & MACH-NC Collaborative Group. (2009). Meta-analysis of chemotherapy in head and neck cancer (MACH-NC): An update on 93 randomised trials and 17,346 patients. *Radiotherapy and Oncology, 92*, 4–14. doi:10.1016/j.radonc.2009.04.014

Polovich, M. (Ed.). (2011). *Safe handling of hazardous drugs* (2nd ed.). Pittsburgh, PA: Oncology Nursing Society.

Polovich, M., Olsen, M., & LeFebvre, K.B. (Eds.). (2014). *Chemotherapy and biotherapy guidelines and recommendations for practice* (4th ed.). Pittsburgh, PA: Oncology Nursing Society.

Rasch, C.R., Hauptmann, M., Schornagel, J., Wijers, O., Buter, J., Gregor, T., ... Hilgers, F.J. (2010). Intra-arterial versus intravenous chemoradiation for advanced head and neck cancer: Results of a randomized phase 3 trial. *Cancer, 116*, 2159–2165. doi:10.1002/cncr.25234

Romesser, P.B., Riaz, N., Ho, A.L., Wong, R.J., & Yee, N.Y. (2014). Cancer of the head and neck. In J.E. Niederhuber, J.O. Armitage, J.H. Doroshow, M.B. Kastan, & J.E. Tepper (Eds.), *Abeloff's clinical oncology* (5th ed.). Philadelphia, PA: Elsevier Saunders.

Romesser, P.B., Romanyshyn, J.C., Schupak, K.D., Setton, J., Riaz, N., Wolden, S.L., ... Lee, N.Y. (2012). Percutaneous endoscopic gastrostomy in oropharyngeal cancer patients treated with intensity-modulated radiotherapy with concurrent chemotherapy. *Cancer, 118*, 6072–6078. doi:10.1002/cncr.27633

Sarris, E.G., Harrington, K.J., Saif, M.W., & Syrigos, K.N. (2014). Multimodal treatment strategies for elderly patients with head and neck cancer. *Cancer Treatment Reviews, 40*, 465–475. doi:10.1016/j.ctrv.2013.10.007

Saunders, D.P., Epstein, J.B., Elad, S., Allemano, J., Bossi, P., van de Wetering, M.D., ... Lalla, R.V. (2013). Systematic review of antimicrobials, mucosal coating agents, anesthetics, and analgesics for the management of oral mucositis in cancer patients. *Supportive Care in Cancer, 21*, 3191–3207. doi:10.1007/s00520-013-1871-y

Schwartz, R.N., Rockey, M., Surati, M., & Gullatte, M.M. (2014). Antineoplastic agents. In M.M. Gullatte (Ed.), *Clinical guide to antineoplastic therapy: A chemotherapy handbook* (3rd ed., pp. 93–502). Pittsburgh, PA: Oncology Nursing Society.

Takenaka, Y., Cho, H., Yamamoto, M., Nakahara, S., Yamamoto, Y., & Inohara, H. (2013). Incidence and predictors of febrile neutropenia during chemotherapy in patients with head and neck cancer. *Supportive Care in Cancer, 21*, 2861–2868. doi:10.1007/s00520-013-1873-9

Tipton, J. (2014). Nausea and vomiting. In C.H. Yarbro, D. Wujcik, & B.H. Gobel (Eds.), *Cancer symptom management* (4th ed., pp. 213–239). Burlington, MA: Jones & Bartlett Learning.

Tortorice, P.V. (2011). Cytotoxic chemotherapy: Principles of therapy. In C.H. Yarbro, D. Wujcik, & B.H. Gobel (Eds.), *Cancer nursing: Principles and practice* (7th ed., pp. 352–389). Burlington, MA: Jones & Bartlett Learning.

Urba, S., van Herpen, C.M.L., Sahoo, T.P., Shin, D.M., Licitra, L., Mezei, K., ... Hong, R.L. (2012). Pemetrexed in combination with cisplatin versus cisplatin monotherapy in patients with recurrent or metastatic head and neck. *Cancer, 118*, 4694–4705. doi:10.1002/cncr.27449

Vermorken, J.B., Psyrri, A., Mesia, R., Peyrade, F., Beier, F., de Blas, B., ... Licitra, L. (2014). Impact of tumor HPV status on outcome in patients with recurrent and/or metastatic squamous cell carcinoma of the head and neck receiving chemotherapy with or without cetuximab: Retrospective analysis of the phase III EXTREME trial. *Annals of Oncology, 25*, 801–807. doi:10.1093/annonc/mdt574

Wilkes, G., & Barton-Burke, M. (2014). *Oncology nursing drug handbook* (18th ed.). Burlington, MA: Jones & Bartlett Learning.

Wilkins, A.C., Rosenfelder, N., Schick, U., Gupta, S., Thway, K., Nutting, C.M., ... Bhide, S.A. (2013). Equivalence of cisplatin and carboplatin-based chemoradiation for locally advanced squamous cell carcinoma of the head and neck: A matched-pair analysis. *Oral Oncology, 49*, 615–619. doi:10.1016/j.oraloncology.2013.02.004

Wu, X., Huang, P.Y., Peng, P.J., Lu, L.X., Han, F., Wu, S.X., ... Zhang, L. (2013). Long-term follow-up of a phase III study comparing radiotherapy with or without weekly oxaliplatin for locoregionally advanced nasopharyngeal carcinoma. *Annals of Oncology, 24*, 2131–2136. doi:10.1093/annonc/mdt163

Wujcik, D. (2014). Mucositis. In C.H. Yarbro, D. Wujcik, & B.H. Gobel (Eds.), *Cancer symptom management* (4th ed., pp. 403–419). Burlington, MA: Jones & Bartlett Learning.

Xu, T., Tang, J., Gu, M., Liu, L., Wei, W., & Yang, H. (2013). Recurrent nasopharyngeal carcinoma: A clinical dilemma and challenge. *Current Oncology, 20*, e406–e419. doi:10.3747/co.20.1456

Zhang, S., Chen, J., Jiang, H., Ma, H., & Yang, B. (2012). Anti-epidermal growth factor receptor therapy for advanced head and neck squamous cell carcinoma: A meta-analysis. *European Journal of Clinical Pharmacology, 68*, 561–569. doi:10.1007/s00228-011-1194-1

Zitella, L.J. (2014). Infection. In C.H. Yarbro, D. Wujcik, & B.H. Gobel (Eds.), *Cancer symptom management* (4th ed., pp. 131–157). Burlington, MA: Jones & Bartlett Learning.

CHAPTER 9

Postoperative Management

Cheryl A. Brandt, RN, ACNS-BC, CORLN, and Tara DiFabio, RN, CNP, CORLN

Introduction

Patients with postoperative head and neck cancer present to the nursing unit with many challenges. The surgery may result in functional and cosmetic alterations. Basic survival functions, such as eating, breathing, and communicating, may be compromised. Patients often present with comorbid conditions, such as alcohol abuse, tobacco use, malnutrition, multiple organ dysfunctions (e.g., liver, lung, kidney), or peripheral vascular disease. These can delay the healing process and prolong recovery time. Nurses caring for postsurgical patients with head and neck cancer must have the skills to manage these challenges. Nurses must have knowledge of normal anatomy and physiology, as well as postsurgical anatomy and physiology alterations. Insight into short- and long-term postoperative goals and rehabilitation needs also is necessary for successful outcomes. Nursing roles, such as caregivers, teachers, advocates, counselors, and care coordinators, are essential throughout the head and neck cancer care continuum.

A well-coordinated multidisciplinary team is needed for optimum outcomes. Staff nurses, advanced practice nurses (nurse practitioner and clinical nurse specialist), social workers, dietitians, speech pathologists, physical and occupational therapists, discharge planners, and surgeons are the key team members. Goals and objectives need to be mutually agreed upon prior to surgical intervention. Available resources for safe discharge need to be assessed. Sharing information and concerns noted during outpatient interactions with the multidisciplinary team will ensure optimum results (Sievers, 2010).

Airway Management

Airway issues are a common problem for patients with head and neck cancer. It is not unusual for patients with head and neck cancer to present to a clinic or emergency department in airway distress. Patients may present with stridor from a tumor obstructing the airway or from vocal cord paralysis. Knowledge of the anatomy and physiology of the upper aerodigestive tract is fundamental to effective nursing management (see Figure 9-1). Interventions should focus on the prevention of problems, prompt action in emergency situations, and calm support and reassurance of patients and families.

Figure 9-1. Anatomy of a Normal Breather

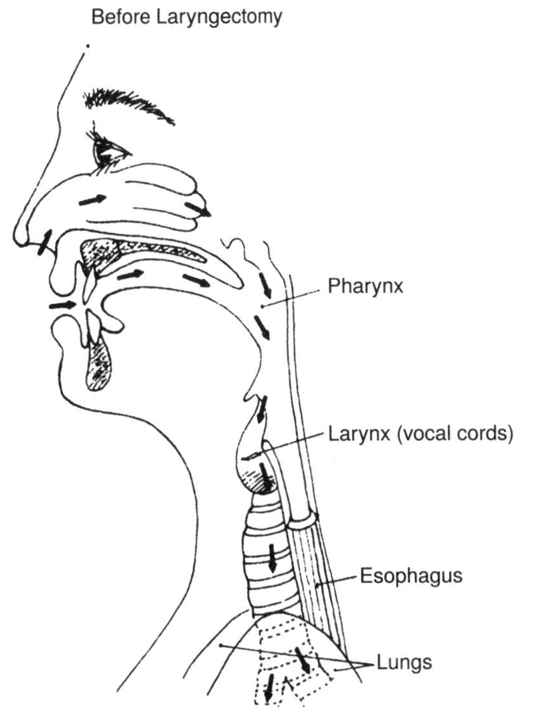

Before Laryngectomy

Pharynx

Larynx (vocal cords)

Esophagus

Lungs

Note. From *Looking Forward: A Guidebook for the Laryngectomee* (3rd ed., p. 9), by R.L. Keith, 1995, New York, NY: Thieme New York. Copyright 1995 by Thieme New York. Reprinted with permission.

Nursing care should focus on positioning patients at a 45° angle or higher to properly align the airway and decrease dependent edema. IV access is necessary for medication administration and adequate hydration. Patients should be kept nil per os (nothing by mouth, or NPO) to prevent aspiration and prepare for radiographic imaging, as well as possible surgical intervention, which may include securing a safe airway. Interventions include the administration of oxygen, nebulizer treatments, epinephrine, slow IV hydration, and heliox (a mixture of helium and oxygen). Fluid balance should be monitored by recording intake and output. Decreasing or limiting patients' activity helps to conserve the work of breathing and promote oxygenation. The increased work of breathing will result in patient fatigue and increased risk of cardiopulmonary arrest (Munday & Semple, 2012). Pulse oximetry is necessary to monitor oxygen saturation. Suction equipment must be available to effectively manage oral secretions. Obtain standard blood chemistry, hematocrit and hemoglobin, and arterial blood gases as ordered. Place a tracheotomy tray or intubation trays with appropriate-sized airways at the bedside. Pain medication, sedation, and anxiolytics should be administered judiciously to prevent further airway compromise.

Prepare patients and caregivers for the possibility of surgical intervention and the need for tracheotomy. If time permits, discuss with patients and families the anatomic and functional changes that will occur following the procedure and alternate methods of communication. Although the capacity to learn during a crisis is limited, the conveyance of knowledge and engagement of trust between the nurse and the adult patient are crucial.

Patients with head and neck cancer often present with a history of chronic obstructive pulmonary disease and chronic bronchitis resulting from a long history of smoking. Tidal volumes may be decreased requiring positive end-expiratory pressure to maintain alveolar ventilation. Chronically ill patients may be anemic and have impaired oxygen-carrying capacity. Comorbid conditions, such as chronic obstructive lung disease, coronary artery disease, and asthma, often require supplemental oxygen to maintain saturations above 95% (Pujade-Lauraine & Gascón, 2004).

Nasal Obstructions

Patients with nasopharyngeal, nasomaxillary, and maxillary orbital tumors presenting with epistaxis and/or nasal obstruction require similar interventions. Patients should be in high Fowler position. Multiple imaging tests, such as computed tomography (CT), magnetic resonance imaging scan, or CT angiography, may be necessary. Interventions to control epistaxis include pinching the nasal ala, applying topical vasoconstrictors (e.g., 0.5% or 1% phenylephrine, 4% cocaine), chemical cautery (e.g., silver nitrate), absorbable hemostatic agents (e.g., absorbable gelatin compressed sponge, oxidized cellu-

lose), nasal packing, and endovascular embolization. If nasal packs are placed, especially posterior nasal packs, risks include nasal trauma, cartilage necrosis, aspiration, infection, and airway obstruction (Jindal, Gemmete, & Gandhi, 2012). Nursing interventions center on airway maintenance, hemodynamic stability, comfort, and pain control.

Tracheotomy

A tracheotomy is a surgical incision into the trachea. The term *tracheostomy* refers to the actual opening into the trachea, or stoma (Mitchell et al., 2013). A tracheotomy often is performed in conjunction with intraoral, pharyngeal, hypopharyngeal, or laryngeal resections to avoid placement of an endotracheal tube in the surgical field and to prevent airway compromise caused by postoperative edema. In this situation, the tracheostomy usually is temporary but may remain in place for the duration of the postoperative course and, if required, through postoperative radiation therapy. A tumor may compromise the airway, resulting in the need for a tracheotomy before initiating definitive cancer treatment. A tracheostomy also can be permanent if airway compromise results in aspiration, dysfunctional larynx, or surgically altered anatomy, such as after a total laryngectomy.

Tracheostomy Tubes

Tracheostomy tubes are selected based on specific patient needs (see Table 9-1). Tracheostomy tubes can be made of plastic (disposable) or stainless steel (reusable) and come in a variety of sizes, lengths, and diameters. The size of the tube (length and diameter) is determined by a patient's anatomy, lung mechanics, upper airway resistance, airway clearance for ventilation, and communication (Mitchell et al., 2013). Some tubes have only a single, outer cannula (no inner tube), whereas most tubes are double cannula with an outer cannula, an inner cannula, and an obturator (see Figure 9-2). The outer cannula remains in the patient at all times, except for routine tube changes. The inner cannula maintains a patent airway and is removed routinely for cleaning (Sievers, 2010). The obturator is used for insertion of the tracheostomy tube and should remain with the patient at all times. A second tracheostomy tube of the same size or one size smaller should be available at the patient's bedside for immediate replacement in the event of inadvertent tube removal.

Tracheostomy tubes may be cuffed or uncuffed. A cuffed tube is placed during the surgical procedure and maintained until mechanical ventilation is no longer required or the patient is no longer at risk for aspiration. When inflated, the cuff seals the space between the tube and the trachea to provide a closed system for positive-pressure ventilation, such as delivery of anesthesia or ventilator support (see Figure 9-3). Cuff pressures should be

	Table 9-1. Tracheostomy Tubes	
Type of Tracheostomy Tube	**Description**	**Reason for Use**
Cuffed	Standard tubes with low-pressure cuff and inner cannula, either reusable or disposable	Initial surgical tubes that are cuff inflated to create a sealed airway for artificial ventilation
Uncuffed	Standard tubes with no cuff; the inner cannula is either reusable or disposable; may be plastic or metal	Interim and permanent tubes used for airway access in the spontaneously breathing patient
Cuffed fenestrated	Standard tubes with cuff and fenestrated outer cannula; only in use when inner cannula is removed (unless inner cannula also is fenestrated)	Used almost exclusively for ventilator patients for speech when a cuff is required to seal the airway
Uncuffed fenestrated	Standard tube, no cuff, fenestrated outer cannula	May be used short term (one to three days) for weaning
Wire-reinforced silicone (also come in endotracheal lengths)	Wire-reinforced silicone-covered tubes that, because of their internal integrity, will not lose their internal diameter in any position; may have adjustable faceplates for exacting placement	Operative tube; used when specific tip placement is required
Extra long	Tubes with longer shafts; usually made of more pliable material; standard tubes but can be custom made in lengths in the proximal or distal portion	Used in patients with excessive skin-to-trachea distance
Sleep apnea	Single-lumen tubes, pliable material; can be capped during the day and opened when asleep for sleep apnea	Used in patients with sleep apnea and patients with head and neck cancer who require slightly longer tubes, possibly because of reconstruction flaps around the airway
Laryngectomy	Shorter but with a larger relative inner diameter; crafted to the shape of a laryngectomy stoma with a more acute curve	After total laryngectomy, in cases where the stoma may be stenotic or obscured by reconstruction flaps or dressings
Laryngectomy buttons	Pliable material used with a pressure fit	For placement in the laryngectomy stoma to keep the airway patent; usually at the skin-trachea suture line
Custom-made	Any of the aforementioned tubes but with custom features to fit a particular patient; extra length, distal or proximal shape, cuff placement, short	Made-to-order tubes designed for a particular patient

checked routinely (Mitchell et al., 2013). Even high-volume, low-pressure cuffs can cause tracheal wall damage by impeding capillary blood flow to the tracheal mucosa, creating necrosis, scarring, and stenosis. An aneroid manometer placed on the cuff inflation valve measures cuff pressure, which should not exceed 20–25 mm Hg (Sievers, 2010). The cuff is deflated when the patient is not on ventilator support or at risk for aspiration.

The tracheostomy tube must be secure and in proper position. Hook-and-loop–type ties or cotton tracheostomy ties secure the tracheostomy tube with the faceplate flush with the neck. Circumferential tracheostomy ties are not indicated in the presence of any type of reconstruction, flap,

graft, or free flap. The tracheostomy tube is sutured in place so as not to put pressure on the reconstruction tissue and the supporting vessels of the flap pedicle (Mitchell et al., 2013; Sievers, 2010). The tube should be positioned in the center of the neck. If the tube is off center, determine the reason, ensure an adequate airway, and discuss the position with a physician.

Tracheostomy Care

Coughing and deep breathing, suctioning, and early ambulation are important aspects of care for the patient with an artificial airway. Tracheostomy care depends on the individual patient's needs and includes saline instillation, suc-

Figure 9-2. Double Cannula Tracheostomy Tube

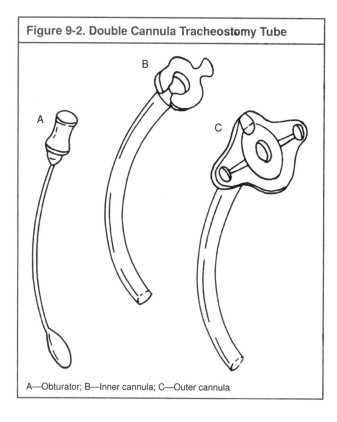

A—Obturator; B—Inner cannula; C—Outer cannula

Figure 9-3. Cuffed Tracheostomy Tube

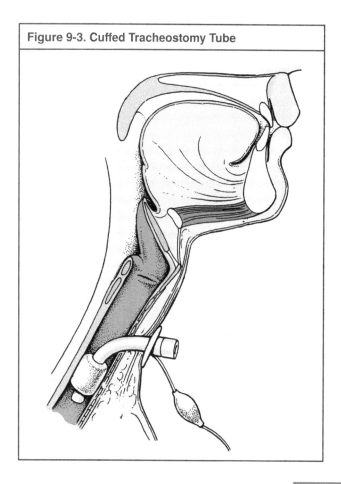

tioning, coughing, surgical incision care, inner cannula care, and patient education directed at self-care. Postoperative head and neck surgery patients often have tenacious, bloody mucus and difficulty mobilizing secretions. Encourage the patient to cough to clear secretions and determine the need for suctioning. Suction when there is audible or visible secretions in the airway, if airway obstruction is suspected, and before and after tracheostomy tube changes (Mitchell et al., 2013). Document the color, amount, and nature of secretions as well as the frequency of suctioning.

Remove and clean the inner cannula of the tube in a solution of equal parts hydrogen peroxide and normal saline. If the inner cannula is disposable, replace it with a clean cannula matching the size of the tracheostomy tube. Clean the stoma site at least every 8–12 hours with half-strength hydrogen peroxide, rinse with normal saline, and dry. Place a tracheostomy dressing or a piece of hydrocolloid dressing under the faceplate of the tube to prevent skin excoriation. Change the dressing when wet or soiled with secretions (Sievers, 2010).

The normal upper airway mechanisms of warming, filtering, and moisturizing inspired air are bypassed when a tracheostomy is present. Supplemental humidity via a mist collar is necessary to protect the normal functioning of the mucociliary blanket and to prevent drying of the tracheal mucosa. Normal saline instillation is used to clear secretions. Slow instillation of 3–5 cc of normal saline or delivery via saline spray bottle will stimulate a cough and help to mobilize secretions (Sievers, 2010). Insufficient clinical evidence is available to definitively support a benefit of saline instillation to patients with tracheostomy, and controversy exists on this practice. Most studies on saline instillation in suctioning focus primarily on critical care patients who are mechanically ventilated. Based on these findings, it is suggested that normal saline instillation not be used (American Association for Respiratory Care, 2010; Caparros, 2014). A study by Hudak and Bond-Domb (1996) with postoperative head and neck surgery patients supported the use of saline following tracheotomy or laryngectomy to increase humidity and stimulate cough. This remains an area of much-needed research to help clarify best evidence-based practice, especially in nonventilated patients with tracheotomy or laryngectomy. Head and neck oncology nurses advocate the use of normal saline instillation and bedside home humidification (Sievers, 2010; Sievers & Donald, 1987).

Self-Care Teaching

Education is a major role for nurses. Patients with head and neck cancer and their families must be taught about the physical changes that have occurred and what they need to do to manage these changes in their day-to-day lives to minimize complications. Teaching should begin early in the postoperative period and, if possible, prior to surgery. Patient and family education regarding tracheostomy will improve outcomes and decrease complications. Recommendations include (Mitchell et al., 2013)

- Develop strategies for teaching and arrange for family members to be present.
- Demonstrate and explain each step of the procedure; assist patients in returning the demonstration.
- Observe patients and families performing the procedures of airway care for 24–48 hours before hospital discharge.
- Make arrangements for patients to have a suction machine and tracheostomy supplies at home and a homecare nurse for support and follow-up.

The goal is for patients to demonstrate competence with tracheostomy care and maintain a patent airway. Patients and caregivers should have a checklist of emergency supplies that remains with them at all times. They should know the type and size of the tracheostomy tube that is in place, as well as have a spare tube of the same type and size. They should know signs and symptoms of respiratory distress, infection, and skin breakdown. Healthcare provider and medical supply company contact information should be provided. Discuss activities of daily living and emergency care with patients and families and provide all instructions in writing (Mitchell et al., 2013).

Tracheostomy self-care teaching includes learning how to change the entire tracheostomy tube. The physician is responsible for the initial tracheostomy tube change. Timing is at the physician's discretion and can vary. The goal is for the tract between the skin and trachea to develop, minimizing complications, such as creation of a false tract, subcutaneous emphysema, mediastinitis, loss of airway, or death (Johnson, 2013). The initial tracheostomy tube change usually occurs on the fifth postoperative day for surgical tracheostomies but can be as early as the third day to facilitate tracheostomy teaching and discharge (Mitchell et al., 2013). Once the airway is stable and a well-formed tract is developed, the entire tracheostomy tube can be changed. Tube changes enhance hygiene, prevent scar stenosis, and minimize the formation of granulation tissue in the stoma area. Ongoing evaluation of patients' ability to safely perform their own care is integral to the education process and safe discharge.

Decannulation

Decannulation, or removal of a temporary tracheostomy tube, is patient dependent. Several questions need to be answered to determine patient readiness (see Figure 9-4). As with all procedures, the process should be explained to patients to ensure understanding. Many physicians also will visually evaluate the integrity of the postsurgical airway by performing a fiber-optic endoscopy. In some instances, weaning patients from a temporary tracheostomy may also be done by downsizing the tube to a smaller, uncuffed tube, allowing for air to flow around the tube into the natural larynx. Patients are taught to cover the tube with a finger

---

Figure 9-4. Prerequisites for Decannulation in Adult Patients

Answer the following to determine readiness of patient for decannulation of tracheostomy tube:

- Have the indications for the tracheostomy placement resolved or significantly improved?
- Is the patient tolerating a decannulation cap on an appropriately sized uncuffed tracheostomy tube without stridor?
- Does fiber-optic laryngoscopy confirm airway patency to the level of the glottis and immediate subglottis?
- Does the patient have an adequate level of consciousness and laryngopharyngeal function to protect the lower airway from aspiration?
- Does the patient have an effective cough while the tracheostomy tube is capped?
- Have all procedures that require general endotracheal anesthesia been completed?

If yes to all, proceed with the following decannulation process:

- Remove the tracheostomy tube.
- Clean the site.
- Cover the site with a dry gauze dressing.
- Instruct the patient to apply pressure over the dressing with fingers when talking or coughing.
- Change dressing daily and as needed if moist with secretions until the site has healed.
- Monitor for decannulation failure.

Note. From "Clinical Consensus Statement: Tracheostomy Care," by R.B. Mitchell, H.M. Hussey, G. Setzen, I.N. Jacobs, B. Nussenbum, C. Dawson, … A. Merati, 2013, *Otolaryngology—Head and Neck Surgery, 148,* p. 16. Copyright 2013 by Sage Publications. Reprinted with permission.

---

when speaking or coughing. Occluding or capping the tracheostomy tube allows patients to breathe through their nose and mouth and to speak. A tracheostomy speaking valve placed on the tube will also permit patients to speak. The return of speech is an acknowledged sign of progress. Patients must be able to coordinate breathing and exhalation with speaking to use either a valve or finger occlusion (Hudak & Hickey, 2008).

When preparing the patient for decannulation, ensure that the tracheostomy tube is capped in the morning to allow for a full day of observation. Monitor oxygen saturation and airway comfort. Uncap the tube if the patient is having any airway distress to allow for unobstructed flow of air. Initially, patients may be uncapped at night, but a trial of capping during sleep is indicated before removing the tube. Remove the tracheostomy tube if the patient tolerates capping for 24 hours.

Place the patient in a sitting position and remove the tube in a downward and curved motion. Place an occlusive dry dressing over the incision and change it when soiled or wet. Instruct the patient to place two fingers over the dressing when talking or coughing to create a seal and promote wound healing. The incision should heal within three to five days. Document the patient's tolerance of the procedure in the chart and monitor for post-decannulation respiratory distress (Mitchell et al., 2013).

Specialty Tracheostomy Tubes

Specialty tracheostomy tubes often are necessary because of alterations in anatomy, either natural or created by a surgical defect. Longer tubes may be required because of anatomic changes, obesity, the presence of reconstruction flaps, or increased skin-to-trachea distance. These usually are single cannula tubes with no inner cannula to remove and clean. Maintain the inner lumen with an increase in humidification using normal saline and mist. Suction the lumen of the tube because secretions often adhere to the distal tip of the tracheostomy tube.

Total Laryngectomy

A total laryngectomy is the removal of the larynx with two to three tracheal rings, resulting in a complete surgical disconnection between the airway and digestive tract. The trachea is sutured to the front of the neck, creating a permanent airway, or stoma (see Figure 9-5). The upper airway (nose and mouth) no longer functions to warm, filter, or humidify air. The patient cannot speak with a normal voice but is able to eat without risk of aspiration once healed. Nursing care focuses on both airway and wound management and communication. The inner wall of the laryngectomy stoma should look similar to the oral mucosa: pink, moist, and glistening. During the healing process, the stoma may be compromised by edema, surgical reconstruction flaps, or the presence of sutures and may require placement of a laryngectomy tube or stoma button.

The nursing focus for patients after a total laryngectomy is to maintain a patent airway. A flashlight or headlight should be at the bedside at all times because proper lighting is imperative to inspect the stoma for crusts and secretions. Bayonet forceps are useful in removing crusts.

When working with patients with a stoma, nurses should protect themselves from secretions by wearing safety eyeglasses, a mask, and gloves. Stoma care will become easier once the sutures are removed.

Self-care teaching begins early in the postoperative period. Patients should begin to perform stoma and wound care as soon as possible. Instruct and support patients in learning to cover the stoma, rather than the mouth, when coughing. Educate patients and families regarding the effects of dry air on the airway. Using a small spray bottle, spray normal saline directly into the stoma. Small particle deposition is an excellent way to add moisture to the airway. At home, bedside humidifiers or cool mist vaporizers can provide additional moisture, particularly with low indoor humidity during the winter. Showers and steam rooms are very helpful for additional moisture. Change of seasons and the inabil-

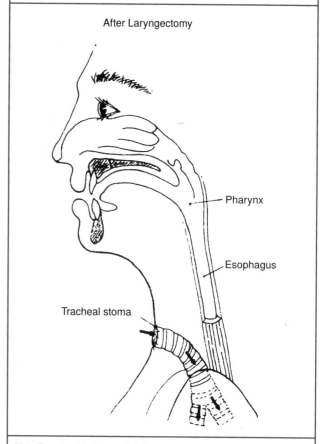

Figure 9-5. Anatomy of a Total Neck Breather (Laryngectomee)

After Laryngectomy

Pharynx

Esophagus

Tracheal stoma

Note. From *Looking Forward: A Guidebook for the Laryngectomee* (3rd ed., p. 9), by R.L. Keith, 1995, New York, NY: Thieme New York. Copyright 1995 by Thieme New York. Reprinted with permission.

ity of patients with a laryngectomy to quickly adapt to dryness may result in tracheitis and an occasional need for hospitalization. The use of humidification, mucolytics, and oral hydration and the avoidance of irritants (e.g., smoking) may prevent further crusting and infection (Hickey & Higgins, 2008).

After total laryngectomy, patients do not have a glottis to close and cannot generate the pressure necessary to produce a normal cough or perform a Valsalva maneuver. This inability to Valsalva, in addition to the use of narcotic analgesics, can lead to constipation. A bowel regimen must become a routine part of life for these patients.

Most airway complications can be prevented by addressing patients' airway needs on a continuous basis (see Table 9-2). Surgical complications include subcutaneous emphysema, bleeding from a slipped ligature, and pneumothorax from a pulmonary bleb rupture or direct injury to the upper lobes of the lung rising above the clavicle and sometimes into the surgical field (Walvekar & Myers, 2008).

Table 9-2. Preventable Airway Complications		
Type	Signs and Symptoms	Nursing Care/Intervention
Obstruction	• Speech without covering tube • "Snoring" with a tracheostomy • Unable to suction via the tube • Patient short of breath or uncomfortable	Humidity, saline, suctioning, inner cannula care, changing the entire tube on a regular basis
Malposition	• Movement of the tube with respiration • Unable to suction via the tube • Patient talking without covering tube • Patient short of breath or uncomfortable	Apply faceplate to the skin, secure with ties or Velcro straps, and resecure often. Ensure tube is appropriate size for the trachea-to-skin distance. Investigate the reason if unable to suction via the tube.
Bleeding	• Frank blood, crusting, clots • Pulsing of the tube	Airway humidification, saline Sign of possible innominate artery rupture
Air in neck	• Subcutaneous air	Decrease pressure if patient is on a ventilator.
Communication with wound	• Saliva via tracheostomy tube or tracheostomy wound	Impeccable wound care and packing
Pneumothorax	• Shortness of breath	Manage chest tube.
Aspiration	• Cough, pneumonia • Change in color of secretions	Cannot occur with a laryngectomy (unless pharyngo-stomal fistula) Reflux precautions, improved airway care, antibiotics

Pain Management

Preoperative Pain

Pain assessment and management, with the goals of improving patient comfort, function, and safety, while minimizing side effects, is an ongoing process (National Comprehensive Cancer Network® [NCCN®], 2015). Pain management begins preoperatively when the patient presents with pain related to the tumor. Symptoms may include sore throat, odynophagia, and unilateral otalgia. Pain can result from the tumor itself compressing on or infiltrating organs, nerves, blood vessels, or connective tissue. Tissue necrosis, infection, edema, surgical effects, or treatment toxicities can also contribute to patient discomfort (McMenamin, 2011). A comprehensive pain assessment considering the location, description, severity, aggravating factors, and relieving factors should be performed. Aggressive pain management and patient and family education help to create a trusting relationship between the patient and nurse that will continue throughout the postoperative course.

Postoperative Pain

Following surgery, patients often describe relief from the pain that was caused by the tumor burden. The causes of postoperative discomfort are edema, numbness, and long immobility. Acute pain results from surgical incisions and tissue manipulation. However, the presence of multiple incisions and the use of flaps and grafts increase the number of potentially painful sites. Pain usually is short term, of moderate to severe intensity, and described as "sharp" or "burning." Pain also can be described as "throbbing head pressure" related to the intracranial rise in spinal fluid pressure that occurs when the jugular vein is sacrificed. Because of the resection of nerve roots of C 2–4, the sensory branches supplying the skin of the neck and scalp, incisional pain is somewhat mediated and better controlled with medications. Patients requiring a skin graft often report that a donor site on the thigh is more painful than an incision on the head and neck. The use of hydrophilic or hydrofiber dressings decreases the amount of pain experienced at the donor site in the early postoperative period (Karlsson, Lindgren, Jarnhed-Andersson, & Tarpila, 2014; Sievers, 2010).

Head and neck surgery often results in alterations in speaking, limiting patients' ability to describe the pain and respond to interventions. Paying attention to nonverbal signs of pain, such as facial grimacing, bracing, and restlessness, is important. Adequate pain control promotes comfort, function, and patient satisfaction, which facilitates recovery and functional abilities.

Postoperative pain management must be individualized to the patient. Administration of opioids for the first few days following surgery can be done intravenously or through the use of patient-controlled analgesia. When patients are cleared to start oral or enteral intake, their medication route should be changed (American Society of Anesthesiologists Task Force, 2012). For narcotic- or opiate-naïve patients, the dosing schedule should be a consistent administration plan of short-acting opioids. The advantage of this is that rapid onset of analgesic effect with route and dosing is decided based on patients' ongoing analgesic needs (NCCN, 2015).

Other concerns in pain management of patients with head and neck cancer are age, comorbidities that may affect medication requirements, and length of surgery with associated positioning. Many patients with head and neck cancer are older adults and present with musculoskeletal disorders, such as arthritis and other degenerative spine and joint conditions (American Geriatrics Society Panel on the Pharmacological Management of Persistent Pain in Older Persons, 2009). No matter the age of the patient, positioning during a lengthy surgery and postoperative bed rest contributes to immobility. Turning and repositioning, ambulation, and upper and lower extremity movement can help relieve stiffness.

As patients recover from surgery, their need for pain medication decreases. Useful analgesic drugs include acetaminophen, acetaminophen with codeine, acetaminophen with hydrocodone, and nonsteroidal anti-inflammatory drugs (NSAIDs). However, caution must be exercised with these medications because they are associated with hepatic and renal toxicity and risk of postoperative and gastrointestinal bleeding. NCCN (2015) guidelines suggest limiting acetaminophen to 3–4 g per day, depending on length of use and patient's liver function. The guidelines also suggest adding a proton pump inhibitor when prescribing NSAIDs.

Caution should be used when prescribing codeine, which is a prodrug. A prodrug is "a class of drugs, initially in inactive form, that are converted into active form in the body by normal metabolic processes" ("Prodrug," n.d.). Codeine is metabolized by cytochrome P450 to morphine. There is evidence that some individuals may be poor metabolizers of codeine, resulting in the drug exhibiting little to no effect on them. Other individuals, however, are rapid metabolizers and may experience toxic effects of the medication (NCCN, 2015). Constipation is a significant problem for patients taking codeine, and its use is discouraged in patients with cancer (McMenamin, 2011).

Consultation with a pain management care team can offer assistance through medication management, alternative medications, and supportive therapies. These teams have been shown to be helpful at decreasing patients' pain; increasing patient satisfaction; and decreasing cost, morbidity, and medication side effects (Bader et al., 2010).

Adjuvant medications, such as antidepressants, anticonvulsants, NSAIDs, steroids, local and topical pain agents, antianxiety agents, and neuropathic agents, are helpful additions to the pain management protocol (NCCN, 2015). Nonpharmacologic supportive therapy is helpful for postoperative patients with head and neck cancer. Shoul-

der dysfunction, fibrosis, fatigue, and neurocognitive deficits can occur as a result of head and neck cancer treatments. Physical and occupational therapy can minimize functional loss and increase quality of life, strength, mobility, balance, endurance, coordination, posture, and ability to perform activities of daily living. Assistive devices help patients support, assist, and adapt to temporary or permanent physical changes through increasing healing and function and decreasing pain (Brown, Yuen, Sulwer, & Lupini, 2013).

Wound Management

Patients with head and neck cancer are at risk for impaired wound healing because of malnutrition, previous radiation therapy, hypothyroidism, smoking, and other existing comorbid conditions, such as diabetes and vascular compromise (Talmi, 2013). A low serum albumin (less than 2 g/dl) is associated with decreased tensile strength and poor wound healing. Preoperative radiation therapy increases the risk of delayed healing through vascular impairment and impaired cellular nutrition. A consequence of radiation therapy in patients with head and neck cancer is hypothyroidism, which is known to increase wound complications (White et al., 2012). Wound management begins with an initial postoperative assessment (see Table 9-3). Assess the suture lines every three to four hours, noting the color, temperature, and adequacy of blood supply. Flaps should be pink in color, feel warm to the touch, and have good capillary refill. A cool, bluish, or dusky flap indicates venous congestion, presence of a hematoma, and impending flap failure; this necessitates immediate notification of the surgical team and preparation of the patient for surgery.

Postoperative patients with head and neck cancer require careful monitoring. Incision care includes cleaning suture lines with half-strength hydrogen peroxide and normal saline to remove crusts. A light coating of antibiotic ointment is applied to the incision during the first few days after surgery. Positioning patients correctly will prevent tension on the wound and vascular compression of the flaps from drains, ventilator tubing, and tracheostomy ties. Avoiding tension, twisting, and kinking of the flap pedicle is critical for successful wound healing (Sievers, 2010).

Drains

Drains are placed during surgery to remove blood, serum, and air; to seal the skin flaps to the underlying wound bed; and to prevent hematoma formation in the surgical wound beds. Drains must be free of kinks for proper functioning and secured at all times to prevent inadvertent removal (see Table 9-3). The integrity of the drains is critical to wound

Table 9-3. University of California, Davis Medical Center Ear, Nose, and Throat (ENT) Intensive Care Unit (ICU) Matrix for the Care of Patients With Head and Neck Cancer

	Topic	Site	Nursing Interventions	Frequency
1	Airway	Tracheostomy	Temporary airway Cuff inflated while on ventilator. Always check cuff pressures Cuff deflated at all other times No ties over reconstruction flaps or grafts Instill saline frequently; suction PRN. Tracheostomy wound care Spare tube at bedside	Q shift and PRN Q 2 hours and PRN Q 4–8 hours and PRN
		Laryngectomy	Permanent airway trachea sutured to anterior skin of neck Stoma care: cotton swabs with hydrogen peroxide and normal saline Remove crusts over suture lines. Instill saline frequently; suction PRN. Goal is shiny glistening mucosa in airway. Bayonet forceps at bedside for secretion removal Stoma button if stoma contracts If tracheoesophageal puncture (TEP), secure tube and alternate left to right side. May feed via TEP if in stomach.	Q 2 hours and PRN Q 2–4 hours and PRN Q shift and PRN Q 2–4 hours and PRN
2	Nutrition	Oral, nasogastric (NG), gastrostomy tube, jejunostomy tube, or via TEP	Do not move NG tube. Secure with Stomahesive® and tape to nares. Do not remove nasal stitch. Do not attempt to replace NG without physician order. Administer feedings by nutrition consult. Chyle leak—feed only nonfat formula (Vivonex® [Novartis, East Hanover, NJ] T.E.N. or similar).	 Change and clean PRN Continuous then bolus
3	Drains	Varidyne® suction vacuum pump, Davol®, Hemovac® or Jackson-Pratt® drain	Secure with Stomahesive and Elastoplast®. Strip to prevent clots. Strict output recording Call house officer if sudden increase or decrease in output or air leaks. Pressure dressing for 24 hours after drain removal	Q 1–2 hours
4	Flaps	Myocutaneous Microvascular free flap • Radial forearm • Fibula • Rectus • Scapula Rotation flap	Color • Venous congestion = red • No arterial supply = white Capillary refill No pressure by lines, drains, or tapes Doppler for arterial and/or venous pulse Keep blood pressure stable at all times to keep microvascular and pedicle vessels patent.	Q 1–2 hours and PRN Q 1–2 hours and PRN Q 1–2 hours and PRN
5	Wound care	Head and neck incisions	Use hydrogen peroxide to remove crusts. Apply light antibiotic ointment to prevent crusts (first three days only).	Q 1–2 hours and PRN
		Split-thickness skin graft/ full-thickness skin graft (usually on thigh)	Change hydrogel (or similar) (not Xeroform). When no longer painful during change, leave open to air. Post-op days 5–7.	Q day and PRN
		Free flap donor site	Do not change dressings. Check neurovascular status—movement, sensation, capillary refill, temperature. • Radial forearm free flap → fingers • Fibular free flap → toes	Q 2 hours advancing to Q 4 hours; then as ordered

(Continued on next page)

Table 9-3. University of California, Davis Medical Center Ear, Nose, and Throat (ENT) Intensive Care Unit (ICU) Matrix for the Care of Patients With Head and Neck Cancer (Continued)

	Topic	Site	Nursing Interventions	Frequency
6	Fistula	Orocutaneous Pharyngocutaneous	Dressing wet to dry, open fluffs and pack carefully. Protect airway.	Q 2 hours then Q 4 hours and PRN
7	Carotid	Internal carotid artery Exposed external or intra-oral	Wet-to-wet to keep carotid in a wet and clean environment Hetastarch in sodium chloride at bedside Type and cross (or hold) two units. Two large-bore IVs Alert operating room that patient is on precautions. If bleed occurs, apply direct pressure and do not remove. Call ENT resident on call for emergency intervention.	Q 2 hours around the clock (ATC) and PRN Give volume expanders, continue pressure, secure airway, and transport to operating room with surgeon.
			If healing, wet with saline, alternating with dressing changes.	Q 2 hours, then Q 4 hours; wet with saline in between.
8	Pain	Post-op management	Regular frequent dosing of opioids Acetaminophen with codeine (or similar) alternating Acetaminophen with codeine for caffeine withdrawal headaches Do not sedate if inadequately medicated for pain. Always check for previous pain medication use—do not assume opiate-naïve. If patients' pain is well managed in ICU, they generally require less pain medication on general ENT floor. Routine bowel care	Q 1–2 hours for the first 24 hours, then PRN but ATC; assess frequently according to pain guidelines.
9	ETOH (alcohol) withdrawal	–	Regular dosing of benzodiazepines Use agitation protocol judiciously. Continue pain medication. Psych/social consults and behavior modification	Restraints for safety PRN
10	Patient teaching	Consistent plan according to policy and patient education records	Begin pre-op; continue post-op and into clinic. Ongoing teaching Reevaluation necessary Documentation	Ongoing

Note. Copyright 2003 by Ann E.F. Sievers, University of California, Davis Medical Center. Adapted with permission.

healing. Strip the drains every one to two hours to prevent obstruction by blood clots and to maintain patency. The drainage should be monitored each shift, noting the color, amount, and consistency of drainage. In the presence of multiple drains, each should be labeled as to its location to permit accurate documentation of output.

Any sudden change in the amount of drainage may indicate bleeding, hematoma, or seroma formation, resulting in a compromise of the vascular bed. Drainage initially is sanguineous but changes to serosanguineous and then serous drainage within a few days. Surgical drains remain in place until output is less than 30 ml in a 24-hour period and usually are removed at postoperative day 3–6. Following drain removal, a pressure dressing is placed over the incision to prevent reaccumulation of fluid under the flap. This dressing usually is in place for 24 hours (Sievers, 2010).

Edema

Patients undergoing head and neck surgery often experience edema of the face and neck caused by removal of lymphatic channels and resection of the jugular vein during neck dissection, both of which impede drainage. Patients who receive radiation therapy are also more at risk for edema (Haas, 2011). Postoperative edema can be significant, and supportive measures are necessary to minimize swelling. Elevate the head of the bed and avoid constricting clothing and tracheostomy ties. Edema of the head and neck usually resolves over time as collateral circulation improves. Cerebral edema may result following radical neck dissection (especially bilateral) and skull base surgery. Cerebral edema is manifested by an alteration in the level of consciousness, confusion, and delirium. Alcohol withdrawal and medication delirium also may occur simultaneously (see Table 9-3) (Sievers, 2010).

Significant edema is frightening to both patients and families. Cognitive and sensory function may be impaired as a result of the edema. Periorbital edema impairs vision; neck edema may impair speech and mobility of the neck; and eustachian tube edema impairs hearing (Harris, 2008). Explaining the rationale for the swelling and offering supportive measures to decrease the edema may alleviate some anxiety. Adequate pain control, limited fluid intake, and the use of antianxiety medications may also help patients (Sievers, 2010).

Negative-Pressure Wound Therapy

Negative-pressure wound therapy (NPWT) is an integrative wound management system used to deliver negative pressure that promotes wound healing, reduces edema, promotes granulation tissue formation and perfusion, helps bolster tissue, prevents tissue shearing, and removes exudate (Kinetic Concepts, Inc., 2014). The most commonly used integrative NPWT system is the vacuum-assisted closure system (Strub & Moe, 2013). This therapy involves placing polyurethane foam over the wound and covering it with an occlusive drape. A suction tubing device is attached that delivers controlled negative pressure to the wound bed when connected to the vacuum device. Fluid is collected into a canister attached to the vacuum device (Asher et al., 2014).

Vacuum-assisted closure therapy is applied in the operating room. The unit applied can be either reusable or disposable (see Figures 9-6 and 9-7). The disposable unit is small and portable, allowing for patients to mobilize easier and possibly be discharged home sooner with the device still applied. Complication rates are low and dependent on proper patient selection, wound preparation, and adequate protection of underlying structures. The most common complications reported are pain and skin irritation (Strub & Moe, 2013). Use of this therapy in head and neck wounds is still new, and much research is warranted.

Flaps and Grafts

Immediate reconstruction of surgical defects usually is performed at the time of tumor resection. The use of microvascular free flaps, or free tissue transfer, has improved the reconstruction of complex surgical defects in patients with head and neck cancer. The development of microvascular instruments and magnification has improved the overall success rates, as well as functional outcomes (Pohlenz et al., 2012).

Successful reconstruction requires a team approach. This team is composed of medical oncologists, extirpative surgeons, and reconstructive surgeons. Important considerations include tumor stage, prognosis, patient age, sex, body

Figure 9-6. V.A.C.® Ultra Negative-Pressure Therapy System

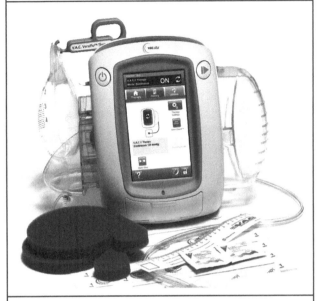

Note. Figure courtesy of Kinetic Concepts, Inc. Used with permission.

Figure 9-7. V.A.C.® VIA

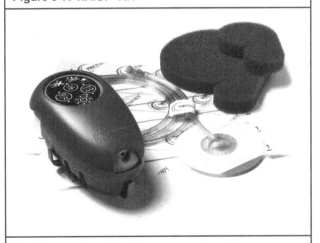

Note. Figure courtesy of Kinetic Concepts, Inc. Used with permission.

habitus, functional status, available donor sites, and psychological status of the patient. The stepwise reconstruction ladder can be as simple as healing by secondary intention. This is followed by primary closure, skin grafting, composite grafts, local flaps, regional pedicle flaps, and free tissue transfer (Lin & Rabie, 2014). Myocutaneous flaps that are used for reconstruction of head and neck defects include pectoralis major myocutaneous flaps, skinless pectoralis flaps, and other flaps designed to repair the defect created by the tumor resection. Microvascular free flaps also are used for reconstruction and require specific expertise by physicians and nurses. Commonly used free flap sites include the radial forearm, fibula, scapula, anterolateral thigh, and rectus abdominis muscle. Specific considerations depend on the site selected. For example, the patient is not permitted any weight bearing for 7–10 days when the fibula is used for reconstruction, and the nondominant arm usually is selected as the donor site when a radial forearm free flap is used. No preoperative blood draws or IVs should be performed in the arm from which the radial forearm free flap is being harvested.

The following are the most common free flaps and their associated defects. For reconstruction of lip defects, the most commonly used technique is rotational or cervicofacial advancement flaps (Lin & Rabie, 2014). For other skin defects that involve the oral cavity soft tissue or the skin of the face or neck, forearm, anterolateral thigh, or cervicofacial advancement flaps are the most commonly used. If the patient has already undergone radiation therapy, a pectoralis major flap is more useful for reconstructing the external coverage. When tumor resection involves the mandible, the fibular free flap is most widely utilized. The fibula flap consists of bone and associated soft tissue pedicle. It obtains its blood supply from branches of the fibular (peroneal) artery. Advantages of this reconstructive option include the amount of bone that can be harvested, extensive vascular support, sturdiness of the bone to accept plates and screws for fixation and dental implants, and potential sensory reinnervation. There are some disadvantages to this approach, such as limited soft tissue and the need for patients to have adequate peripheral vasculature. This can be a challenge in patients with peripheral vascular disease. Other reconstructive options for the mandible include iliac crest flap, scapular flap, anterolateral thigh flap, or rectus abdominis free flap. When the oral cavity resection structures are needed for function, two free flaps are more useful (Lin & Rabie, 2014).

Split-thickness skin graft is most frequently used to close the donor site defect from the harvest for reconstruction of oral cavity resections when large amounts of tissue and bone are not required. Alternative methods of closure also include full-thickness skin graft from the forearm, inner arm, and abdomen. A layer of skin is harvested from the anterior thigh using a Padgett® dermatome at a thickness of 0.35–0.45 mm and placed over the wound (Jaquet, Enepekides, Torgerson, & Higgins, 2012). Problems can occur at the donor site, such as graft loss, scar contracture, loss of elasticity, sensory impairment, adhesions of flexor tendons, and unpleasant aesthetic results. Because of superficial nerve fiber exposure, the donor site is painful. In order to prevent these issues, various skin-grafting techniques to the donor site and postoperative wound site care are necessary (Orlik et al., 2014). Placing a hydrocolloid dressing over the wound to protect the area markedly decreases

the pain and improves wound healing. The dressing over the graft donor site remains in place for five to seven days. Once the dressing has been removed, it can be changed daily until the site is no longer painful. At this time, the donor site is exposed and should have neurovascular assessments each hour. Assess the fingers (radial forearm free flap) or the toes (fibular free flap) for color, temperature, and ability to sense touch and to move on command. The flap site should be monitored hourly for the first 24–48 hours (Wax, 2014).

The gold standard for flap monitoring continues to be direct clinical observation of the flap. The use of an implantable Doppler probe, which is secured around the vessel adventitia of a vascular pedicle, provides specific information about the patency of arteries and veins (Learned, Malloy, & Loevner, 2012). A Doppler sound device assesses the microvascular anastomosis for patency. It is capable of measuring blood flow in both the arterial and venous systems accurately. External Dopplers are used in the postoperative setting to map the vascular pedicle by placing a suture on the external skin to identify where the signal is best detected (Wax, 2014). Evaluate the site with a Doppler every hour. If the blood flow by Doppler is stable and the reconstruction flap maintains a pink color after the first three days, the assessment can take place every four to six hours, progressing to every shift until discharge. A stable blood pressure, with a mean arterial pressure of approximately 60–80 mm Hg, is necessary to sustain blood flow through the vascular pedicle. The effect of arterial blood pressure on blood flow is significant. An increase in arterial pressure decreases vascular resistance by increasing the force with which blood is pushed through the vessels while simultaneously distending the vessels. This decreases vascular resistance (Schrey et al., 2011).

To avoid internal vessel factors leading to the failure of flaps, the patient is traditionally kept warm and vasodilated with external heaters, optimal fluid infusion, and vasoactive infusions, such as dobutamine, where necessary. Various drugs, such as IV dextran, have been recommended to reduce the risk of anastomotic thrombosis to prevent platelet aggregation (Marsh, Elliott, Anand, & Brennan, 2009). Postoperative subcutaneous heparin was found to reduce incidence of thrombotic occlusion in the flap anastomosis sites (Pattani, Byrne, Boahene, & Richmon, 2010).

All flaps should be assessed for color, temperature, and integrity. Bulging of the flap, increase in drain output, fullness of the flap, and color changes may be signs of vascular compromise and must be reported immediately to the reconstructive surgeon. Significant changes in the flap may require additional surgery to decompress the vascular compromise, artery, or vein.

Physical therapy and occupational therapy are consulted for patients who have undergone free flap reconstruction. Direct each therapy to the disability from the resections and the reconstruction, such as stability in ambulation after fibula grafts, hand range of motion after forearm flaps, and shoulder exercises after neck dissection. One of the most common complications that stems from a neck dissection is shoulder dysfunction, which can lead to atrophy of the trapezius muscle. This is caused by damage to the accessory nerve (cranial nerve XI) and can be monitored by electromyography immediately postoperatively (de Lima, Amar, & Lehn, 2011).

Eye Care

Following a neck dissection, temporal bone dissection, parotidectomy, or extensive ear surgery, the function of the facial nerve must be evaluated. The facial nerve, cranial nerve VII, may be resected or injured, resulting in a temporary or permanent paresis. Each of the five branches of the nerve is important to the structure and function of the facial musculature. Patients with facial nerve paralysis may experience many, often severe, limitations. There may be significant ophthalmic complications secondary to the inability to blink, retraction of the upper and lower lid, and lagophthalmos. Also, the loss of orbicularis tone predisposes patients to dry eye symptoms and corneal abrasions resulting from corneal exposure. It is imperative to protect the corneas (Rofagha & Seiff, 2010). A protocol for eye care should be started for anyone with facial nerve dysfunction in which the eye is affected. If the cornea is visible with the dysfunction or if the blink is absent, patients should instill lubricating eye drops every two hours and apply an ointment at bedtime. Patients also should wear a clear eye shield or tape the eye closed while sleeping. Eye care continues until the facial nerve function returns or surgery is performed to insert a gold weight in the upper eyelid to allow for closure.

Damage can also occur to cranial nerves III, IV, and VI, affecting movement of the eye, the response of pupils to light, or both. Therefore, a thorough cranial nerve examination should be performed on all postoperative patients.

Oral Care

The focus of oral health treatment plans for patients with head and neck cancer prior to treatment should be on identifying and managing existing dental disease and infection. This will help to prevent and minimize oral side effects caused by cancer treatment. The oral cavity assessments should be conducted at least two to three weeks prior to the start of treatment. This assessment includes a thorough dental examination, periodontal evaluation, and any necessary dental x-rays to assess for the presence of infection. It has been found that patients who receive periodontal debridement and oral care instruction prior to surgery were less likely to develop an infection of the surgical

site than patients who did not receive either debridement or instruction (Rhodes-Nessert & Laronde, 2014). Basic oral care is important in maintaining a clean oral cavity and consists of brushing with a soft toothbrush, flossing, using bland rinses, such as normal saline or sodium bicarbonate solution, and using oral moisturizers. This will also, in turn, reduce the risk of oral infection from normal or abnormal flora, minimize trauma-induced mucosal tissue injury, and promote comfort. An oral rinse that is known to have specific antimicrobial properties is chlorhexidine (McGuire et al., 2013).

Head and neck cancer surgery increases the risk of wound infection because bacterial flora commonly contaminates the upper aerodigestive tract. It is imperative to identify the risk factors responsible for wound complication to minimize the rate of infection. Preoperative dental scaling, good oral hygiene, and maintenance of operating room asepsis should be ensured to prevent wound infection (Chaukar et al., 2013). It is very important to irrigate oral wounds, especially those created from surgical resection of tumors. Adequate irrigation is essential to ensure good hygiene, promote comfort and healing, and minimize the risk of infection. Conventional oral irrigation units are commonly used, such as Waterpik®. The spray settings on these units can sometimes be too forceful for new postsurgical patients and can damage the tissue or impede the suture lines. Using disposable syringes with connective tubing and a saliva ejector tip can be an easier and more cost-effective way to irrigate fresh oral cavity surgical wounds because it allows flushing with moderate pressure or pulsing in to the wound for effective washing (Chambers, Lemon, & Martin, 2003).

Many patients with oral cancer will undergo radiation with or without chemotherapy after surgery, and some will undergo these therapies prior to their surgical resection. Complications from radiation and chemotherapy include hyposalivation, loss of taste, trismus (limited jaw opening), infection, mucositis, dental caries, and osteoradionecrosis. Patients who undergo a partial glossectomy will have restricted movement of the remaining tongue. The restricted movement will result in decreased self-cleansing and higher biofilm levels. Trismus may impede oral hygiene self-care and the ability to deliver dental hygiene therapy (Rhodes-Nessert & Laronde, 2014).

Radiation therapy may also cause changes to the gingiva, leading to hypovascularization and hypoxic tissue that affects the healing process. Surgical patients who have undergone radiation therapy preoperatively are at a higher risk for infection and complications. Patients who have undergone primary chemotherapy can have weakened immune systems. Common hemodynamic side effects of systemic treatment can cause an increased risk of infection and prolonged bleeding times (Rhodes-Nessert & Laronde, 2014).

Postsurgical Complications

Postoperative Hemorrhage

Most hemorrhagic symptoms occur early in the postoperative period, usually within the first 24 hours. Causes of postoperative bleeding after neck surgery are retching and bucking during recovery, the Valsalva maneuver, and increased blood pressure. Bleeding also can be brought on after extubation, vomiting, or coughing. The following events can cause an increase in venous return pressure: slipping of the ligature on major vessels, reopening of cauterized veins, and oozing from the area of incision (Nambu et al., 2013). Signs and symptoms of postoperative hemorrhage include tense and bulging flaps, expansion of the flap, oozing at the suture line, a drop in blood pressure, restlessness, possibly hypoxia, and blood in the surgical drains. Because each drain is placed in a specific anatomic area, increased bleeding from an individual drain helps to locate the area of bleeding.

It is important to note that vital signs can remain stable, especially in the younger patient population, until shock ensues. Drains may become blocked, kinked, or malpositioned. The bleeding may be remote from the site of surgery and may accumulate in an undrained compartment. Physical examination findings that are important to integrate are tachycardia, diminished cardiac output, decreased central venous pressure, reduced urine output, and abnormal capillary refill. The search for an occult cause of the bleeding should occur regularly and repeatedly until the patient is stable and the bleeding has stopped. Appropriate imaging scans, such as CT, magnetic resonance imaging, magnetic resonance angiogram, and ultrasound, may need to be employed to identify the source of the bleeding (Dagi, 2005).

The usual management of head and neck bleeding is local pressure, suture closure, nasal packing, surgical ligation, cautery, and transfusion of blood products, as indicated. When these conventional methods fail, transarterial embolization therapy can be considered. Major postoperative bleeding of the head and neck may not be amenable to traditional surgical approaches (Bachar et al., 2013).

Carotid Artery Rupture

In most cases, hemorrhage in patients with advanced cancer usually occurs at the site of the malignancy. The carotid artery rupture is the most common in head and neck tumors (Harris & Noble, 2009). Predisposing factors that can lead to carotid exposure and rupture include surgery, radiation therapy, poor nutrition, diabetes mellitus, and prolonged corticosteroid use. Carotid blowout, or rupture, is a devastating complication of head and neck cancer treatment. This occurs when a compromised arterial wall is weakened by loss of overlying soft tissue with resultant desiccation, by infection from a pharyngocutaneous fistula or deep neck abscess, direct tumor involvement, or a combination of these factors. Rupture of the common carotid artery is a life-threatening oncologic emergency. Nurses must be aware of the risk factors, signs, and symptoms and establish a consistent, standard plan of care (see Table 9-3). Carotid exposure can occur externally through the neck or internally from the oropharynx. Internal bleeding is much more difficult to control because of limited access to the bleeding site (McDonald, Moore, & Johnstone, 2012).

The overall goal is to prevent drying of the carotid adventitia, the outermost layer of the artery. The adventitia dries and forms an eschar. If the eschar is disrupted, hemorrhage will occur. A small sentinel, or herald, bleed may precede arterial rupture. It is usually a small prodromal bleeding that occurs 24–48 hours before the rupture of an artery. It can either resolve spontaneously or with packing or pressure (Harris & Noble, 2009).

In patients who are identified as being at risk for carotid artery rupture, various measures should be considered to control early signs of bleeding. These may be local measures or systemic, and their use should be individualized to the patient. Local measures include compressive dressings, hemostatic agents (e.g., absorbable gelatin compressed sponge, calcium alginate, 1% sucralfate paste), vasoconstrictor agents, and surgery. Systemic measures include vitamin K, antifibrinolytic agents, and transfusion of blood products (see Figure 9-8) (Harris & Noble, 2009). The patient who is at risk for carotid artery rupture is placed on "carotid precautions," and emergency supplies are placed at the bedside. Emergency supplies include gloves, plastic aprons, goggles, face shields, large sterile dressings, saline, oxygen, dark-colored towels, wide-bore IV cannula, artificial airways and syringes to inflate the tracheostomy cuff, drugs for sedation and pain relief, and clinical waste disposal bags (Frawley & Begley, 2005). Patients should occupy a room close to the nursing station to allow for constant observation, and nurses should monitor vital signs, airway, responsiveness, and pain. IV access is maintained with a wide-bore IV cannula to allow for immediate infusion of fluids and blood in the event of rupture. Wound care includes gentle packing of the wound with saline-soaked nonadhering dressings to keep the exposed carotid artery moist and the wound bed clean. Wet-to-wet dressings are changed every two hours. Dressing changes advance to every four hours, and normal saline solution is applied every two hours between dressing changes as the wound heals. This also will provide a longer period of uninterrupted sleep for patients.

In the event of carotid artery rupture, aggressive and immediate treatment is paramount to saving the patient's life. A nurse must remain with the patient and immediately apply digital pressure to the carotid. Dressings that allow direct point pressure to the site of the rupture should be used. Avoid use of bulky dressings, which impair the ability to localize the site of bleeding. Initial management involves establishing an airway and obtaining large-bore IV access, allowing for rapid volume resuscitation. Inflate the cuff immediately to seal the airway if an artificial airway is in place. Attention should then focus on controlling the hemorrhage to prevent rapid exsanguination. Maintain pressure over the carotid until surgery is available to manage the bleeding. Historically, open surgical intervention has been the standard of care by either repairing the artery primarily, grafting, oversewing, or ligating. In recent years, the approach has shifted to managing carotid ruptures with

---

Figure 9-8. Carotid Artery Rupture

Identify Patient at Risk

General Risk Factors	**Specific Risk Factors for Carotid Artery Rupture**
Thrombocytopenia	Surgery (e.g., radical neck dissection)
Large head and neck carcinomas	Radiotherapy
Large centrally located lung cancers	Poor postoperative healing
Refractory acute and chronic leukemia	Visible arterial pulsation
Myelodysplasia	Pharyngocutaneous fistula
Metastatic liver disease and deranged clotting	Fungating tumors
	Systemic factors (e.g., diabetes, age over 50 years, loss of 10%– 15% body weight, immunodeficiency malnourishment)

Multidisciplinary Team Discussion

May include oncologist, surgeon, nursing staff, pharmacist, chaplain
Proactive preparation and advance planning
Factors to consider:
• Patient's prognosis
• Patient's performance status
• Patient's perceived quality of life and preferences

Discussion With Patient and Family

Level of discussion may depend upon:
How likely the MDT feels that terminal hemorrhage may occur
Patient and family's knowledge and acceptance of diagnosis and prognosis
How much information the patient and carer want to receive
Patient and family's desired level of participation in discussions about their care
Patient's and family's coping strategies

In event of hemorrhage, use measures to a level appropriate to the individual patient

General Supportive Measures:	**General Resuscitative Measures:**	**Specific Intervention to Stop the Bleeding:**
Call for assistance	Volume and fluid replacement with colloid fluid or blood products	Surgical ligation of an artery
Ensure a nurse stays with the patient		
Provide psychological support		
Apply pressure if bleeding externally visible		
Use of dark towels to camouflage blood loss		
Use of suction if possible		
Use of sedative medication: currently no consensus regarding drug, dose, or route		

After the Event

Debrief and support for relatives/carers AND staff after the event
Consider whether counseling is needed

MDT—multidisciplinary team

Note. From "Management of Terminal Hemorrhage in Patients With Advanced Cancer: A Systematic Literature Review," by D.G. Harris and S.I.R. Noble, 2009, *Journal of Pain and Symptom Management, 38,* p. 918. Copyright 2009 by U.S. Cancer Pain Relief Committee. Reprinted with permission.

endovascular coils, balloons, or stents. Following ligation, the patient should be observed for neurologic deficits or signs of stroke from cerebral hypoxia (McDonald et al., 2012).

It is recommended that the multidisciplinary team assess patients' and their families' knowledge of the prognosis and risk for carotid artery rupture. This discussion should take place in the event of a herald bleed and should include patient preference with regard to aggressive attempts to prolong life or supportive care. The event is unlikely to be painful, and patients might find comfort in this fact. They should be aware that sedation will be available (Harris & Noble, 2009). A debriefing session is valuable to support the staff following this traumatic event. Consultation with a social worker or psychiatric liaison also may be helpful.

Chyle Leak

A chyle leak can occur during a neck dissection and is a rare complication. It results from damage to the thoracic duct or right lymphatic duct. A leak of up to one liter per day may be tolerated for one to two days before an electrolyte imbalance occurs. Leaks that are prolonged can lead to protein loss (Brennan, Blythe, Herd, Habib, & Anand, 2012). The appearance of copious amounts of milky white, opaque drainage may indicate the presence of a chyle fistula. The best time to diagnose a chyle leak and manage thoracic duct damage is at the time of surgery. Because preoperative fasting can cause a reduced volume of chyle in the thoracic duct, this is sometimes difficult. A chyle leak usually presents as swelling in the neck, skin erythema, and increased output in the drains. It often becomes more apparent as the patient begins feeding again. The drainage is analyzed for the presence of amylase, increased triglycerides, and lymphocytes. Management of chyle leaks can include intraoperative management, conservative postoperative management, management using interventional radiology, and re-exploration of the wound with repair. The basic management of a leak that has an output of less than one liter per day can be accomplished with local pressure dressings, although this has limited efficacy. The most beneficial management of low-output leaks is to adopt a modified medium-chain triglyceride (MCT) or low-fat diet. A low-fat MCT diet reduces a chyle leak, but fat does not fully bypass the digestive tract, nor does it provide adequate essential nutrients. Therefore, total parenteral nutrition has been suggested as a better alternative (Brennan et al., 2012).

Fistula

A fistula is a breakdown in tissue that causes communication between two sites. Orocutaneous (between the oral cavity and the neck) and pharyngocutaneous (between the pharynx and the neck) fistulas occur postoperatively with a variable rate that is dependent on many factors. The type of surgery, prior irradiation and/or chemotherapy, poor nutri-

tional status, and other comorbidities can all attribute to fistula formation. Pharyngocutaneous fistulas are the most common surgical complication after a total laryngectomy. They occur when there is a failure in the pharyngeal repair, resulting in salivary leakage. The consequences of a fistula include delay in oral intake, higher incidence of morbidity, increased length of hospital stay, and increased medical costs. These can all result in life-threatening infection or vascular rupture and can even cause a delay in the start of radiation treatments (Dedivitis, Aires, Cernea, & Brandão, 2015).

The standard of care is to open the suture line widely to facilitate drainage, debride the wound, pack the wound with sterile wet dressings to promote granulation and healing, and administer IV antibiotics. Diversion of the salivary stream away from the wound and the airway facilitates wound healing. The use of a tonsil-tip oral suction device helps to control the saliva. In an attempt to prevent the development of a pharyngocutaneous fistula, patients who have undergone a total laryngectomy should not reintroduce oral feedings until 7–10 days after the surgery. Patients are NPO and receive enteral feedings to prevent food from entering the wound while still ensuring good nutrition. Pain medication and topical anesthetic agents may be used to minimize the pain associated with dressing changes and debridement. A fistula heals naturally, from the wound bed outward. Once granulation tissue is established in the wound, the patient or family may be taught how to change the dressing in preparation for home care (Dedivitis et al., 2015).

Cranial Nerve and Neurologic Impairment

Following head and neck surgery, neurologic impairment may result from tumor involvement, surgical resection, or perioperative hypotension. Symptoms include delirium, dementia, depression, cranial nerve dysfunction, and vascular impairment resulting in stroke. An accurate preoperative assessment is crucial to establishing a baseline for comparison because patients may have preexisting dementia or depression or suffered previous strokes. Delirium complicates 15%–50% of major operations in the older adult population and can be associated with other major postoperative complications, prolonged length of stay, poor functional recovery, dementia, and death. Delirium may be predictable in up to 80% of the cases. It is an acute state of confusion characterized by inattention, an abnormal level of consciousness, and thought disorganization. Any delirium that occurs after surgery may be called *postoperative delirium*. Most cases of delirium develop in the first two postoperative days, with a peak incidence on the first postoperative day. Later onset of delirium is usually associated with a major postoperative complication or withdrawal from alcohol or sedatives. Delirium is strongly associated with poor surgical outcomes, including an increased risk of death. Patients who develop delirium have a two- to five-day increased length of hospital stay (Marcantonio, 2012).

Delirium requires assessment by care providers postoperatively. Nurses, in particular, should be aware of acute changes in patients' mental status and fluctuating course, inattention and disorganized thinking, and/or an altered level of consciousness. Simple tests of attention include having patients repeat a sequence of random numbers in forward or backward order, recite the days of the week or months of the year backward, or raise their hand whenever they hear a certain letter or number in a list (Marcantonio, 2012).

Also in the immediate postoperative period, it is essential to assess cranial nerves and cognitive function (see Table 9-4). Isolated cranial nerve deficits can affect the facial nerve (cranial nerve VII), hypoglossal nerve (cranial nerve XII), glossopharyngeal nerve (cranial nerve IX), and vagus nerve (cranial nerve X), leading to dysphagia. Cranial nerve VII affects the manipulation and control of bolus in the oral cavity. Cranial nerve XII deficits lead to poor oral manipulation and transport of bolus toward the pharynx. Cranial nerve IX deficits result in limited bolus propulsion/clearance and delayed trigger of the pharyngeal reflex secondary to diminished tongue base and pharyngeal sensitivity. Cranial nerve X has two components: the sensory division (superior laryngeal nerve), which provides sensation to the epiglottis, false vocal folds, and pyriform sinus, and the motor division (recurrent laryngeal nerve), which controls motor skills of the larynx and contributes to the pharyngeal plexus. Unilateral palsies of cranial nerves IX and X can cause altered voice quality, dysphagia, and dysarthria. Vocal fold paralysis is often reported and can persist after the dysphagia resolves. Both the altered glottic closure and pharyngeal paralysis cause dysphagia (Pizzorni et al., 2014).

A very common cranial nerve injury that can occur in patients with head and neck cancer is cranial nerve XI, the spinal accessory nerve. This nerve is vulnerable to injury because of its long and superficial course in the posterior cervical region. It is considered to contribute most innervation to the trapezius muscle. Damage to the spinal accessory nerve results in shoulder dysfunction that can affect overall quality of life. Injury most commonly occurs following lymph node dissections, posterior neck node excisions or biopsies, parotidectomies, carotid vessel surgery, and even face-lifts. The most common presenting symptoms in this nerve injury are shoulder pain, limited or loss of sustained abduction of the shoulder, scapular winging, and drooping of the ipsilateral shoulder (Walvekar, 2014).

Nutritional Management

Patients who have been or are being treated for head and neck cancer are at high risk for malnutrition and compro-

mised nutritional status. These nutritional deficits have a high impact on morbidity, mortality, and overall quality of life. More than 50% of patients with advanced head and neck cancer have impaired nutrition and associated involuntary weight loss prior to any treatment and often are malnourished at the time of diagnosis (Chasen & Bhargava, 2009). Physiologic functions and changes contribute to long-term nutritional complications. Altered taste and smell can occur with chemotherapeutic agents. Saliva is important for preparing food for mastication and swallowing, as well as for normal taste perception. With decreased saliva, eating can be difficult. Radiation to the head and neck region can cause dry mouth, mucositis, nausea, vomiting, and pain in the oral cavity. Dysphagia, the most common nutrition-related problem resulting from head and neck cancer, can occur from surgical ablation of muscular and nervous structures or could be the effect of radiation or chemotherapy (Chasen & Bhargava, 2009).

Enteral feeding is an essential factor for maintaining a good quality of life for patients with head and neck cancer. Percutaneous endoscopic gastrostomy (PEG) tubes are well tolerated for long-term nutrition supplementation and limit disorders of intestinal motility by maintaining gastrointestinal tract function. PEG tubes are beneficial in facilitating adequate hydration and nutrition prior to, during, and after cancer treatment because they do not result in taste changes and irritation to the mucosa. They are preferred over NG tubes because they reduce discomfort and provide a cosmetic improvement (Fujita et al., 2013).

Prophylactic placement of a PEG tube is common practice before, during, and after treatment. There are risks associated with PEG tube placement, such as local site infection, tube blockage, and migration or dislodgment. More serious complications, although uncommon, include abscess, peritonitis, or development of a fistula. PEG tubes can be placed during the treatment in patients who develop severe swallowing difficulty. There is some concern that PEG tube placement leads to prolonged tube dependency and long-term dysphagia (Brown et al., 2014). The timing of placement is not standardized; it is guided mostly by patient and family preferences and may vary depending upon the practice setting. Patients with head and neck cancer also have a significant insensible water loss caused by suctioning of the mouth and artificial airway. This requires special attention to fluid replacement along with nutrition replacement. Improving patients' nutritional state is challenging and requires a multidisciplinary approach for optimal success.

Head and neck cancer directly impairs oral intake, and the associated treatments increase the risk for severe malnutrition. Unlike simple malnutrition, patients with cancer suffer from a negative energy balance and profound skeletal muscle wasting that are caused by reduced food

Table 9-4. Cranial Nerve Impairments and Associated Nursing and Patient Issues

Cranial Nerve	Name	Cause or Reason for Impairment	Target	Nursing and Patient Issues
I	Olfactory Sensory	Rhinectomy Anterior skull base tumor Laryngectomy	Olfactory bulb	Safety issues resulting from loss of smell
II	Optic Sensory	Resection Tumor, stroke	Eye	Blindness
III	Oculomotor Motor	Anterior cranial facial resection Tumor, stroke	Eye movement	Visual field limitations
IV	Trochlear Motor	Anterior cranial facial resection Tumor, stroke	Eye movement	Visual field limitations
V	Trigeminal Sensory Motor	Anterior cranial facial resection Tumor, stroke	Muscles of mastication	Numbness, so decreased post-operative pain
VI	Abducent Motor	Anterior cranial facial resection Tumor, stroke	Eye movement	Visual field limitations
VII	Facial Motor	Temporal bone resection Acoustic neuroma Parotidectomy	Five branches for facial movement/oral competence	Eye protection and safety drops Lubrication at night Moisture chamber Oral drooling
VII	Facial Chorda tympani Sensory	Temporal bone resection Acoustic neuroma Parotidectomy	Taste (anterior two-thirds of the tongue)	Pleasure and safety
VIII	Acoustic or vestibulocochlear Sensory Cochlear Vestibular	Acoustic neuroma Lateral skull base Lateral temporal bone	Hearing Balance	Hearing Safety and balance issues
IX	Glossopharyngeal Motor Sensory	Base of tongue Laryngectomy	Taste (posterior third of the tongue)	Pleasure Safety
X	Vagus Motor Sensory	Resection of recurrent laryngeal nerve, superior laryngeal nerve	Vocal function Sensation of the larynx	Airway, speech Oral nutrition without aspiration
XI	Spinal accessory Motor	Radical neck dissection	Paralysis of the trapezius "Winging" of the scapula Frozen shoulder	Physical therapy Compliance with exercises Prevention of frozen shoulder
XII	Hypoglossal Motor	Base of tongue resection	Speech and swallowing	Speech therapy Safety in nutrition
C 2-3-4	Cervical plexus Sensory	–	Numbness in ear Scalp sensitivity Supraclavicular numbness	No feeling for injury Pain on combing hair

Note. Copyright 2002 by Ann E.F. Sievers, University of California, Davis Medical Center. Adapted with permission.

intake and abnormal metabolism (elevated energy expenditure, insulin resistance, lipolysis, and proteolysis). These alterations in metabolism require specific interventions to enable anabolism and to reduce inflammation and catabolic processes. Patient assessments should be performed weekly or more frequently as warranted, and special attention should be paid to weight changes, ability to swallow, hydration status, electrolytes, and albumin to ensure early detection of malnutrition and intervention. Weight loss of more than 1%–2% per week, or 5% in less than a month, should prompt more intensive assessment, nutritional counseling, and intervention (Dechaphunkul et al., 2013). Before treatment, a clinical dietitian performs a baseline nutritional assessment and provides dietary counseling, giving advice about a high-caloric diet and recommendations for nutritional supplements. To develop a nutritional plan of care, patients' body weight should be regularly assessed, as well as physical examination results, anthropometric measurements, and laboratory data. Objective measurements include height, weight, pre-illness weight, weight change over time, and body mass index (Ehrsson, Langius-Eklöf, & Laurell, 2012).

Postoperatively, the patient will be NPO until edema subsides, suture lines are healed, and the patient demonstrates the ability to swallow without aspiration. The patient will receive enteral therapy during this time to prevent stress on the suture lines and reduce the risk of aspiration. The choice and location of the enteral feeding tube are critical to the method of feeding. A small-bore nasogastric tube (NGT) is used for short-term feedings (less than seven days). A PEG tube is preferable for patients who require long-term enteral support, as well as postoperative radiation therapy. A jejunostomy tube (JT) is selected when a PEG is contraindicated and for patients who have had gastric procedures. Tubes that have been surgically placed will result in discomfort at the site for several days. Administer pain medication as needed and assist patients with positioning and mobility until the pain subsides. Assess the tube site daily for the presence of drainage and skin breakdown. Clean the site with half-strength hydrogen peroxide to remove crusting. Use a gauze dressing if the area is draining (Arbogast, 2002).

Administer NGT and PEG feedings by bolus or continuous feedings as tolerated by patients. Deliver JT feedings continuously to prevent dumping syndrome. Patients restarting nutrition with high-carbohydrate feedings after a prolonged period of malnutrition are at risk for refeeding syndrome. Refeeding syndrome is a severe fluid and electrolyte shift in malnourished patients during oral, enteral, or parenteral feeding. The metabolic shift from starvation to feeding increases cellular uptake of potassium, glucose, phosphate, and magnesium and lowers the serum concentration of electrolytes. Early signs of refeeding syndrome include severely low serum electrolyte concentrations

of serum phosphate, potassium, and magnesium. If left untreated, this can progress to acute circulatory fluid overload, respiratory compromise, and cardiac failure. Severe hypophosphatemia has been described as the hallmark of refeeding syndrome (Rio, Whelan, Goff, Reidlinger, & Smeeton, 2013).

The choice of nutritional support for enteral feeding is based on caloric density, protein, fiber, osmolality, and fluid needs (see Figure 9-9). Continuous, slow feedings are initiated using a feeding pump, and the volume and rate are gradually increased. The patient may advance to a bolus feeding as tolerated. Administer feedings three to four times daily, similar to normal meal times. Smaller feedings can be considered for patients who have slight to moderate intolerance to larger quantities.

Weigh the patient on a regular schedule and record weights to determine progress. Documentation of caloric intake as well as fluid intake and output is necessary to ensure adequacy of the feeding regimen. Monitor patients closely for complications and intolerance problems. Potential complications of enteral feedings include blockage of the tube and signs of intolerance, such as fullness, nausea, vomiting, and dumping syndrome. If intolerance occurs, decrease the amount and strength of feeding and consult a dietitian for further recommendations, as the patient is at nutritional risk (Mueller, Compher, & Druyan, 2011).

Aspiration, the passage of liquid or food through the vocal folds, can be a serious consequence of dysphagia and may cause chronic coughing, choking, airway obstruction, and aspiration pneumonia. It is of particular concern for patients following head and neck surgery. In some cases, patients have a decreased sensation where aspiration does not elicit a cough response. This is a particularly dangerous situation (Pizzorni et al., 2014).

To prepare for home enteral feeding, teach patients and families to administer the feedings. Supervise the adminis-

---

Figure 9-9. Targets for Nutritional Goals for Postsurgical Head and Neck Cancer Patients—Estimated Macronutrient Guidelines

- Calories: 25–30 kcal/kg
- Protein: 1–1.5 g protein/kg
- Water: 30–40 ml/kg or 1 ml/kcal
- Vitamins and minerals: Recommended daily allowance requirements

For weight gain, increase calories and protein:
- 30–35 kcal/kg or greater
- 1.5–2.5 g protein/kg

Patients with severe malnutrition should be fed 15–20 kcal/kg for the first several days then gradually advance calorie goals.

Note. Based on information from Fessler, 2008.

tration of feedings until the patients and families are proficient.

Swallowing

Excision of a tumor of the head and neck may result in a surgical defect with loss of structures that can result in difficulty swallowing. The bolus of food or liquid in the oropharynx starts a chain reaction that begins with relaxation of the upper esophageal sphincter followed by peristaltic waves that move the bolus to the lower esophagus and then through the relaxed lower esophageal sphincter into the stomach. Effects of radiation or chemotherapy may cause surgical ablation of muscular and nervous structures, potentially disrupting this process. The severity of the deficit depends upon the size and location of the tumor, the extent of surgical resection and nature of the reconstruction, and the side effects of medical treatments (Chasen & Bhargava, 2009). Normal swallowing is divided into four phases: oral preparation, oral, pharyngeal, and esophageal. During the oral preparatory phase, food is chewed and mixed with saliva to form a bolus. During the oral phase, the bolus is transported to the pharynx. The swallowing reflex is triggered in the pharyngeal phase, which then forces the larynx to close to prevent aspiration. This is followed by contraction of the pharyngeal constrictor muscles, laryngeal elevation, epiglottic inversion, and finally, relaxation of the cricopharyngeus that allows the bolus to pass into the esophagus. In the final phase, peristalsis moves the bolus into the stomach (Murphy & Gilbert, 2009).

Tissue loss, transection of muscles and nerves, scar formation, and loss of sensation can cause dysphagia in patients undergoing tumor resection. These can all result in significant alteration in function that is vital for normal swallowing (Murphy & Gilbert, 2009).

Radiation therapy can also cause acute and late-effect dysphagia. This causes damage to the mucosa and soft tissue within the radiation field. Patients develop mucositis, edema of the soft tissue, radiation dermatitis, pain, thickened and excessive mucus production, xerostomia, and edema, which can all attribute to acute dysphagia. Late-effect dysphagia is caused by ongoing effects of radiation, causing tissues to become fibrotic and firm with resultant loss or impedance of function (Murphy & Gilbert, 2009).

Transoral robotic surgery (TORS) has been used in the treatment of benign and malignant lesions of the oropharynx, hypopharynx, supraglottis, glottis, and parapharyngeal space. TORS is more widely used in early T-stage tumors of the upper aerodigestive tract and most frequently for oropharyngeal and tongue base tumors. TORS has significant advantages to the pharynx by avoiding large neck incisions, mandibulotomies, pharyngotomies, and the resultant morbidities associated with those approaches. It is a minimally invasive approach and provides the surgeon with a three-dimensional, high-definition view of the operative field. The maneuverability of the endoscope affords a wide field of vision that allows for precise bimanual tissue manipulation and en bloc excision of tongue base and other oropharyngeal tumors (Richmon et al., 2014).

Patients undergoing TORS resection should have a formal preoperative swallowing evaluation to establish baseline function. This is done with functional endoscopic evaluation of swallowing (FEES) or modified barium swallow study. Postoperatively, patients should receive 24 hours of IV steroids and antibiotics to manage edema of the airway, nausea, pain, and bacterial overgrowth within the pharyngeal wound. Patients should be closely monitored and placed in an observation ward to assess airway edema. Patients who undergo TORS should have a bedside swallowing evaluation the next morning to determine if the NG tube can be removed and the patient initiated on a clear liquid diet and allowed to advance as tolerated. If oral feeding cannot be initiated, enteral feedings should begin. If patients also have a concurrent neck dissection and a drain is placed, they will either be discharged after the drain is removed or sent home with drain care instructions. If patients are discharged with a temporary NG tube, they should follow up with speech pathology and swallowing evaluation approximately 10 days postoperatively. TORS has associated risks such as hemorrhage, prolonged intubation, dehydration, oral thrush, and aspiration (Richmon et al., 2014).

For patients experiencing abnormalities in their swallowing, the speech-language pathologist will recommend safe swallowing strategies emphasizing the avoidance of aspiration, therapeutic postures and exercises that help improve function over time, and ways to modify diet to ensure adequate oral intake. Patients, families, and their healthcare teams should all be aware of the recommendations (see Table 9-5) (Murphy & Gilbert, 2009).

Oral realimentation can be started six hours after surgery with first a liquid diet, followed by a normal diet within 13 hours after surgery. Enteral realimentation by PEG includes 500 ml of sterile saline solution between hours 7 and 13 postoperatively, followed by progressive enteral nutrition. It is important to maintain nutrition for wound healing and protect the airway from aspiration while rehabilitating patients' ability to swallow an oral diet. Videofluoroscopic swallowing assessment should be performed to evaluate specific changes in patients' swallowing mechanism. Some of the changes may include decreased base of tongue retraction, resulting in reduced propulsion of the bolus into the pharynx, as well as reduced laryngeal elevation. In addition, decreased pharyngeal contraction has been known to result in bolus residue in the pharynx after swallowing (Zuercher, Grosjean, & Monnier, 2011).

After a partial laryngectomy, significant alterations in swallowing are inevitable, and compensatory mechanisms

Table 9-5. Examples of Exercises and Maneuvers for Dysphagia Therapy

Mendelsohn maneuver	Voluntary prolongation of laryngeal excursion and cricopharyngeal opening during swallowing. Participants initiate the swallow and "hold" the larynx in the elevated position for five seconds, using the muscles of the neck.
Shaker exercises	Targets upper esophageal sphincter dysphagia. Patients lie flat on their back and lift the head four inches and look at their toes without lifting the shoulders. Extended or repetitive format.
Effortful swallow	Targets reduced pharyngeal peristalsis with residue after swallow. Participant swallows hard, squeezing the walls of the throat together.
Supraglottic swallow	Targets decreased airway protection, aspiration by increasing airway protection with closure of true vocal folds; dispels residue above the glottis after the swallow.
Compensatory positions	Chin tuck/chin to chest: help with reduced bolus control, premature spillage into larynx, decreased tongue base movement. Head rotation to affected side: compensatory measure for unilateral pharyngeal paresis or unilateral vocal fold dysfunction or cricopharyngeal dysmotility
Oral stage exercises	Includes lip closure, lingual and jaw range of motion
Base of tongue exercises	Includes tongue retraction, yawn/gargle, Masako maneuver. This maneuver is performed by protruding your tongue between the front teeth, holding it in place by gently biting down on the anterior portion of the tongue, and maintaining this posture while swallowing saliva.

Note. From "Dysphagia in Head and Neck Cancer Patients Treated With Radiation: Assessment, Sequelae, and Rehabilitation," by B.A. Murphy and J. Gilbert, 2009, *Seminars in Radiation Oncology, 19,* p. 37. Copyright 2009 by Elsevier. Reprinted with permission.

are necessary to restore the function. The laryngeal anatomy is severely modified and glottis closure is impaired as a result of tumor resection. Dysphagia is mainly related to impairment of airway protection, caused by insufficient glottis closure during the pharyngeal phase of swallowing. Laryngeal sensation can also be reduced because of superior laryngeal nerve impairment. After a total laryngectomy, the swallowing is usually well preserved because the digestive and respiratory tracts are entirely separated (Pizzorni et al., 2014).

Patients who have undergone composite resections for oral cavity tumors are at higher risk for aspiration because of the alteration of the oral cavity and the presence of an intact and vulnerable larynx (see Figures 9-10 and 9-11).

Swallowing Evaluation

Although it should be standard of care to assess swallowing function in patients with head and neck cancer, the treating practitioners should be aware of triggers that suggest aspiration. These triggers are inability to control food or liquid in the oral cavity; storing of food in the cheek; excessive chewing, drooling, coughing, or choking during or after swallowing; a "wet" or "gurgly" voice after swallowing; complaints of difficulty swallowing, food sticking, or globus sensation; nasal regurgitation; and weight loss (Murphy & Gilbert, 2009).

Swallowing assessment and therapy should be performed by a certified speech-language pathologist who is

Figure 9-10. Risk Factors for Aspiration

- Decreased level of consciousness
- Supine position
- Presence of a nasogastric tube
- Tracheal intubation and mechanical ventilation
- Bolus or intermittent feeding delivery methods
- Malpositioned feeding tube
- Vomiting
- High-risk disease and injury conditions
- Neurologic disorders
- Major abdominal and thoracic trauma/surgery
- Diabetes mellitus
- Poor oral health
- Inadequate RN staffing levels
- Advanced age

Note. Based on information from Metheny, 2002.

trained in the care of patients with head and neck cancer. The speech-language pathologist should be consulted early in the treatment of these patients, and routine follow-up should be part of the treatment plan so that intervention can be accomplished when necessary (Murphy & Gilbert, 2009). The evaluation should include assessment of the swallowing function to determine any preexisting swallowing abnormalities, determine whether further testing is needed to diagnose a swallowing disorder, create a plan of treatment that includes swallowing therapy and patient education, communicate with nutritionists to establish an adequate diet, and

Figure 9-11. Methods for Decreasing Risk of Aspiration Pneumonia

- Elevate head of bed 30°–45°, unless contraindicated.
- Limit use of sedatives.
- Assess feeding tube placement every four hours.
- Avoid bolus feeding in patients at high risk for aspiration.
- Suction subglottic secretions.
- Assess swallowing before initiating oral feedings for recently extubated patients.
- Maintain tracheal cuff pressures, as appropriate.

Note. Based on information from Bell, 2011.

identify patients at risk for aspiration (Murphy & Gilbert, 2009).

A number of methods are used to assess swallowing function. The most common is modified barium swallow study (MBSS), a videofluoroscopic test that assesses oral and pharyngeal function. This helps to identify swallowing impairments, aspiration, and patients' ability to maintain adequate nutrition and hydration (Murphy & Gilbert, 2009).

FEES, another common assessment tool, allows direct visualization of the nasopharynx, tongue base, hypopharynx, and larynx. This allows evaluation of sensory deficits, muscular function, and management of secretions. This is a safe procedure that can be done at the bedside or in the outpatient setting. Because FEES does not assess the oral cavity and the upper esophageal sphincter function, it should be used as a complementary assessment tool to MBSS (Murphy & Gilbert, 2009).

Of the current methods used to treat dysphagia, deep pharyngeal neuromuscular electrical stimulation (NMES) is a technique in which controlled neuromuscular stimulation is used to build strength in swallowing muscles and improve laryngeal elevation. The primary goal of using NMES in the pharynx or larynx is to utilize electrical current to stimulate the pharyngeal and laryngeal muscles through intact peripheral nerves. Electrodes are simultaneously activated over the laryngeal and submental regions and produce simultaneous contraction of the mylohyoid to elevate the hyoid bone and then the thyrohyoid to elevate the larynx to the hyoid bone (Ryu et al., 2009).

NMES therapy continues to be a popular treatment mode, with the goal to strengthen and re-educate muscles and ultimately improve motor control of the swallowing mechanism. NMES improves blood flow to the muscles being stimulated and can slow down muscular atrophy (DeFabrizio & Rajappa, 2010).

Communication

But the most traumatic result of the surgery was the loss of voice, even though I had known it was coming. My doctor had said that . . . it is more shattering to the patient than coming out of an operation blind. (Dresden, 1978, p. 46)

Treatments for head and neck cancers are associated with temporary or permanent loss of voice, or speechlessness, which limits patients' ability to communicate critical information to their care team immediately postoperatively. Some patients undergo radical surgeries, such as total laryngectomy and glossectomy; these result in a permanent loss of speech. Other patients experience temporary speechlessness secondary to upper airway edema, extended intubation, or tracheostomy. Patients with head and neck cancer are typically able to vocalize prior to surgical intervention but have varying degrees of voice changes or voicelessness postoperatively (Rodriguez & Blischak, 2010). The alterations to communication following head and neck surgery pose a unique challenge to most patients. Preoperative teaching by both the nurse and the speech-language pathologist about the loss of normal communication, even if temporary, is essential to postoperative adaptation and recovery.

The sudden inability to communicate is a common problem that negatively affects patient-nurse communication in the acute care setting. Sudden speechlessness often results from surgeries that impair structures needed for speech or conditions that require respiratory support with airway intubation or artificial airways. This is not only abrupt and frightening for patients but can also be a challenge for nurses helping these patients to communicate their needs effectively. The means in which the patients attempt to communicate is with mouthing words, hand gestures, and written communication (Rodriguez, Spring, & Rowe, 2015). Nurses should provide their patients with writing tools, dry-erase boards, or word-alphabet boards. For patients with decreased mobility from free flap graft donor sites or impaired vision, these options for communication are not feasible. A speech-language pathologist is someone who is specially trained in augmentative and alternative communication and can be a very valuable resource to assist in the assessment and intervention of nonspeaking patients (Radtke, Baumann, Garrett, & Happ, 2011).

Complete loss of laryngeal function, including the loss of the natural voice, is one of the most important consequences of a total laryngectomy because it affects both the physical and psychological quality of life in these patients. The primary options for voice restoration are artificial larynx (electrolarynx), esophageal speech, and tracheoesophageal puncture (TEP). The initiation of these methods will vary greatly and are patient dependent. Immediate postoperative conditions could inhibit the use of an electrolarynx, such as fibrotic soft tissue in the neck or the presence of copious amounts of secretions. Esophageal speech is very difficult to teach and learn and requires a lot of practice, making it not feasible immediately postoperatively.

TEP is the most commonly used form of voice restoration and is considered the gold standard because of its superiority in most phoniatric measures. The procedure involves a surgically created puncture made to the posterior tracheal wall via the esophagus. A valve prosthesis is then inserted (see Figure 9-12). To achieve a successful TEP, it is essential that the speech-language pathologist educate patients beforehand. The timing of the TEP is multifactorial and dependent on the philosophies and practices of the treating surgeon and team and the patient's desire (Moon et al., 2014).

Patients' ability, method, and preferences for communication need to be assessed, as well as their ability to read and write. Knowledge of a patient's native language and level of education also is essential. The speech-language pathologist evaluates patients' ability to articulate and use facial communication and hand gestures. Patients who are more naturally animated speakers usually will cope and communicate better after surgery.

Understanding patients' specific needs is essential in supporting postoperative communication. Nurses must take the time to listen and understand an individual's speech pattern and focus on articulation as well as context. The investment of time and patience will result in patient confidence and appreciation.

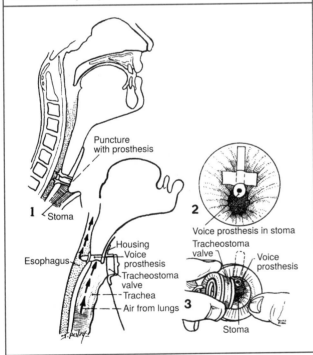

Figure 9-12. Anatomy of a Total Neck Breather With Tracheoesophageal Puncture

Note. From *Looking Forward: A Guidebook for the Laryngectomee* (3rd ed., p. 9), by R.L. Keith, 1995, New York, NY: Thieme New York. Copyright 1995 by Thieme New York. Reprinted with permission.

Body Image Disturbance

Body image is a critical psychosocial issue for patients with head and neck cancer, as the disease and its treatment can significantly alter physical appearance and result in loss or impairment in function. The face plays an important role in an individual's sense of self. It is the most visibly prominent area of anatomy that reflects animation and emotion and serves as the primary means of communicating with others. Facial disfigurement can profoundly affect social interactions, self-perceptions, and overall emotional well-being. This can cause patients to feel isolated and restricted in their social activities (Penner, 2009). Patients usually present later in their illness and require more aggressive forms of treatment, such as radical resections of bone and soft tissue, resulting in physical and psychological symptoms and dysfunction, such as dysphagia, disfigurement, anxiety, and depression. Those with greater deformities have higher levels of depression. Gender is widely recognized to be a strong predictor of body image dissatisfaction in the general population, with women experiencing higher levels of difficulties and concerns in this area. Visible physical changes are often associated with negative self-image, low self-esteem, isolation, and fear of rejection in interpersonal and romantic relationships (Valente, 2009). Multimodal treatment introduces additional body image changes that can further compromise quality of life (Penner, 2009). Some studies have shown that interventions such as self-help materials, cognitive behavioral therapy, group-based person-centered therapy, social skills training, and support groups can be helpful. Social support is an important factor in alleviating social dysfunction and emotional distress that patients with facial disfigurement experience (Penner, 2009).

Nurses need to provide informational, practical, and emotional support to these patients to help them develop effective coping skills and increase confidence in social settings. Nurses should use good eye contact and leisurely conversation with these patients to demonstrate to them that their appearance is socially acceptable. Nurses should be present the first time their patients look in the mirror and allow them to express their feelings, as well as answer their questions in a sensitive manner. Furthermore, educating the patients in self-care activities, such as applying makeup or shaving, can help facilitate coping skills and encourages independence (Penner, 2009).

Impairment in the ability to eat and drink in a socially acceptable manner often poses difficulties for patients with head and neck cancer. Dysphagia has a profound effect on the lives of patients and their families. It causes alterations in the physical, emotional, and social aspects of normal life routines, which changes the meaning that these patients attribute to food. They may require additional time to eat or experience oral incontinence, causing them to avoid eating in public or around others in general. This leads to embarrassment and feelings of social isolation and ultimately a significantly lower quality of life. Swallowing rehabilitation is a crucial part of care from both a functional and psychosocial perspective (Penner, 2009).

Associated with challenges with eating are rapid or significant changes in weight. This not only affects patients' well-being, strength, and energy, but also impacts their appearance, body image, and self-perception. Although treatment, either by surgical resection and reconstruction or radiation with or without chemotherapy, causes obvious physical changes to the face and neck, most of these changes are temporary. Changes in the body related to weight loss, difficulty regaining weight or living with losses related to eating, swallowing, and managing food make the rite of passage from illness back to health more difficult. The drastic changes in weight and body may serve as a constant reminder of illness and cancer, making a return to health difficult (McQuestion, Fitch, & Howell, 2011).

Sexuality can be a major concern for patients with head and neck cancer. Reduced libido and sexual enjoyment are common in patients who undergo surgery for laryngeal and hypopharyngeal cancer. Ensure that patients' concerns regarding sexuality are met by bringing up the topic of sexual function early, allowing patients to know that this is a valid concern and appropriate to discuss (Penner, 2009).

Patients face significant challenges in relation to physical, emotional, and social functioning. It is imperative to assess how these patients are coping with these challenges. Ineffective coping strategies are strongly associated with depression. Hopelessness, helplessness, anxiety, and fatalism are feelings that should be monitored, as they can lead to a lower quality of life. Screening for depression at the time of diagnosis is part of health promotion and evaluation for nurses and other licensed professionals (Valente, 2009).

Tobacco Use in Patients

Smoking accounts for at least 30% of all cancer deaths and nearly 90% of all lung cancer deaths annually. Almost 62% of all patients recently diagnosed with cancer are reportedly current smokers or former smokers or have quit in the past 12 months. Smoking cessation and prevention of relapse are important areas needed to improve cancer survival rates, reduce the risk of cancer treatment complications, and improve quality of life. Prognosis, tumor site, and the effect of cancer treatment itself can influence tobacco cessation rates. The overall prevalence of current smoking among cancer survivors is approximately 23% in the first year after diagnosis. After this period, smoking rates drop gradually. This suggests that the first year after diagnosis is a crucial time to initiate relapse prevention interventions. To treat a tobacco use disorder, clinicians must be aware of its presence. It is recommended that systematic screening for tobacco use be performed. In 2013, the U.S. government began mandating systematic screening of tobacco and alcohol use as part

of a "meaningful use" of electronic health records. In order to treat tobacco use disorders, the biologic, psychological, and social aspects of the disorder should be addressed. The main pillars of screening and interventions for tobacco use and dependence are summarized in the "5 A's" model, which was recommended in the 2008 Clinical Practice Guidelines Update by the U.S. Public Health Service. This directs clinicians to ask and document smoking status, advise all smokers to quit, assess patients' readiness to quit, assist them with more intensive counseling and resources for tobacco cessation, and arrange follow-up and any necessary referrals (Karam-Hage, Cinciripini, & Gritz, 2014).

Patients need psychological support preoperatively and postoperatively by means of education about the process, as well as outcomes of surgery. Patients need support to cope with their fears, worries, and depressive symptoms related to their disease and symptoms related to the treatment. Nurses who evaluate emotional responses provide support and use therapeutic interventions and appropriate referrals to enhance treatment for their patients. It is appropriate to involve family practitioners to target and address patients' physical and psychosocial needs after discharge from the hospital or cancer treatment center. All healthcare providers need to continue to proactively assess the psychosocial needs of cancer survivors and intervene accordingly. In addition, caregivers and family members are in a unique position of both giving and needing support (Valente, 2009). Social support strategies need to be tailored to patients experiencing head and neck cancer, their caregivers, and family members to improve perceived support and well-being (McQuestion et al., 2011).

Summary

Postoperative management of patients with head and neck cancer takes a team of skilled healthcare professionals to assess, manage, and educate patients and families, and nurses play an integral role. Nurses must have a clear understanding of the anatomic and physiologic changes, comorbid conditions, and psychosocial needs of this patient population. Staying educated on current research, advances in treatment, and care is key to guiding the patients and families along the head and neck cancer care continuum.

The authors would like to acknowledge Ann E.F. Sievers, RN, MA, CORLN, for her contribution to this chapter that remains unchanged from the first edition of this book.

References

American Association for Respiratory Care. (2010). AARC clinical practice guidelines: Endotracheal suctioning of mechanically ventilated patients with artificial airways 2010. *Respiratory Care, 55*, 758–764. Retrieved from http://www.rcjournal.com/cpgs/pdf/06.10.0758.pdf

American Geriatrics Society Panel on the Pharmacological Management of Persistent Pain in Older Persons. (2009). Pharmacological management of persistent pain in older persons. *Pain Medicine, 10*, 1062–1083. doi:10.1111/j.1526-4637.2009.00699.x

American Society of Anesthesiologists Task Force on Acute Pain Management. (2012). Practice guidelines for acute pain management in the perioperative setting: An updated report by the American Society of Anesthesiologists Task Force on Acute Pain Management. *Anesthesiology, 116*, 248–273. doi:10.1097/ALN.0b013e31823c1030

Arbogast, D. (2002). Enteral feedings with comfort and safety. *Clinical Journal of Oncology Nursing, 6*, 275–280. doi:10.1188/02.CJON.275-280

Asher, S.A., White, H.N., Golden, J.B., Magnuson, J.S., Carroll, W.R., & Rosenthal, E.L. (2014). Negative pressure wound therapy in head and neck surgery. *JAMA Facial Plastic Surgery, 16*, 120–126. doi:10.1001/jamafacial.2013.2163

Bachar, G., Esmat, N., Stern, S., Litvin, S., Knizhnik, M., Perlow, E., ... Belenky, A. (2013). Transarterial embolization for acute head and neck bleeding: Eight-year experience with emphasis on rebleeding risk in cancer patients. *Laryngoscope, 123*, 1220–1226. doi:10.1002/lary.23996

Bader, P., Echtle, D., Fonteyne, V., Livadas, K., De Meerleer, G., PaezBorda, A., ... Vranken, J.H. (Eds.). (2010). *Guidelines on pain management*. Arnhem, Netherlands: European Association of Urology.

Bell, L. (2011). American Association of Critical Care Nurses practice alert: Prevention of aspiration. Retrieved from http://www.aacn.org/wd/practice/docs/practicealerts/prevention-aspiration-practice-alert.pdf?menu=aboutus

Brennan, P.A., Blythe, J.N., Herd, M.K., Habib, A., & Anand, R. (2012). The contemporary management of chyle leak following cervical thoracic duct damage. *British Journal of Oral and Maxillofacial Surgery, 50*, 197–201. doi:10.1016/j.bjoms.2011.02.001

Brown, D.D., Yuen, H.K., Sulwer, M.R., & Lupini, J. (2013). Physical and occupational therapy. In G. Har-El, C.O. Nathan, T.A. Day, & S.A. Nguyen (Eds.), *A multidisciplinary approach to head and neck neoplasms* (pp. 186–195). Noida, Uttar Pradesh, India: Thieme.

Brown, T., Banks, M., Hughes, B., Kenny, L., Lin, C., & Bauer, J. (2014). Protocol for a randomized controlled trial of early prophylactic feeding via gastrostomy versus standard care in high risk patients with head and neck cancer. *BMC Nursing, 13*, 17. doi:10.1186/1472-6955-13-17

Caparros, A.C. (2014). Mechanical ventilation and the role of saline instillation in suctioning adult intensive care unit patients: An evidence-based practice review. *Dimensions of Critical Care Nursing, 33*, 246–253. doi:10.1097/DCC.0000000000000049

Chambers, M.S., Lemon, J.C., & Martin, J.W. (2003). How I do it: A technique for oral wound irrigation following maxillectomy and mandibulectomy. *ORL—Head and Neck Nursing, 21*(4), 27–28.

Chasen, M.R., & Bhargava, R. (2009). A descriptive review of the factors contributing to nutritional compromise in patients with head and neck cancer. *Supportive Care in Cancer, 17*, 1345–1351. doi:10.1007/s00520-009-0684-5

Chaukar, D.A., Deshmukh, A.D., Majeed, T., Chaturvedi, P., Pai, P., & D'Cruz, A.K. (2013). Factors affecting wound complications in head and neck surgery: A prospective study. *Indian Journal of Medical and Paediatric Oncology, 34*, 247–251.

Dagi, T.F. (2005). The management of postoperative bleeding. *Surgical Clinics of North America, 85*, 1191–1213. doi:10.1016/j.suc.2005.10.013

Dechaphunkul, T., Martin, L., Alberda, C., Olson, K., Baracos, V., & Gramlich, L. (2013). Malnutrition assessment in patients with cancers of the head and neck: A call to action and consensus. *Critical Reviews in Oncology/Hematology, 88*, 459–476. doi:10.1016/j.critrevonc.2013.06.003

Dedivitis, R.A., Aires, F.T., Cernea, C.R., & Brandão, L.G. (2015). Pharyngocutaneous fistula after total laryngectomy: Systematic review of risk factors. *Head and Neck, 37*, 1691–1697. doi:10.1002/hed.23804

DeFabrizio, M.E., & Rajappa, A. (2010). Contemporary approaches to dysphagia management. *Journal for Nurse Practitioners, 6*, 622–630. doi:10.1016/j.nurpra.2009.11.010

de Lima, L.P., Amar, A., & Lehn, C.N. (2011). Spinal accessory nerve neuropathy following neck dissection. *Brazilian Journal of Otorhinolaryngology, 77*, 259–262. doi:10.1590/S1808-86942011000200017

Dresden, D. (1978, November 26). Speechless. *The Washington Post Magazine*, pp. 46–52.

Ehrsson, Y.T., Langius-Eklöf, A., & Laurell, G. (2012). Nutritional surveillance and weight loss in head and neck cancer patients. *Supportive Care in Cancer, 20*, 757–765. doi:10.1007/s00520-011-1146-4

Fessler, T.A. (2008). Enteral nutrition for patients with head and neck cancer. *Today's Dietitian, 10*(6), 46. Retrieved from http://www.todaysdietitian.com/newarchives/tdjune2008pg46.shtml

Frawley, T., & Begley, C.M. (2005). Causes and prevention of carotid artery rupture. *British Journal of Nursing, 14*, 1198–1202. doi:10.12968/bjon.2005.14.22.20173

Fujita, T., Tanabe, M., Kobayashi, T., Washida, Y., Kato, M., Iida, E., ... Matsunga, N. (2013). Percutaneous gastrostomy tube placement using a balloon catheter in patients with head and neck cancer. *Journal of Parenteral and Enteral Nutrition, 37*, 117–122. doi:10.1177/0148607111435264

Haas, M.L. (2011). Radiation therapy: Toxicities and management. In C.H. Yarbro, D. Wujcik, & B.H. Gobel (Eds.), *Cancer nursing: Principles and practice* (7th ed., pp. 312–351). Burlington, MA: Jones & Bartlett Learning.

Harris, D.G., & Noble, S.I.R. (2009). Management of terminal hemorrhage in patients with advanced cancer: A systematic literature review. *Journal of Pain and Symptom Management, 38*, 913–927. doi:10.1016/j.jpainsymman.2009.04.027

Harris, L.L. (2008). Nursing diagnosis. In L.L. Harris & M.B. Huntoon (Eds.), *Core curriculum for otorhinolaryngology and head-neck nursing* (2nd ed., pp. 401–415). New Smyrna Beach, FL: Society of Otorhinolaryngology and Head-Neck Nurses.

Hickey, M.M., & Higgins, T.S. (2008). Trachea and esophagus. In L.L. Harris & M.B. Huntoon (Eds.), *Core curriculum for otorhinolaryngology and head-neck nursing* (2nd ed., pp. 275–304). New Smyrna Beach, FL: Society of Otorhinolaryngology and Head-Neck Nurses.

Hudak, M., & Bond-Domb, A. (1996). Postoperative head and neck cancer patients with artificial airways: The effect of saline lavage on tracheal mucus evacuation and oxygen saturation. *ORL—Head and Neck Nursing, 14*(1), 17–22.

Hudak, M., & Hickey, M.M. (2008). Nursing management of the patient with a tracheostomy. In E.N. Myers & J.T. Johnson (Eds.), *Tracheotomy airway management, communication, and swallowing* (2nd ed., pp. 147–168). San Diego, CA: Plural Publishing.

Jaquet, Y., Enepekides, D.J., Torgerson, C., & Higgins, K.M. (2012). Radial forearm free flap donor site morbidity: Ulnar-based transposition flap vs split-thickness skin graft. *Archives of Otolaryngology—Head and Neck Surgery, 138*, 38–43. doi:10.1001/archoto.2011.216

Jindal, G., Gemmete, J., & Gandhi, D. (2012). Interventional neuroradiology applications in otolaryngology, head and neck surgery. *Otolaryngologic Clinics of North America, 45*, 1423–1449. doi:10.1016/j.otc.2012.08.010

Johnson, W.A. (2013). Tracheostomy tube change. Retrieved from http://emedicine.medscape.com/article/1580576-overview

Karam-Hage, M., Cinciripini, P.M., & Gritz, E.R. (2014). Tobacco use and cessation for cancer survivors: An overview for clinicians. *CA: A Cancer Journal for Clinicians, 64*, 272–290. doi:10.3322/caac.21231

Karlsson, M., Lindgren, M., Jarnhed-Andersson, I., & Tarpila, E. (2014). Dressing the split-thickness skin graft donor site: A randomized clinical trial. *Advances in Skin and Wound Care, 27*, 20–25. doi:10.1097/01.ASW.0000437786.92529.22

Kinetic Concepts, Inc. (2014). V.A.C. therapy clinical guidelines: A reference source for clinicians. Retrieved from http://www.kci1.com/cs/Sat

ellite?blobcol=urldata&blobheader=application%2Fpdf&blobkey=id&
blobtable=MungoBlobs&blobwhere=1226689404554&ssbinary=true

Learned, K.O., Malloy, K.M., & Loevner, L.A. (2012). Myocutaneous flaps and other vascularized grafts in head and neck reconstruction for cancer treatment. *Magnetic Resonance Imaging Clinics of North America, 20,* 495–513. doi:10.1016/j.mric.2012.05.004

Lin, S.J., & Rabie, A.N. (2014). Head and neck cancer—Reconstruction. Retrieved from http://emedicine.medscape.com/article/1289799-overview

Marcantonio, E.R. (2012). Postoperative delirium: A 76-year-old woman with delirium following surgery. *JAMA, 308,* 73–81. doi:10.1001/jama.2012.6857

Marsh, M., Elliott, S., Anand, R., & Brennan, P.A. (2009). Early postoperative care for free flap head and neck reconstructive surgery—A national survey of practice. *British Journal of Oral and Maxillofacial Surgery, 47,* 182–185. doi:10.1016/j.bjoms.2008.06.004

McDonald, M.W., Moore, M.G., & Johnstone, P.A. (2012). Risk of carotid blowout after reirradiation of the head and neck: A systematic review. *International Journal of Radiation Oncology, Biology, Physics, 82,* 1083–1089. doi:10.1016/j.ijrobp.2010.08.029

McGuire, D.B., Fulton, J.S., Park, J., Brown, C.G., Correa, M.E., Eilers, J., … Lalla, R.V. (2013). Systematic review of basic oral care for the management of oral mucositis in cancer patients. *Supportive Care in Cancer, 21,* 3165–3177. doi:10.1007/s00520-013-1942-0

McMenamin, E. (2011). Cancer pain management. In C.H. Yarbro, D. Wujcik, & B.H. Gobel (Eds.), *Cancer nursing: Principles and practice* (7th ed., pp. 685–712). Burlington, MA: Jones & Bartlett Learning.

McQuestion, M., Fitch, M., & Howell, D. (2011). The changed meaning of food: Physical, social, and emotional loss for patients having received radiation treatment for head and neck cancer. *European Journal of Oncology Nursing, 15,* 145–151. doi:10.1016/j.ejon.2010.07.006

Metheny, N.A. (2002). Risk factors for aspiration. *Journal of Parenteral and Enteral Nutrition, 26*(Suppl. 6), S26–S31. doi:10.1177/014860710202600605

Mitchell, R.B., Hussey, H.M., Setzen, G., Jacobs, I.N., Nussenbaum, B., Dawson, C., … Merati, A. (2013). Clinical consensus statement: Tracheostomy care. *Otolaryngology—Head and Neck Surgery, 148,* 6–20. doi:10.1177/0194599812460376

Moon, S., Raffa, F., Ojo, R., Landera, M.A., Weed, D.T., Sargi, Z., & Lundy, D. (2014). Changing trends of speech outcomes after total laryngectomy in the 21st century: A single-center study. *Laryngoscope, 124,* 2508–2512. doi:10.1002/lary.24717

Mueller, C., Compher, C., & Druyan, M.E. (2011). A.S.P.E.N. clinical guidelines: Nutritional screening, assessment, and intervention in adults. *Journal of Parenteral and Enteral Nutrition, 35,* 16–24. doi:10.1177/0148607110389335

Munday, D., & Semple, C.J. (2012). Palliative and psychosocial issues in advanced head and neck cancer. In H.M. Mehanna & K.K. Ang (Eds.), *Head and neck cancer recurrence* (pp. 277–293). New York, NY: Thieme.

Murphy, B.A., & Gilbert, J. (2009). Dysphagia in head and neck cancer patients treated with radiation: Assessment, sequelae, and rehabilitation. *Seminars in Radiation Oncology, 19,* 35–42. doi:10.1016/j.semradonc.2008.09.007

Nambu, J., Sugino, K., Oishi, K., Yano, M., Nishihara, M., & Dohi, K. (2013). Characteristics of postoperative bleeding after neck surgery. *Surgical Science, 4,* 192–195. doi:10.4236/ss.2013.43036

National Comprehensive Cancer Network. (2015). *NCCN Clinical Practice Guidelines in Oncology (NCCN Guidelines®): Adult cancer pain* [v.2.2015]. Retrieved from http://www.nccn.org/professionals/physician_gls/pdf/pain.pdf

Orlik, J.R., Horwich, P., Bartlett, C., Trites, J., Hart, R., & Taylor, S.M. (2014). Long-term functional donor site morbidity of the free radial forearm flap in head and neck cancer survivors. *Journal of Otolaryngology—Head and Neck Surgery, 43.* doi:10.1186/1916-0216-43-1

Pattani, K.M., Byrne, P., Boahene, K., & Richmon, J. (2010). What makes a good flap go bad? A critical analysis of the literature of intraoperative factors related to free flap failure. *Laryngoscope, 120,* 717–723. doi:10.1002/lary.20825

Penner, J. (2009). Psychosocial care of patients with head and neck cancer. *Seminars in Oncology Nursing, 25,* 231–241. doi:10.1016/j.soncn.2009.05.008

Pizzorni, N., Ginocchio, D., Mozzanica, F., Roncoroni, L., Scarponi, L., & Schindler, A. (2014). Head and neck diseases and disorders causing oropharyngeal dysphagia. *Journal of Gastroenterology and Hepatology Research, 3,* 1272–1280. Retrieved from http://www.ghrnet.org/index.php/joghr/article/view/884

Pohlenz, P., Klatt, J., Schön, K.G., Blessmann, M., Li, L., & Schmelzle, R. (2012). Microvascular free flaps in head and neck surgery: Complications and outcome of 1000 flaps. *International Journal of Oral and Maxillofacial Surgery, 41,* 739–743. doi:10.1016/j.ijom.2012.02.012

Prodrug. (n.d.). In *The American Heritage Stedman's medical dictionary.* Retrieved from http://dictionary.reference.com/browse/prodrug

Pujade-Lauraine, E., & Gascón, P. (2004). The burden of anaemia in patients with cancer. *Oncology, 67*(Suppl. 1), 1–4. doi:10.1159/000080702

Radtke, J.V., Baumann, B.M., Garrett, K.L., & Happ, M.B. (2011). Listening to the voiceless patient: Case reports in assisted communication in the intensive care unit. *Journal of Palliative Medicine, 14,* 791–795. doi:10.1089/jpm.2010.0313

Rhodes-Nessert, S., & Laronde, D.M. (2014). Dental hygiene care of the head and neck cancer patient and survivor. *Canadian Journal of Dental Hygiene, 48*(10), 20–26. Retrieved from http://www.researchgate.net/publication/262035954_Dental_hygiene_care_of_the_head_and_neck_cancer_patient_and_survivor

Richmon, J.D., Feng, A.L., Yang, W., Starmer, H., Quon, H., & Gourin, C.G. (2014). Feasibility of rapid discharge after transoral robotic surgery of the oropharynx. *Laryngoscope, 124,* 2518–2525. doi:10.1002/lary.24748

Rio, A., Whelan, K., Goff, L., Reidlinger, D.P., & Smeeton, N. (2013). Occurrence of refeeding syndrome in adults started on artificial nutrition support: Prospective cohort study. *BMJ, 13.* doi:10.1136/bmjopen-2012-002173

Rodriguez, C.S., & Blischak, D.M. (2010). Communication needs of nonspeaking hospitalized postoperative patients with head and neck cancer. *Applied Nursing Research, 23,* 110–115. doi:10.1016/j.apnr.2008.04.001

Rodriguez, C.S., Spring, H.J., & Rowe, M. (2015). Nurses' experiences of communicating with hospitalized, suddenly speechless patients. *Qualitative Health Research, 25,* 168–178. doi:10.1177/1049732314550206

Rofagha, S., & Seiff, S.R. (2010). Long-term results for the use of gold eyelid load weights in the management of facial paralysis. *Plastic and Reconstructive Surgery, 125,* 142–149. doi:10.1097/PRS.0b013e3181c2a4f2

Ryu, J.S., Kang, J.Y., Park, J.Y., Nam, S.Y., Choi, S.H., Roh, J.L., … Choi, K.H. (2009). The effect of electrical stimulation therapy on dysphagia following treatment for head and neck cancer. *Oral Oncology, 45,* 665–668. doi:10.1016/j.oraloncology.2008.10.005

Schrey, A., Kinnunen, I., Vahlberg, T., Minn, H., Grénman, R., Taittonen, M., & Aitasalo, K. (2011). Blood pressure and free flap oxygenation in head and neck cancer patients. *Acta Oto-Laryngologica, 131,* 757–763. doi:10.3109/00016489.2011.554438

Sievers, A.E.F., & Donald, P.J. (1987). The use of bolus normal saline instillations in artificial airways: Is it useful or necessary? *Heart and Lung, 16,* 342–343.

Sievers, A.E.F. (2010). Nursing care of the complex head and neck cancer patient. In P.J. Donald (Ed.), *The difficult case in head and neck cancer surgery* (pp. 468–484). New York, NY: Thieme.

Strub, G.M., & Moe, K.S. (2013). The use of negative-pressure therapy in the closure of complex head and neck wounds. *Facial Plastic Surgery Clinics of North America, 21,* 137–145. doi:10.1016/j.fsc.2012.11.005

Talmi, Y.P. (2013). Indications and modifications of neck dissection. In G. Har-El, T. Day, C.A. Nathan, & S.A. Nguyen (Eds.), *A multidisciplinary approach to head and neck neoplasms* (pp. 167–176). Noida, Uttar Pradesh, India: Thieme.

Valente, S.M. (2009). Visual disfigurement and depression. *Plastic Surgical Nursing, 29,* 10–16. doi:10.1097/01.PSN.0000347719.75285 .6a

Walvekar, R.R. (2014). Accessory nerve injury. Retrieved from http://emedicine.medscape.com/article/1298684-overview

Walvekar, R.R., & Myers, E.N. (2008). Technique and complications of tracheostomy in adults. In E.N. Myers & J.T. Johnson (Eds.), *Tracheot-*

omy: Airway management, communication, and swallowing (2nd ed., pp. 35–67). San Diego, CA: Plural Publishing.

Wax, M.K. (2014). The role of the implantable Doppler probe in free flap surgery. *Laryngoscope, 124,* S1–S12. doi:10.1002/lary.24569

White, H.N., Golden, B., Sweeny, L., Carroll, W.R., Magnuson, J.S., & Rosenthal, E.L. (2012). Assessment and incidence of salivary leak following laryngectomy. *Laryngoscope, 122,* 1796–1799. doi:10.1002/lary.23443

Zuercher, B.F., Grosjean, P., & Monnier, P. (2011). Percutaneous endoscopic gastrostomy in head and neck cancer patients: Indications, techniques, complications and results. *European Archives of Otorhinolaryngology, 268,* 623–629. doi:10.1007/s00405-010-1412-y

CHAPTER 10

Survivorship

Penelope Stevens Fisher, MS, RN, CORLN

There is no profit in curing the body, if in the process we destroy the soul.

Inscription on the Gate
City of Hope National Medical Center
Duarte, California

Introduction

Cancer survivorship begins when a person learns of a cancer diagnosis and reaches out for information, a treatment plan, and hope. The National Coalition for Cancer Survivorship (NCCS, n.d.) defines a cancer survivor as "any individual that has been diagnosed with cancer, from the time of discovery and for the balance of life." According to the American Cancer Society (ACS), an estimated 14.5 million cancer survivors in the United States were alive in January 2014, and the overall five-year survival rate is 68% (ACS, 2015).

At the milestone of completion of cancer treatment, survivors once again face untraveled ground and unknown expectations. It is well documented in the literature that cancer survivorship has many challenges that result from the disease process and treatment. Head and neck cancer survivors may experience many of the same sequelae as other survivors, but additional concerns may arise as a result of the anatomic location of the disease and area of treatment. Whether the survivors receive curative or palliative care, optimizing quality of life is paramount. Enhancing survivorship outcomes requires an expanded role and expertise for the oncology nurse, as well as increased multidisciplinary research to support reliable and valid interventions.

History of Survivorship

To understand the evolution of survivorship care, it is helpful to look at early survivorship concepts. The literature (Mellon, Northouse, & Weiss, 2006) reports that many cancer survivors experience psychosocial and physiologic challenges, financial concerns, short- and long-term treatment effects, and lengthy rehabilitation. Survivors must put forth effort in maintaining quality of life. This often requires assistance from family members and friends to maintain balance. Mellon et al. also concluded that finding positive meaning in the dimensions of survivorship experiences improved the quality of life for both survivors and their families and decreased stress over the chronic fear of recurrence.

Survivors may feel troubled and burdened by treatment effects. Problems and concerns may include costly alterations to lifestyle because of treatment, short- and long-term complications, prolonged rehabilitation or no access to rehabilitation services, fear of recurrence, economic burden, spiritual effects, physical changes, fatigue, loss of self-determination, pain, indecision, difficult end-of-life decisions, and inability to locate supportive care resources.

Nursing practice considerations include the following.
- Exercise increased assessment and listening skills.
- Apply expert communication, coordination, and documentation skills.
- Use collaborative interprofessional referrals to obtain resources.
- Maintain and provide knowledge and ongoing education for nurses, survivors, and caregivers.

Cancer survivorship had a historic turning point in 2005. The Institute of Medicine (IOM) assembled to review, discuss, and plan for the needs of cancer survivors. The number of survivors had increased, disease and treatment sequelae had been studied, disease-free intervals were longer, and survivors wanted more options to achieve the best quality of life possible. Many survivors required improved interventions for success to enhance life after cancer. The outcomes presented in this report introduced guidelines for programs, resources, systems, and mandates related to cancer survivorship (Hewitt, Greenfield, & Stovall, 2006).

Nursing history is rich in the art and science of care. The contribution of nurses is well recognized by survivors and among multidisciplinary teams. In 2003, the National Cancer Policy Board and IOM commissioned Ferrell, Virani, Smith, and Juarez to examine oncology nursing care for cancer survivors. The outcome was a review of existing oncology nursing standards, textbooks, research-based articles, nursing education, certification, and professional organizations that addressed issues of cancer survivors, caregivers, and nurses. The data gathered from this work set a nursing education framework for the future. Elements of this framework included increasing, supporting, and promoting the following: nursing professional groups' focus on survivorship; specialty education within graduate programs and continuing education for all; education curricula on all levels to include survivorship; basic and advanced certification; integrative survivorship content among educational levels of nurses; and oncology nursing research in survivorship. It additionally called for exploring opportunities for nursing research in clinical trials and with cooperative groups. Today, many of these elements are in effect and actively contribute to the improvement of cancer survivorship care. The work of many nursing leaders devoted to cancer survivorship will be cited in this chapter.

Susan Leigh is an oncology nurse, three-time cancer survivor, founding member of NCCS, and noted author on cancer survivorship. She described survivorship as a process with three stages: acute, extended, and permanent. The survivorship process, although linear, is fraught with unique physical and psychosocial needs. Leigh (2001) described the culture of cancer survivorship for these phases. A summary can be found in Table 10-1.

Leigh (2007) noted the relationship of cancer care and nursing, the emergence of survivorship programs, and the role of nurses in relation to survivorship and long-term care. She identified nurses as the most qualified oncology professionals but noted that there must be a framework shift from disease management to wellness promotion, a model previously adopted in pediatric oncology.

Cancer Rehabilitation and Survivorship: Transdisciplinary Approaches to Personalized Care was published after a major undertaking by the Oncology Nursing Society to facilitate a comprehensive view of cancer survivorship (Lester & Schmitt, 2011). In the chapter titled "From Anecdote to Evidence: The Survivor's Perspective," Leigh (2011) described the history of cancer survivorship and the potential impact of the IOM survivorship treatment summaries and survivor treatment plans. Storytelling is also highlighted as a valuable strategy for survivorship success.

Nursing practice considerations include the following.
* Explore, read, and share literature inclusive of research in survivorship care.
* Integrate awareness of the patient as surviving into personal practice.
* Determine what needs to be added to nurses' practice to assist each patient and optimize independence.
* Ask what is important for the patient population and apply valid and reliable research findings to patients' needs.
* Establish research questions for the patient population that will improve care and initiate research projects.
* Reach out to colleagues, professional nursing groups, interprofessional healthcare team members, and nurse educators for survivor care strategies.

Head and Neck Cancer

The incidence of head and neck cancer in the United States is predicted as accounting for 3% of all malignancies in 2015, with an estimated 60,000 new cases and 12,000 deaths annually (Siegel, Miller, & Jemal, 2015). Head and neck cancer may not be as prevalent as other malignancies, but the disease and treatment present unique challenges to survivors and uniquely affect their quality of life. The general cancer survivor's troubles and concerns have been previously addressed, but head and neck cancer survivors may experience additional challenges because of the association

Table 10-1. The Culture of Cancer Survivorship				
Stage	**Time Frame**	**Facing/Coping**	**Needs**	**Culture**
Acute	• Diagnosis through care	• Fear, losses • Acute side effects of therapy	• Acute care • Management • Education	• Erroneous information, myths • Language barriers
Extended	• End of initial treatment	• Adjusting to compromises	• Rehabilitation • Support	• Lack of understanding
Permanent	• Remission • Potentially cured	• Adaptation • Long-term/late effects of therapy	• Insurance/financial security • Managing late effects of treatment	• Conflicting attitudes, beliefs, values

Note. Based on information from Leigh, 2001.

of treatment modalities related to body image, aesthetics, and function.

Survival Rates

Overall, the five-year survival rate for head and neck cancer in the United States is 56% in Whites and 34% in Blacks (Ridge, Mehra, Lango, & Feigenberg, 2014). Survival rates are affected by histopathology, aggressiveness of the tumor, and tumor-node-metastasis stage. The patient's age, comorbidities, and lifestyle behaviors also contribute to survival. Table 10-2 provides five-year survival rates for head and neck cancer reported by the National Cancer Institute (NCI) Surveillance, Epidemiology, and End Results Program (SEER) (Howlader et al., 2013).

Treatment Sequelae of Head and Neck Cancer

Treatment modalities for head and neck cancer include one or more of the following: surgery, radiation, chemotherapy, and biotherapy. The disease and its treatment may result in late or long-term side effects that may affect both the survivor's perceived and actual well-being. These outcomes may negatively influence the head and neck cancer survivors' quality of life. Figure 10-1 provides a list of known treatment sequelae.

The burden of disease for patients with head and neck cancer, which is affected by the cancer, treatment, care, and survivorship issues, has been described by healthcare providers, researchers, patient advocacy organizations, and regulatory agencies. Symptoms include anxiety, depression, cognitive dysfunction, inability to exercise, fatigue, pain,

Figure 10-1. Head and Neck Cancer Disease and Treatment Sequelae That May Affect Survivors' Quality of Life

- Aphonia: difficulty with speech
- Body image impairment
- Difficulty sleeping
- Difficulties with eating: dysphagia, esophageal strictures, taste, difficulty eating in public, feeding tube dependence
- Distress: worry about becoming a burden for family and/or caregiver, fear of death, fear of suffering, depression, suicide or suicide ideation
- Fatigue
- Financial burden
- Impaired relationships: problems with intimacy, sexual dysfunction, family disruptions
- Musculoskeletal dysfunction (neck and shoulder dysfunction)
- Oral cavity impairments: mucositis, xerostomia, trismus, periodontitis, caries
- Pain
- Tracheal stenosis
- Treatment side effects and complications

sexual dysfunction, sleep disturbances, social isolation, disfigurement, anorexia, dysphagia, dyspnea, aphonia, unintelligible speech, diminished sense of or loss of self, and others.

Funk, Karnell, and Christensen (2012) reported outcomes of a five-year prospective and observational study of health-related aspects of quality of life in 337 head and neck cancer survivors. A Likert scale was developed to assess the key elements affecting patients with head and neck cancer (e.g., eating, speech, aesthetics, social disruption, physical and mental depressive symptoms, overall quality of life). In this group, the most evident concerns were with eating (50%), depressive symptoms (28.5%), and persistent pain (17.3%). Additionally, the researchers noted that 13.6% of the patients continued to smoke, and 38.9% continued to use alcohol. These finding suggest that early interventions are needed in each of the areas to improve quality of life. The authors also proposed that more attention should be given to education and management of tobacco and alcohol cessation in head and neck cancer survivors.

Dropkin (2012) applied the findings from Funk et al. (2012) to the four dimensions of care—physical, functional, cognitive, and emotional—as outlined in Scott and Eisendrath's (1986) survivorship model. Using the concepts of both research and evidence-based nursing practice described by Fawcett and Garity (2009), Dropkin identified interventions for each of the survivorship model dimensions and concluded that these interventions could lead to useful evidence-based protocols.

The psychosocial challenges of living with head and neck cancer have been the focus of many studies over the years. Lang, France, Williams, Humphris, and Wells (2013) reviewed 46 qualitative studies that focused on head and

Table 10-2. Head and Neck Cancer Five-Year Survival Rates (2005–2011)

Site	Survival Rate (%)
Floor of the mouth	51.4
Larynx	60
Lip	89.5
Nasopharynx	59.2
Oropharynx	41.7
Salivary gland	72.4
Thyroid	97.9
Tongue	62.7
Tonsil	70.8

Note. Based on information from Howlader et al., 2013.

neck cancer survivor experiences. This meta-analysis resulted in the identification of six core concepts: (1) uncertainty and waiting, (2) disruption to daily life, (3) the diminished self, (4) making sense of the experience, (5) sharing the burden, and (6) finding a path. The authors concluded that healthcare professionals must focus on patients' actual needs rather than on assumed needs and adopting a holistic approach. Supporting head and neck cancer survivors requires an understanding of the disruption to their sense of self and daily life as well as an acknowledgment of the uncertainty that is part of their present and future.

These findings illustrate the complexity of the work every multidisciplinary head and neck cancer team must tackle to improve education and care. It is only then that head and neck cancer survivors will reach a higher level of satisfaction in the quest to find quality of life again.

Nursing practice considerations include the following.

- Use heightened specialty assessment and communication skills.
- Implement creative communication skills for survivors with sensory and functional losses.
- Build expertise and seek ongoing education and validated skills for specialty physiologic, psychosocial, and spiritual care.
- Increase ability to coordinate, facilitate, and advocate for initiation of interprofessional specialty team members' referrals.
- Obtain current strategies for successful tobacco and alcohol cessation to mentor and support survivors.
- Mentor survivors to instill self-confidence and comfort in ability of self-expression.

Survivorship Planning

The IOM committee consensus report *From Cancer Patient to Cancer Survivor: Lost in Transition* was a landmark description of the need for systems and strategies to improve the quality of life for cancer survivors (Hewitt et al., 2006). It examined several existing fact sheets on survivor needs and called upon stakeholders to begin developing plans for the growing population of survivors. Increased awareness stimulated survivorship education and research. This led to the development of survivorship care delivery systems and tools to support care. Treatment summary forms, survivorship care plans (SCPs), survivorship clinics, and health promotion became a reality. Because of their unique skills and education, nurses are often the best prepared professionals to coordinate survivorship care.

In light of the IOM recommendation for survivorship care plans, Salz, Oeffinger, McCabe, Layne, and Bach (2012) reviewed publications exploring the perspectives of cancer survivors, primary care providers, and oncology care providers regarding the content and use of SCPs. The NCI-designated cancer centers were surveyed to learn the extent that SCPs were being used for two of the most common

cancer types—breast and colorectal—and to determine the alignment of these plans with IOM's recommendations. While cancer survivors and healthcare providers agree that SCPs are useful tools, there is little knowledge of what information should be included. Oncology care providers have identified significant resource challenges associated with implementation of SCPs. Only 43% of the NCI-designated cancer centers provided SCPs to breast or colorectal cancer survivors, and when SCPs were provided, none were found to address all of the components identified by IOM. Continued education of healthcare providers and cancer survivors in the use and value of SCPs is still needed.

Hahn and Ganz (2011) published a qualitative study that examined four cancer survivorship programs and SCP use. The clinical settings included an academic medical center, a community hospital, a primary care medical group, and a county hospital in a large metropolitan city. Interviews were conducted with each institution's survivorship providers. Each had a diverse approach to establishing the survivorship program and care plans.

The academic center program evaluated adult survivors in one visit through a multidisciplinary team that used several quality-of-life and symptom scales to identify which consultations and services were needed. The nurse practitioner (NP) was then responsible for documenting the team consensus, building the SCP, and following the survivors' progress.

The community hospital chose to focus on patients with breast cancer. A survivorship team followed up with the cancer survivors at specific predetermined points during the care continuum. The team was led by a clinical nurse specialist (CNS), who conducted classes, provided transition education related to survivorship, and documented prepublished American Society of Clinical Oncology (ASCO) SCPs. The CNS ordered care consults as the survivors' needs were identified during ongoing evaluations.

The primary care medical group partnered with a community oncologist for decisions about survivors' needs. The oncologist met and communicated with the primary care physicians and the group's social worker. Together the oncologist and the social worker developed the SCP. The social worker communicated with the survivors via telephone and mail and documented on the ASCO SCPs.

The fourth group, a county hospital, was more challenging because of the wide variety of tertiary care needs of survivors with more advanced disease, cultural diversity, and greater socioeconomic diversity. The hospital also adopted the ASCO SCPs with a focus on primary care needs, particularly chronic comorbidities, in addition to cancer survivor needs. To identify the survivorship needs of breast cancer survivors, a breast surgeon and NP established the program using a consultation approach. The NP documented on the SCP and ordered consultations. All of the programs prepared patient education print materials, with the academic center providing the most comprehensive patient information packet.

Each of the four oncology programs concluded that the SCP was a flexible tool for survivorship care and an important element for success. Three of the four sites planned to expand their survivorship programs and use of SCPs. While each of these models differs, the role of the advanced practice nurse was pivotal in documenting the survivorship plan and requesting consultations to ensure the survivors' needs were met. A number of published resources for SCPs can be found in Figure 10-2.

Nursing practice considerations include the following.
• Prepare to understand, collect information, and document the SCP for the multidisciplinary team.
• Serve as the validator and educator of information for the survivor.
• Be knowledgeable of available resources and facilitate connections.

Survivorship Clinics

SCPs do not stand alone but rather are one of many tools for survivorship care. The IOM consensus report called for an organized delivery system for patients with cancer who were exiting the acute care phase; this led to the development of survivorship clinics or programs (Hewitt et al., 2006). Many of these programs have established a formal system of survivor visits for follow-up care. These programs have heightened awareness and further defined the care that is provided for cancer survivors, providing systematic monitoring and surveillance, long-term care, health promotion, and management of long-term and late effects of cancer treatment. Several models of survivorship programs exist today, and models of survivorship care delivery continue to be explored.

As the number of survivorship programs and clinics develop and mature, ongoing evaluation will help to improve survivorship care and enhance the quality of life for cancer survivors. Because of the variety of impairments they face, head and neck cancer survivors will surely benefit. Table 10-3 provides a listing of some of the established survivorship clinics and programs.

Nursing practice considerations include the following.
• Serve as the lead professional in the program.
• Develop leadership skills and apply to specialty survivorship care.
• Educate and mentor nursing and oncology teams.

• Participate in development and revisions of survivorship programs.
• Establish a coexisting educational and support group for the survivor.
• Assist in identifying key indicators or quality improvement efforts.

Health Promotion

Health promotion is a key principle embraced by many institutions, such as the World Health Organization (WHO), National Institutes of Health, and Centers for Disease Control and Prevention. Cancer screening and regular monitoring intervals of cancer survivors have been identified through research. The National Comprehensive Cancer Network® (NCCN®), ACS, and other oncology specialty groups have identified cancer screening recommendations and cancer preventive measures as important health promotion activities. Health promotion measures have been included in SCPs, which often use terms such as *healthy living, live well, stay well, well-being,* and *wellness.* Beckjord et al. (2008) surveyed 1,040 cancer survivors two to five years after their diagnosis. They reported 71% of cancer survivors felt that more information related to tests and treatments was needed, and 68% requested more knowledge about health promotion strategies. SCPs can be an important tool to capture health promotion information for head and neck cancer survivors. Some of the published SCPs provide health promotion as one of the elements to be addressed, monitored, and documented. Monitoring cancer survivors' healthy living behaviors and alignment of compliance with screening and follow-up recommendations may help to identify recurrent disease or second malignancies in the early stages, allowing for earlier intervention and better outcomes.

Nursing practice considerations include the following.
• Develop educational tools to outline the recommended screening and cancer prevention strategies.
• Monitor test results and obtain necessary consultations and referrals as needed.
• Provide patient education and support within scope of practice.
• Allay fears of new disease or recurrence through education, attend to individual needs, and facilitate timely medical appointments for evaluation.

Figure 10-2. Published Tools for Survivorship Care Planning

• American Cancer Society: www.cancer.org/treatment/survivorshipduringandaftertreatment/survivorshipcareplans/index
• American Society of Clinical Oncology: www.cancer.net/survivorship/asco-cancer-treatment-summaries
• Institute of Medicine: www.iom.edu/Reports/2005/From-Cancer-Patient-to-Cancer-Survivor-Lost-in-Transition
• Journey Forward: www.journeyforward.org
• Livestrong Foundation: www.livestrongcareplan.org
• OncoLink: www.oncolink.org/oncolife

Table 10-3. Survivorship Clinics in the United States (Limited List)			
Institution	Location	Population	Providers
Fox Chase Cancer Center	Philadelphia, PA	Adult head and neck cancer	NP, CNS, PA
John Stoddard Cancer Center Survivorship Program	Des Moines, IA	Adult cancer and wellness	Multidisciplinary
Mayo Clinic	Rochester, MN	Adult cancer	Multidisciplinary
Memorial Sloan Kettering Cancer Center	New York, NY	Adult cancer	NP
Providence Cancer Center	Portland, OR	Adult cancer	NP
Sylvester Comprehensive Cancer Center	Miami, FL	Adult head and neck cancer	Multidisciplinary
University of Alabama at Birmingham Comprehensive Cancer Center	Birmingham, AL	Adult cancer	Multidisciplinary
University of Texas MD Anderson Cancer Center	Houston, TX	Adult supportive care	Multidisciplinary

CNS—clinical nurse specialist; NP—nurse practitioner; PA—physician assistant

Rehabilitation

Lester and Schmitt (2011) wrote about the future of cancer survivorship and listed rehabilitation as its foundation: "A primary goal of rehabilitation is intended to help patients restore and achieve maximum levels of function ... in life" (p. 420). Additionally, they proposed that rehabilitation address and include all life domains while "minimizing the limitations imposed by the disease or cancer treatment" (Lester & Schmitt, 2011, p. 420).

Textbooks, such as *Essentials of Head and Neck Oncology* (Close, Larson, & Shah, 1998), raised awareness of survivors' needs nearly 20 years ago. The authors categorized rehabilitation into three groups: functional, prosthetic, and psychosocial. The *functional* category included addressing dysfunctions of swallowing and speech and shoulder impairment. The *prosthetic* category included restoration, reconstruction, and cosmesis of missing anatomic areas of the head and neck. The *psychological* category highlighted coping and adjustment strategies. The healthcare team began to address elements such as depression, pain, body image, dry mouth, enduring tubes, and the effects of surgery, chemotherapy, and radiation.

An additional approach to managing rehabilitation of head and neck cancer survivors is the use of the WHO International Classification of Functioning, Disability, and Health (ICF) model. The ICF model defines functions and disabilities in body function, structure, personal activities of life, and environment. The model was developed using a multidisciplinary and cross-cultural process with the goal to become internationally accepted terminology to classify function and disability and facilitate multidisciplinary coop-

eration. Tschiesner, Rogers, Dietz, Yueh, and Cieza (2010) published a head and neck cancer survivor ICF core set using a consensus procedure of 21 international experts in head and neck cancer. Qualifiers from the general ICF were reviewed and categorized into head and neck cancer survivor concerns. All participants were trained to understand and use the ICF tools and qualifiers. Inter-rater agreement served to support validity and feasibility of the qualifiers. The questions and qualifiers were formatted into short and long versions of the head and neck cancer ICF. Leib, Cieza, and Tschiesner (2012) reported head and neck expert physician validation as a third step in validating the head and neck cancer ICF. The authors noted that validation had earlier been completed with psychologists and physiotherapists. The importance of the multidisciplinary approach to care was highlighted in the validation exercise of the head and neck cancer ICF. Physicians tend to focus on body functions and structures, and this was complemented by the focus of psychologists and physiotherapists. The body functions not addressed by physicians, such as exercise tolerance, mobility, and muscle power, were the focus of physiotherapists. Body image, temperament, personality, intellect, sleep, and sexual functions were not identified as a focus for physicians and were instead addressed by psychologists. Psychologists also focused on many more categories, such as activities, participation, and environment factors.

The complexity of rehabilitation of head and neck cancer survivors can be realized from the research efforts reported here. However, rehabilitation requires an extraordinarily committed team that is multidisciplinary and includes processes for physical therapy, nutrition, speech and swallowing therapy, prosthetics, occupational rehabilitation, and psychosocial support. Nurses play a pivotal role, as they often coordinate the team, review or write orders, and document or complete the SCP.

Nursing practice considerations include the following.
• Have knowledge in specialty nursing care skills.
• Monitor survivors' responses to disease and treatment in all life domains.
• Provide education and strategies to aid in wellness.
• Communicate identified needs to the multidisciplinary team and assist with strategies and evaluation of progress.
• Assist survivors in building a useful toolbox.
• Sit with survivors and guide them in complex self-care elements.
• Provide resources within the institution and community.

Costs

The cost of quality cancer care may strain the finances of survivors and may require that they undergo financial rehabilitation to reestablish economic stability. Mariotto, Yabroff, Shao, Feuer, and Brown (2010) used the SEER-Medicare database to estimate cancer costs. Using the 2010 value of a dollar, the authors estimated head and neck cancer costs to total $3.64 billion in 2010 and projected this to increase to $4.65 billion by 2020. These costs include expenses for diagnostic testing, hospitalization for surgery, and chemotherapy and radiation. The annualized mean net cost for head and neck cancer is depicted in Table 10-4. The authors noted that head and neck cancer care is the 11th most costly cancer in the United States.

The cost of treatment is dependent on the tumor location, stage, and treatment modalities for the specific cancer. Cost of survivorship relates to the management of treatment side effects and rehabilitation. This economic burden can be measured in direct and indirect costs. Indirect costs might include transportation, time off work, loss of wages, payment to others to perform household chores, and increased utility bills as a result of running durable medical equipment. Direct costs include monies needed for health care, such as institutional and professional fees, medications, and durable

medical equipment. Using statistics from the 2008 Medical Expenditure Panel Survey, Rascati, Park, and Rascati (2011) evaluated the economic burden of disease for 25 head and neck cancer survivors. Of the 25 survivors, 11 were age 65 or older and 14 were under the age of 65. Direct medical expenditure by service was $9,414 per survivor. There were an average of 11.3 outpatient clinic visits per survivor, which accounted for 79% of the expenditures. The remaining costs were distributed across inpatient care (18%), home health (3%), and emergency department care and pharmacy (1%). The payer mix for cost of this care included private insurance (69%), Medicare (15%), self-pay (9%), veteran benefits (3%), Medicaid (2%), and public health and other insurance policies (1%). Genther and Gourin (2012) conducted a retrospective study of 36,948 older adult head and neck cancer survivors, reviewing inpatient discharge data from a nationwide sample spanning from 2003–2008. Survivors were 65 years of age or older who underwent surgery for cancer of the oral cavity, larynx, hypopharynx, or oropharynx. Survivors with two or more comorbidities were referred to as *frail elderly*. The frail elderly were 80 years of age or older, required more transfers to short-term rehabilitation institutions or long-term skilled nursing centers, had more acute medical complications, and demonstrated higher rates of mortality. While the rate of postoperative surgical complications was not increased in the frail elderly, they experienced significantly longer hospital stays and higher hospital costs. The authors concluded that as the population ages more, additional resources will be needed to care for older adult survivors with head and neck cancer.

Jacobson et al. (2012) explored the cost of oral, oral pharyngeal, and salivary gland malignancies in selected insurance groups through the review of claim documents from Medicare (n = 2,003), Medicaid (n = 585), and private insurance (n = 3,918) to compare and analyze expenditures. These data were compared to patients without head and neck cancer from similar demographic and socioeconomic groups in relation to insurance experience, types of insurance, cost of care, missed work time, and compensated short-term disability. The cost analysis for head and neck cancer for one-year post-diagnosis was tabulated from the insurance data.

Table 10-4. Head and Neck Cancer Annualized Mean Net Cost by Phase of Care in 2010			
Population	Initial Cost of Care	Continuing Costs	Cost at Death
Men younger than age 65	$47,015	$4,001	$125,493
Women younger than age 65	$50,376	$4,826	$129,903
Men age 65 and older	$39,179	$4,001	$83,662
Women age 65 and older	$41,980	$4,826	$86,602
Note. Based on information from Mariotto et al., 2011.			

Propensity scoring technique matched the groups, finding a significantly higher cost for head and neck cancer survivors treated for oral, oral pharyngeal, and salivary gland cancers and that multimodality therapy was nearly twice as much as single modality therapy. These findings were similar across all insurance groups, suggesting that the cost of care is greater for advanced-stage head and neck cancer survivors because this patient population is most likely to be treated with multiple modalities. The authors postulate that earlier detection should help control costs.

The cost of head and neck cancer care requires ongoing evaluation. Earlier detection of head and neck cancer should help to control costs, as can the use of clinical pathways, evidence-based treatment guidelines, and systems monitoring.

Nursing practice considerations include the following.
• Obtain referrals for interprofessional assistance.
• Explain the value of insurance case managers and patient advocacy organizations.
• Provide a list of contact information for organizations.

Insurance and Employment

Health insurance is important to all cancer survivors. O'Hara and Caswell (2013) reported that in 2012, an estimated 48 million people, 15.4% of the U.S. population, did not have health insurance. The government-covered health insurance programs Medicaid and Medicare insured 50.9 million people (16.4%) and 48.9 million people (15.5%), respectively. For head and neck cancer survivors who engage in functional, prosthetic, psychosocial, and economic rehabilitation, understanding and dealing with insurance policies, inquiries, and disclosures may become overwhelming. While it is too early to evaluate long-term outcomes from healthcare reform, measures have been introduced by the Patient Protection and Affordable Care Act of 2010. This important legislation outlined consumers' rights and brought coverage for preventive care, preexisting illness protection, employer-shared responsibility, essential health benefits with government subsidized insurance plans, and an end to lifetime coverage limits (U.S. Department of Health and Human Services, 2014). Insurance and case managers, financial counselors, and patient advocacy groups may provide assistance (see Table 10-5).

Maintaining prediagnosis employment during treatment or at any survivorship stage may pose challenges to survivors. Early literature focused on survivors' employment rights, such as employment discrimination, concerns about layoffs, promotions, duty changes, and merit raises. The Affordable Care Act and the Patient's Bill of Rights help to protect survivors from insurance discrimination (ACS, 2014).

Taylor et al. (2004) found that 52% of the head and neck cancer survivors studied were unable to return to work because of cancer treatment–related disabilities. In 2007,

Table 10-5. Community Economic Rehabilitation and Insurance Resources (Limited List)

Resource	Website
Financial	
CancerCare	www.cancercare.org
Cancer Financial Assistance Coalition	www.cancerfac.org
Life Credit Company	www.lifecreditcompany.com
National Foundation for Credit Counseling	www.nfcc.org
Partnership for Prescription Assistance	www.pparx.org
Insurance	
American Cancer Society Booklet; Health Insurance and Financial Assistance for the Cancer Patient	www.cancer.org
America's Health Insurance Plans	www.ahip.org
National Council on Aging	www.ncoa.org

Buckwalter, Karnell, Smith, Christensen, and Funk studied employment after treatment, reviewing 666 head and neck cancer survivor cases, 239 of whom continued to work during therapy. Evaluation continued over time with testing at diagnosis and at three, six, nine, and 12 months postdiagnosis. Ninety-one additional survivors stopped working during this time. Eighty-two of these 91 survivors who left work identified the factors leading to the termination of their employment. The five factors in rank order were fatigue, speech challenges, eating challenges, pain or discomfort, and appearance. It is important to note that 37 of the 82 (40.7%) did return to work.

Jacobson et al. (2012) found that 48% of the 6,812 survivors of oral, pharyngeal, and salivary gland cancer that they studied returned to work. However, head and neck cancer survivors missed 48.3 days of work compared to the 44 days other cancer survivors were absent. The authors noted that head and neck cancer survivors with commercial insurance were older and had higher wages. This was thought to be because of employees' length of service and specialized skills that could lead to employers needing to spend more on resources to cover the absenteeism. Table 10-6 provides a list of several resources for community assistance with legal rights. NCCS published an employment legal rights booklet for cancer survivors and their families titled *Working It Out: Your Employment Rights as a Cancer Survivor* (Hoffman, 2008).

Table 10-6. Community Legal Rights for Survivors (Limited List)		
Laws/Governing Forces/Alliances	Purpose	Details
Consolidated Omnibus Budget Reconciliation Act (COBRA), 1986	Continues insurance	Must request within 60 days of leaving workplace
Health Insurance Portability and Accountability Act (HIPAA), 1996	Ensures insurance portability and accountability	Protects from denial of insurance based on preexisting health problems and sets guidelines for waiting period of coverage when changing employer group insurance
Family and Medical Leave Act (FMLA), 1993	Allows family and medical leaves	Provides up to 12 weeks of job-protected leave
Americans With Disabilities Act (ADA), 1990	Protects Americans with disabilities	Helps to prevent discrimination for disabilities and provides accommodations
Affordable Care Act (ACA), 2010	Ensures healthcare insurance	Numerous provisions to protect patients with cancer
National Coalition for Cancer Survivorship (NCCS)	Supports action through education and advocacy for employment challenges and existing laws	*Working It Out: Your Employment Rights as a Cancer Survivor*

Nursing practice considerations include the following.
- Seek resources for patients, such as applications for public insurance from social services.
- Obtain referral for vocational rehabilitation through social services.
- Provide a list of community agencies that may assist, as well as advocacy groups.

Support Groups

Support programs throughout the continuum of the head and neck cancer journey provide additional opportunities for the survivor, family, and nursing staff. Building networks with others who have faced the same diagnosis and challenges can help survivors develop healthy coping strategies and benchmark positive outcomes. Being able to talk to other head and neck cancer survivors about the similarities and differences of their cases may help to reinforce self-confidence and motivation (Leigh, 2011). Advocacy is often fostered through support groups and conversations among survivors, caregivers, and care providers. Table 10-7 lists available advocacy groups.

Use of the Internet for survivorship support is a topic of study and controversy. Historically, literature supported the value and success of the face-to-face support groups, but little research existed regarding outcomes of Internet groups. Klemm and Hardie (2002) compared the traditional face-to-face support group method to the use of contemporary Internet support groups. Using a reliable and validated scale, they evaluated a common concern in survivorship: depression. They studied multiple variables and found a significant level of depression in the treatment phase. The Internet support group participants had significantly higher depres-

sion scores than the face-to-face group participants. Depression was less evident in survivor groups that had face-to-face interaction, was run by a facilitator, and met on a regular schedule.

Cancer survivors are becoming increasingly more Internet savvy and dependent. Internet-based support groups may be the only viable option for survivors who are unable to attend in-person meetings for various reasons, such as remote location or lack of transportation. This newer venue for support may require a shift in thinking for oncology nurses in the assessment and delivery of supportive interventions. Nurses are instrumental in establishing support groups. Their teaching and coordination skills promote partnering of survivors with social services, other healthcare providers, and community leaders to maximize resources for support group development. Table 10-8 provides a list of online and community resources for survivor support.

Nonprofit advocacy agencies, such as ACS and Support for People With Oral and Head and Neck Cancer, offer

Table 10-7. Advocacy Groups for Survivors (Limited List)	
Group	Website
American Cancer Society	www.cancer.org
CancerCare	www.cancercare.org
National Coalition for Cancer Survivorship	www.canceradvocacy.org
Patient Advocate Foundation	www.patientadvocate.org
Support for People With Oral and Head and Neck Cancer	www.spohnc.org

Table 10-8. Support Resources for Head and Neck Cancer Survivors	
Support Resource	**Website**
American Cancer Society	www.cancer.org
American Academy of Otolaryngology—Head and Neck Surgery	www.entnet.org
CancerCare	www.cancercare.org
Head and Neck Cancer Alliance	www.headandneck.org
I Had Cancer	www.ihadcancer.com
International Association of Laryngectomees	www.theial.com
Oncology Nursing Society	www.ons.org
Society of Otorhinolaryngology and Head-Neck Nurses	www.sohnnurse.com
Support for People With Oral and Head and Neck Cancer	www.spohnc.org
Tobacco information and support links	www.tobacco.org

several supportive programs for head and neck cancer survivors. Literature on specific cancers, programs for transportation, self-help books, and classes to help with coping are often provided through local facilities. Figure 10-3 lists self-help reading material for head and neck cancer survivors.

Nursing practice considerations include the following.
• Provide survivors with community resources.
• Serve as a guest lecturer to a support group.
• Volunteer to facilitate a support group.
• Encourage head and neck cancer survivors, when ready, to engage in groups or share with another head and neck cancer survivor.
• Connect survivors and caregivers with others.

Second Primary Cancer or Recurrence

One common fear among survivors is cancer recurrence. Ghazali et al. (2013) investigated the prevalence for significant fear of recurrence (FoR) among 189 post-therapy survivors of head and neck cancer. Survivors attended 456 clinic visits and completed three outcome tools to measure perceived quality of life and a FoR questionnaire. A significant FoR was reported by 35% of the survivors at least once. Of these survivors, 30% reported significant consistent FoR from one visit to the next, and 20% experienced significant FoR at one visit. The remaining 50% did not report significant FoR. The authors felt the FoR experienced by head and neck cancer survivors negatively affected quality of life.

Chuang et al. (2008) studied patients with first primary cancers of the head and neck. They reviewed 10 years of follow-up after diagnosis across 13 cancer registries and noted that 36% of head and neck cancer survivors had a 20-year cumulative risk of developing a second primary head and neck cancer. The most frequent second primaries after head and neck cancer were of the head and neck (35%–73%), lung (15%–32%), and esophagus (9%).

Prudent follow-up care, scheduled surveillance, and health promotion are outlined in the NCCN clinical guidelines for head and neck cancer (NCCN, 2015a). Ongoing provider and survivor education is essential. Survivors must understand and embrace the need to comply with surveillance protocols and be mindful of reporting changes to care providers.

Nursing practice considerations include the following.
• Allay fears when new symptoms appear by timely care and appointments.
• Provide education and information in a supportive, matter-of-fact approach.
• Offer supportive services when appropriate.
• Obtain orders for testing, if appropriate.
• Assist in obtaining clinical information and coordination of follow-up care.

Palliative Care

The goal of palliative care is to maintain quality of life. The loss of quality of life is a fear shared by patients, caregivers, and survivors. Disease and treatment may interrupt and interfere with the balance of life. Pain, suffering, and loss of self or lifestyle impairs coping and living through or with the disease. The multiple dimensions of being a head and neck cancer survivor can be complex and overwhelming. Supportive care is needed throughout the trajectory of the disease and is often paramount if the disease recurs or if the patient presents with advanced disease with a low probability of cure.

WHO (2012) developed a definition for palliative care and identified key components, which include attention to pain, distress, support systems, psychological support, spiritual needs, bereavement care, and affirmed life and dying processes. Traditionally, the term *palliative care* has been perceived as equating with end-of-life care. Transition from use of *palliative care* to *supportive care* has been associated with earlier implementation of supportive therapy in the course of disease (Dalal et al., 2011). The National Consensus Project for Quality Palliative Care published the third edition of its multidisciplinary guidelines for quality palliative care in 2013. The guidelines emphasize patient- and family-centered care, promoting access to palliative care. Addi-

---

Figure 10-3. Self-Help Resources for Head and Neck Cancer Survivors

- CancerCare. (2012). *Coping with Cancer: Tools to Help You Live.* Available at http://media.cancercare.org/publications/original/3-ccc _coping.pdf
- CancerCare. (2015). *Caregiving for Your Loved One With Cancer.* Available at www.cancercare.org/publications/1-caregiving_for _your_loved_one_with_cancer
- Leupold, N.E., & Sciubba, J.J. (2011). *Meeting the Challenges of Oral and Head and Neck Cancer: A Guide for Survivors and Caregivers* (2nd ed.). Locust Valley, NY: Support for People With Oral and Head and Neck Cancer.
- Livestrong Foundation. (2006). *The Survivorship Journey: Living After Cancer Treatment.* Available at http://images.livestrong.org/down loads/flatfiles/what-we-do/our-actions/protools/lact/PacificIslanderBrochure.pdf
- National Cancer Institute. (2014). *Caring for the Caregiver.* Available at www.cancer.gov/publications/patient-education/caring-for-the -caregiver.pdf
- Sampedro-Iglesia, M. (2011). *The Heroes Among Us.* Bloomington, IN: WestBow Press.

---

tionally, NCCN has published guidelines for palliative care for patients with cancer, which are regularly reviewed and revised as needed (NCCN, 2015b).

Comfort and safety measures for head and neck cancer survivors often must be intense and require creative approaches. Cancer-related symptoms and treatment sequelae may require implementation of multiple interventions. Appropriate management of the airway, nutrition, prevention of hemorrhage, and physical dysfunctions that may negatively impact quality of life is foremost. Additionally, invasive tumors may result in complicated wounds because of bleeding, disfigurement, drainage, odor, or infection. The combination of these symptoms may cause the acuity of care to become too burdensome for the family. Patients and families may need assistance in the home to manage care. Home health agencies and hospices have become invaluable in supervising or providing care, providing durable medical equipment, and coordinating the multidisciplinary team to meet patients' needs.

Pimentel, Yennurajalingam, Brown, and Castro (2012) evaluated a nurse-led supportive care phone triage program that provided frequent communications to patients with advanced disease. Survivor self-reported symptom burden was measured with the Edmonton Symptom Assessment Scale (ESAS). The patients and families were provided instruction about the program, which was included in the SCP. Interventions to manage symptoms were provided by the nurses. Symptoms related to fatigue and emotional distress had the highest score. One month later, a significant decrease was noted in emotional distress, fatigue, depression, and anxiety, and the feeling of wellness had significantly improved. These findings support nurse-led supportive care triage programs, use of the ESAS, awareness to symptom management, and survivor satisfaction with supportive care. Head and neck cancer survivors require supportive care at any stage of disease, phase of treatment, and period of survivorship, including the end of life.

Support systems for survivors and families are essential. Home healthcare agencies and hospices provide support to both and often include services such as volunteer sitters, shopper services, housekeeping, transportation, and grief and bereavement counseling. Some hospices also have inpatient facilities that offer respite services. The *MD Anderson Supportive and Palliative Care Handbook* (4th ed.) lists helpful information and strategies for palliative care. Table 10-9 provides a limited list of resources for supportive care.

Nursing practice considerations include the following.
- Foster a positive, supportive approach.
- Provide interprofessional team support.
- Obtain, facilitate, and coordinate appropriate supportive orders.
- Provide a list of resources.
- Be present to listen and, if survivors have needs, assist in verbalizing needs.
- Support survivors' self-determination while maximizing their safety.

Summary

Throughout this book, nursing care has been addressed. When relating it to a survivor of head and neck cancer, it seems appropriate to correlate nursing care with the survi-

Table 10-9. Resources for Palliative and Supportive Care and End-of-Life Decisions

Organization	Website
Center to Advance Palliative Care	www.capc.org
Hospice and Palliative Nurses Association	www.hpna.org
International Association for Hospice and Palliative Care	www.hospicecare.com
National Comprehensive Cancer Network®	www.nccn.org
National Hospice and Palliative Care Organization	www.nhpco.org

vorship model described by Leigh (2001). The acute stage of survivorship is the assessment process. It is the proving ground for the novice to identify his or her needs and abilities and understand the challenges. Nurses provide, direct, and instruct survivors in their care, which is the beginning of rehabilitation. The extended stage relates to intermediate survivors who accept the challenge and demand excellence in rehabilitation. In the third stage, permanency, survivors are now expert strategists who have regained function and confidence. Their lives have returned to near normal, and they now can begin to give back to others. Yet even with self-confidence restored, the fear of cancer recurrence remains with survivors. To that end, the role of the nurse shifts to instilling hope and promoting health maintenance behaviors.

Nurses serve as caregivers, teachers, mentors, facilitators, validators, supporters, evaluators, and coordinators of their multidisciplinary team and help guide head and neck cancer survivors through the complex journey. Mastering these many roles requires nurses to arm themselves with all available tools and resources—most importantly, the resource of self. Nursing is the art and science of caring for people with healthcare needs. It is the happy nurse who finds a place within a specialty, but it is the committed, dedicated, and fulfilled nurse who continues to learn, listen, and love the role.

References

American Cancer Society. (2014). Patient's bill of rights. Retrieved from http://www.cancer.org/treatment/findingandpayingfortreatment/understandingfinancialandlegalmatters/patients-bill-of-rights

American Cancer Society. (2015). Cancer treatment and survivorship facts and figures, 2015. Retrieved from http://www.cancer.org/acs/groups/content/@editorial/documents/document/acspc-044552.pdf

Beckjord, E.B., Arora, N.K., McLaughlin, W., Oakley-Girvan, I., Hamilton, A.S., & Hesse, B.W. (2008). Health-related information needs in a large and diverse sample of adult cancer survivors: Implications for cancer care. Journal of Cancer Survivorship, 2, 179–189. doi:10.1007/s11764-008-0055-0

Buckwalter, A.E., Karnell, L.H., Smith, R.B., Christensen, A.J., & Funk, G.F. (2007). Patient-reported factors associated with discontinuing employment following head and neck cancer treatment. Archives of Otolaryngology—Head and Neck Surgery, 133, 464–470. doi:10.1001/archotol.133.5.464

Chuang, S.C., Scelo, G., Tonita, J.M., Tamaro, S., Jonasson, J.G., Kliewer, E.V., … Brennan, P. (2008). Risk of second primary cancer among patients with head and neck cancers: A pooled analysis of 13 cancer registries. International Journal of Cancer, 123, 2390–2396. doi:10.1002/ijc.23798

Close, L.G., Larson, D.L., & Shah, J.P. (Eds.). (1998). Essentials of head and neck oncology. New York, NY: Thieme.

Dalal, S., Palla, S., Hui, D., Nguyen, L., Chacko, R., Li, Z., … Bruera, E. (2011). Association between a name change from palliative care to supportive care and the timing of patient referrals at a comprehensive cancer center. Oncologist, 16, 105–111. doi:10.1634/theoncologist.2010-0161

Dropkin, M.J. (2012). Review of "Long-Term Health Related Quality of Life in Survivors of Head and Neck Cancer." ORL—Head and Neck Nursing, 30(1), 24–26.

Fawcett, J., & Garity, J. (2009). Evaluating research for evidence-based nursing practice. Philadelphia, PA: F.A. Davis.

Ferrell, B.R., Virani, R., Smith, S., & Juarez, G. (2003). The role of oncology nursing to ensure quality care for cancer survivors: A report commissioned by the National Cancer Policy Board and Institute of Medicine [Online exclusive]. Oncology Nursing Forum, 30, E1–E11. doi:10.1188/03.ONF.E1-E11

Funk, G.F., Karnell, L.H., & Christensen, A.J. (2012). Long-term health-related quality of life in survivors of head and neck cancer. Archives of Otolaryngology—Head and Neck Surgery, 138, 123–133. doi:10.1001/archoto.2011.234

Genther, D.J., & Gourin, C.G. (2012). Head and neck cancer surgery in the elderly. Otolaryngology—Head and Neck Surgery, 147(Suppl. 2), 159–160. doi:10.1177/0194599812451426a110

Ghazali, N., Cadwallader, E., Lowe, D., Humphris, G., Ozakinci, G., & Rogers, S.N. (2013). Fear of recurrence among head and neck cancer survivors: Longitudinal trends. Psycho-Oncology, 22, 807–813. doi:10.1002/pon.3069

Hahn, E.E., & Ganz, P.A. (2011). Survivorship programs and care plans in practice: Variations on a theme. Journal of Oncology Practice, 7, 70–75. doi:10.1200/JOP.2010.000115

Hewitt, M., Greenfield, S., & Stovall, E. (Eds.). (2006). From cancer patient to cancer survivor: Lost in transition. Washington, DC: National Academies Press.

Hoffman, B. (2008). Working it out: Your employment rights as a cancer survivor (8th ed.). Retrieved from http://www.canceradvocacy.org/resources/employment-rights

Howlader, N., Noone, A.M., Krapcho, M., Garshell, J., Miller, D., Altekruse, S.F., … Cronin, K.A. (Eds.). (2013). SEER cancer statistics review, 1975–2012. Retrieved from http://seer.cancer.gov/csr/1975_2012

Jacobson, J.J., Epstein, J.B., Eichmiller, F.C., Gibson, T.B., Carls, G.S., Vogtmann, E., … Murphy, B. (2012). The cost burden of oral, oral pharyngeal, and salivary gland cancers in three groups: Commercial insurance, Medicare, and Medicaid. Head and Neck Oncology, 4(15), 1–17.

Klemm, P., & Hardie, T. (2002). Depression in Internet and face-to-face cancer support groups: A pilot study [Online exclusive]. Oncology Nursing Forum, 29, E45–E51. doi:10.1188/02.ONF.E45-E51

Lang, H., France, E., Williams, B., Humphris, G., & Wells, M. (2013). The psychological experience of living with head and neck cancer: A systematic review and meta-synthesis. Psycho-Oncology, 22, 2648–2663. doi:10.1002/pon.3343

Leib, A., Cieza, A., & Tschiesner, U. (2012). Perspective of physicians within a multidisciplinary team: Content validation of the comprehensive ICF core set for head and neck cancer. Head and Neck, 34, 956–966. doi:10.1002/hed.21844

Leigh, S.A. (2001). The culture of survivorship. Seminars in Oncology Nursing, 17, 234–235. doi:10.1053/sonu.2001.27910

Leigh, S.A. (2007). Cancer survivorship: A nursing perspective. In P.A. Ganz (Ed.), Cancer survivorship: Today and tomorrow (pp. 8–13). New York, NY: Springer.

Leigh, S.A. (2011). From anecdote to evidence: The survivor's perspective. In J.L. Lester & P. Schmitt (Eds.), Cancer rehabilitation and survivorship: Transdisciplinary approaches to personalized care (pp. 7–14). Pittsburgh, PA: Oncology Nursing Society.

Lester, J.L., & Schmitt, P. (2011). Cancer survivorship care in the future. In J.L. Lester & P. Schmitt (Eds.), Cancer rehabilitation and survivorship: Transdisciplinary approaches to personalized care (pp. 417–425). Pittsburgh, PA: Oncology Nursing Society.

Mariotto, A.B., Yabroff, K.R., Shao, Y., Feuer, E.J., & Brown, M.L. (2010). Projection of the cost of cancer care in the United States: 2010–2020. Journal of the National Cancer Institute, 103, 117–128. doi:10.1093/jnci/djq495

Mellon, S., Northouse, L.L., & Weiss, L.K. (2006). A population-based study of quality of life of cancer survivors and their family caregivers. *Cancer Nursing, 29,* 120–131. doi:10.1097/00002820-200603000-00007

National Coalition for Cancer Survivorship. (n.d.). NCCS mission. Retrieved from http://www.canceradvocacy.org/about-us/our-mission

National Comprehensive Cancer Network. (2015a). *NCCN Clinical Practice Guidelines in Oncology (NCCN Guidelines®): Head and neck cancer* [v.1.2015]. Retrieved from http://www.nccn.org/professionals/physician_gls/pdf/head-and-neck.pdf

National Comprehensive Cancer Network. (2015b). *NCCN Clinical Practice Guidelines in Oncology (NCCN Guidelines®): Palliative care* [v.2.2015]. Retrieved from http://www.nccn.org/professionals/physician_gls/PDF/palliative.pdf

O'Hara, B., & Caswell, K. (2013). *Health status, health insurance, and medical services utilization: 2010.* Retrieved from https://www.census.gov/prod/2012pubs/p70-133.pdf

Pimentel, L.E., Yennurajalingam, S., Brown, E.D., & Castro, D.K. (2012). Challenges of managing advanced cancer patients through phone triaging at an outpatient supportive care clinic: A case series of palliative care patients. *Palliative Care: Research and Treatment, 6,* 9–14. doi:10.4137/PCRT.S10733

Rascati, M.E., Park, H., & Rascati, K.L. (2011, November). *Direct costs of head and neck cancer in the U.S.: An analysis using 2007–2008 Medical Expenditure Panel Survey (MEPS) data.* Poster session presented at the ISPOR 14th Annual European Congress, Madrid, Spain.

Retrieved from https://www.utexas.edu/pharmacy/research/posters/ispor11/park2.pdf

Ridge, J.A., Mehra, R., Lango, M.N., & Feigenberg, S. (2014). Head and neck tumors. In D.G. Haller, L.D. Wagman, K.A. Camphausen, & W.J. Hoskins (Eds.), *Cancer management: A multidisciplinary approach.* Retrieved from http://www.cancernetwork.com/cancer-management/head-and-neck-tumors

Salz, T., Oeffinger, K.C., McCabe, M.S., Layne, T.M., & Bach, P.B. (2012). Survivorship care plans in research and practice. *CA: A Cancer Journal for Clinicians, 62,* 101–117. doi:10.3322/caac.20142

Scott, D.W., & Eisendrath, S.J. (1986). Dynamics of the recovery process following the initial diagnosis of breast cancer. *Journal of Psychosocial Oncology, 3*(4), 53–66. doi:10.1300/J077v03n04_06

Siegel, R.L., Miller, K.D., & Jemal, A. (2015). Cancer statistics, 2015. *CA: A Cancer Journal for Clinicians, 65,* 5–29. doi:10.3322/caac.21254

Taylor, J.C., Terrell, J.E., Ronis, D.L., Fowler, K.E., Bishop, C., Lambert, M.T., … Duffy, S.A. (2004). Disability in patients with head and neck cancer. *Archives of Otolaryngology—Head and Neck Surgery, 130,* 764–769. doi:10.1001/archotol.130.6.764

Tschiesner, U., Rogers, S., Dietz, A., Yueh, B., & Cieza, A. (2010). Development of ICF core sets for head and neck cancer. *Head and Neck, 32,* 210–220. doi:10.1002/hed.21172

U.S. Department of Health and Human Services. (2014). About the law. Retrieved from http://www.hhs.gov/healthcare/rights

World Health Organization. (2012). WHO definition of palliative care. Retrieved from http://www.who.int/cancer/palliative/definition/en

CHAPTER 11

Nursing Research

David Anthony (Tony) Forrester, PhD, RN, ANEF, FAAN, and
Raymond Scarpa, DNP, APNC, AOCN®

Introduction

The purpose of this chapter is to present an overview of the head and neck cancer nursing research evidence published over the past decade, summarize the research findings, and identify future directions for head and neck cancer nursing research. An international literature search was conducted on both research studies/reports and significant research-related articles (published in English) using the Rutgers George F. Smith Library of the Health Sciences, MEDLINE®, Cumulative Index of Nursing and Allied Health Literature, and Dissertation Abstracts International.

This chapter is organized according to the Oncology Nursing Society's (ONS's) 2009–2013 Research Agenda (ONS, 2011). The purpose of the ONS Research Agenda "is to provide guidance for research initiatives to meet the ONS mission to promote excellence in oncology nursing and quality cancer care" (ONS, 2011, p. 1). The ONS Research Agenda is revised every two years and "provides important and timely direction for research and evidence-based practice" (ONS, 2011, p. 2). In 2009–2013, the content areas and priority topics for oncology nursing research were as follows: symptoms, late effects of cancer treatment and survivorship care, palliative and end-of-life care, self-management, aging, family and caregivers, improving healthcare systems, and risk reduction.

The ONS Research Agenda content leaders and experts identified four broad categories as "cross-cutting themes" throughout the Agenda (ONS, 2011, pp. 1–2).
- **Individual/population issues**—including cultural sensitivity, health disparities, life span orientation, family as the care recipient, global health issues, ethics, and personalized medicine
- **Design/methods issues**—including models outside oncology nursing, mechanisms underlying responses to cancer and treatment (e.g., biologic, psychological, behavioral, sociocultural), longitudinal, multisite or multilevel designs, intervention work, targeted interventions, behavioral change, informatics/technologic innovations, outcomes evaluation (i.e., implementation/service outcomes), and strengthening measurement science
- **System issues**—including interdisciplinary teams; mentored grants (to optimize capacity building simultaneously with knowledge generation); partnerships and team building with other professional organizations; partnerships among researchers, clinicians, and regulators; workforce issues of medical oncologists and oncology-certified advanced practice nurses; cost and cost-effective measures; partnerships joining researchers and service organizations to promote implementation; health policy implications; and healthcare reform

Studies reviewed in this chapter are grouped according to two of the aforementioned three themes: individual/population issues and system issues. No studies were found for the past decade that directly addressed the design/methods issues theme as identified by the ONS Research Agenda (ONS, 2011). The 2009–2013 Agenda content areas and priority topics for oncology nursing research are identified for each study reviewed.

As previously stated, the ONS Research Agenda is revised every two years. In 2014, a new Research Agenda was published to guide research and evidence-based practice initiatives for 2014–2018 (ONS, 2014). The content areas, priority topics, and cross-cutting themes of this updated Agenda are described in the "Future Directions" section later in this chapter.

Individual/Population Issues

General Symptom Assessment

ONS Research Agenda Content Areas and Priority Topics: *Cancer symptoms and side effects, late effects of cancer* *treatment and long-term survivorship issues, psychosocial and family issues, nursing-sensitive patient outcomes, translation science*

Williams et al. (2006) conducted a descriptive study of the self-reported symptoms and associated self-care by 37 adults receiving chemotherapy (primarily for leukemia, lymphomas, or breast cancer) or radiation therapy (primarily for head and neck or lung cancers). Study instruments included the Therapy-Related Symptom Checklist (TRSC) for Adults, a demographic data form, and an interview form regarding self-care for identified symptoms. Severe symptoms on the TRSC results for chemotherapy included severe symptoms of fatigue, eating difficulties, nausea, pain, numbness in fingers and toes, hair loss, and constipation. Patients receiving radiation therapy experienced severe symptoms of eating difficulties, fatigue, skin changes, mucosal changes to the oropharynx, and constipation. Using complementary medicine as a framework, Williams et al. studied the self-care strategies in the categories of diet, nutrition, and lifestyle change (e.g., use of nutritional supplements; modifications of food and of eating habits; naps, sleep, rest); mind and body control (e.g., relaxation methods, prayer, music); biologic treatments (e.g., vitamins); herbal treatments (e.g., green mint tea); and ethno-medicine (e.g., lime juice and garlic). The first category was predominantly used by patients in both treatment types. Medications were also prescribed to help control symptoms, such as pain and nausea.

Williams et al. concluded that symptom monitoring and self-care for the symptoms identified may be facilitated by the TRSC. Based on reported symptom severity, care providers may prioritize interventions. The authors recommended that larger studies be done regarding the use of the TRSC as a clinical tool to assess symptoms that patients with cancer experience during therapy. In addition, the TRSC should assess whether care providers, based on patient-reported symptom severity, can prioritize interventions and how this might influence the efficiency of care; the self-care strategies used by patients on chemotherapy, radiation therapy, or both; and how useful these strategies are in alleviating symptoms.

Lymphedema Assessment and Management

ONS Research Agenda Content Areas and Priority Topics: *Cancer symptoms and side effects, late effects of cancer treatment and long-term survivorship issues, translation science*

Deng, Ridner, Dietrich, Wells, and Murphy (2013) noted that early identification and accurate documentation of head and neck lymphedema are critically important to prevent the progress of lymphedema. These investigators compared four grading and staging scales used to measure external lymphedema in patients with head and neck cancer. Their study sample consisted of 103 head and neck cancer survivors being treated in a comprehensive cancer center. They used a cross-sectional design to compare four scales that were being used to evaluate study participants' external lymphedema status and assessed problems and gaps related to the scales. These four tools included the Common Terminology Criteria for Adverse Events (CTCAE) Lymphedema Scale, the American Cancer Society (ACS) Lymphedema Scale, Stages of Lymphedema (Földi Scale), and CTCAE Fibrosis Scale. The main research variables studied included the occurrence rate and severity of lymphedema, as well as the components and descriptors of each scale.

Deng et al. (2013) found that the prevalence and severity of external lymphedema differed significantly based on the tools used to assess lymphedema. Each tool had an identified limitation, and existing grading criteria failed to capture important characteristics of external head and neck lymphedema. The investigators noted that current theory postulates a continuum between lymphedema and fibrosis, but only the Földi scale adequately reflected that concept. They concluded that none of the four scales studied clearly captured all the important characteristics of external lymphedema in patients with head and neck cancer. They recommended that a clearly defined and validated scale of external lymphedema in the head and neck cancer population needs to be developed. The implications they identified for nursing are that oncology nurses should take an active role in addressing issues related to lymphedema assessment in patients with head and neck cancer post-treatment, new assessment tools need to be developed for clinical nurses to use, and more research efforts need to be made to address this underrecognized issue.

Deng, Ridner, and Murphy (2011) conducted a comprehensive literature review to describe the current state of the science on secondary lymphedema in patients with head and neck cancer. Data sources included published journal articles and books, websites, and data from the National Cancer Institute, ACS, and other healthcare-related professional associations.

Synthesis of these data indicated that survivors of head and neck cancer may develop secondary lymphedema as a result of the cancer or its treatment. Secondary lymphedema may involve external (e.g., submental area) and internal (e.g., laryngeal, pharyngeal, oral cavity) structures. Although lymphedema affects highly visible anatomic sites (e.g., face, neck) and profoundly influences critical physical functions (e.g., speech, breathing, swallowing, cervical range of motion), research regarding lymphedema in patients with head and neck cancer is lacking. They concluded that secondary lymphedema in patients with head and neck cancer is a significant but understudied issue. Among the implications for nursing, there exists a need to systematically examine secondary lymphedema related to treatment for head and neck cancer and address gaps in the current literature, such as symptom burden, effects on body functions, and influences on quality of life (QOL). They further concluded that new studies are needed to address a variety of vital questions, including incidence and prevalence, optimal measurement techniques, associated symptom burden, functional loss, and psychosocial impact (Deng et al., 2011).

Deng et al. (2011) reported that empirical evidence would be needed to support oncology nurses and other healthcare professionals in the management of lymphedema after head and neck cancer treatment. They noted that there is a lack of empirical evidence, making specific recommendations for nursing interventions difficult. They suggested that nurses should look for face and neck swelling along with tissue fibrosis; assess symptom and functional deficiencies related to lymphedema and document; collaborate with the surgeon, radiation oncologist, and medical oncologist to reduce the impact of secondary lymphedema in patients with head and neck cancer; and facilitate suitable referrals for specific services and follow-up.

Appetite Assessment

ONS Research Agenda Content Areas and Priority Topics: *Cancer symptoms and side effects, late effects of cancer treatment and long-term survivorship issues, translation science*

Ogama and Ogama (2013) conducted a study to develop an oral assessment tool for evaluating the appetite of patients with head and neck cancer receiving radiation therapy and who had dysgeusia, xerostomia, and/or oral mucositis. They also wanted to verify the assessment tool's validity and reliability. Based on an interview survey of 30 patients, the authors prepared a draft oral assessment tool, which included a five-point scale and 19 items. The resultant questionnaire survey was administered to 209 participants. A factor analysis of construct validity revealed three factors: (a) dysgeusia and loss of flavors, (b) salivation abnormality and loss of moisture in the oral cavity, and (c) pain in the oral cavity and lack of motivation. These factors contributed to 14 items that were adopted for the final oral assessment tool. During a review of criteria validity, a correlation was found between the scores of the three factors and the overall oral assessment tool, including the scores on taste sensitivity, xerostomia, oral mucositis, and appetite with a correlation coefficient of $r = 0.41–0.89$ ($p < 0.01$). According to test–retest study results, and with regard to reliability, stability was determined as 0.87 ($p < 0.01$). Internal consistency was confirmed by a Cronbach's alpha coefficient of 0.83 ($p < 0.01$) and an interclass correlation coefficient of 0.80 ($p < 0.01$). These investigators concluded that, based on the validity and reliability of the new oral assessment tool, it is practical for use in the assessment of appetite of patients with head and neck cancer.

Smoking Cessation

ONS Research Agenda Content Areas and Priority Topics: *Health promotion, psychosocial and family issues, translation science*

Duffy, Scheumann, Fowler, Darling-Fisher, and Terrell (2010) conducted a cross-sectional study to determine the predictors of participation in a smoking cessation program among patients with head and neck cancer. This was a substudy of a larger, randomized trial of patients with head and neck cancer that determined the predictors of smokers' participation in a cessation intervention. The authors studied 286 patients who had smoked within six months of the screening survey and who were eligible for a smoking cessation intervention. Forty-eight percent of the patients who were eligible for inclusion participated. Their study setting included three otolaryngology clinics located in three different Veterans Affairs medical centers. Descriptive statistics and bivariate and multivariate logistic regression were used to determine the independent predictors of smokers' participation in an intervention study. The main research variables studied were perceived difficulty quitting (as a construct of self-efficacy), health behaviors (e.g., smoking, excessive drinking), clinical characteristics (e.g., depression, cancer site/stage), and various demographic variables.

Duffy et al. found that a perceived high difficulty of quitting smoking was the only statistically significant predictor of participation, whereas alcohol abuse, lower depressive symptoms, and laryngeal cancer site approached significance. They concluded that special outreach may be needed to contact patients with head and neck cancer who are problem drinkers, are overly confident in quitting smoking, or have been diagnosed with laryngeal cancer. They also noted that oncology nurses are in an opportune position to assess patients' perceived difficulty in quitting smoking and to motivate them to enroll in cessation programs, ultimately improving QOL, reducing risk of recurrence, and increasing survival for the head and neck cancer population.

Silent Aspiration

ONS Research Agenda Content Areas and Priority Topics: *Cancer symptoms and side effects, late effects of cancer treatment and long-term survivorship issues, translation science*

To increase nurses' awareness of the diagnostic pathology groups associated with silent aspiration, Garon, Sierzant, and Ormiston (2009) conducted a retrospective study of aspiration and the lack of a protective cough reflex at the vocal folds (termed *silent aspiration*) on a wide variety of hospitalized patients. Of the 2,000 patients evaluated in this study, 51% aspirated during their videofluoroscopic evaluation. Of the patients who aspirated, 55% had no protective cough reflex. The diagnostic pathology groups with the highest rates of silent aspiration were brain cancer, brainstem stroke, head and neck cancer, pneumonia, dementia/Alzheimer, chronic obstructive lung disease, seizures, myocardial infarcts, neurodegenerative pathologies, right hemisphere stroke, left hemisphere stroke, and closed head injury. These investigators concluded that the diagnostic groups identified in this research as having the highest risk of silent aspiration should be viewed as "red-flag" patients by the nurses caring for them. They recommended early nursing dysphagia screening with close attention to the clinical symptoms associated with silent aspiration, and they stressed the importance of early referral for formal dysphagia evaluation.

Depression

ONS Research Agenda Content Areas and Priority Topics: *Cancer symptoms and side effects, late effects of cancer treatment and long-term survivorship issues, end-of-life issues, psychosocial and family issues, nursing-sensitive patient outcomes, translation science*

In order to establish a knowledge base for future head and neck cancer research, Haisfield-Wolfe, McGuire, Soeken, Geiger-Brown, and De Forge (2009) conducted a comprehensive summary of the existing research literature related to prevalence and correlates of depression in adult patients with head and neck cancer. Their data sources included quantitative studies in English measuring depression or mood in adults with head and neck cancer published in 1986–2008. They found that a substantial body of knowledge exists regarding prevalence, correlates, and predictors of depression in patients with head and neck cancer. In addition, prevalence rates of depression are highest at diagnosis, during treatment, and in the first six months following treatment, and mild to moderate depression may continue for three to six years after diagnosis. The authors also noted that certain patient demographic characteristics (e.g., marital status, education), symptoms, and specific time points in the illness trajectory (e.g., time of treatment) are correlated with depression. Specific patient variables at the time of diagnosis, such as depression, can predict depression at later time points.

The authors suggested that evidence-based information contained in their comprehensive summary of the research literature regarding the prevalence and correlates of depression among adult patients with head and neck cancer may be useful to oncology nurses in their practice with this population.

Haisfield-Wolfe et al. concluded the following.

• Additional research should assess depressive symptoms using consistent depression instruments or clinical interviews based on specific criteria in patients with head and neck cancer. Multisite studies should be conducted with increased sample sizes.

• Research related to symptom clusters and the effect of clusters on patients is needed.

• Longitudinal studies that examine depression and patient characteristics, symptoms, type of treatments, and the correlates of depression across the trajectory of illness are important.

• Replication of existing research using multiple patient and clinical characteristics to explore predictors of depression may reveal profiles for patients most at risk of developing depression.

Taste Dysfunction

ONS Research Agenda Content Areas and Priority Topics: *Cancer symptoms and side effects, late effects of cancer treatment and long-term survivorship issues, psychosocial and family issues, nursing-sensitive patient outcomes, translation science*

McLaughlin (2013) conducted an exploratory cross-sectional study to describe the prevalence of issues with taste function in head and neck cancer survivors. She studied 92 outpatient survivors. The sample was heterogeneous in terms of cancer site, treatment type, and time post-treatment, ranging from three months to more than 28 years after completion of therapy. She assessed taste discrimination using high, medium, and low concentrations of sweet-, salty-, sour-, and bitter-tasting solutions. Of the 92 study participants, 85 were found to have some measurable level of taste dysfunction. Confusion between bitter and sour and the inability to discriminate among differing concentrations of sweet solutions were common taste dysfunctions. Statistically significant weight loss was found to be associated with diminished taste sensation (hypogeusia) and discrimination (dysgeusia).

McLaughlin concluded that taste alteration was a persistent problem across all categories of head and neck cancer treatments, sites, and stages; those with loss of one or more specific modality did poorly on the taste test; and participants could not accurately determine which taste was most severely impaired. Flavor recognition is changed by any alteration in one or more of the sensory experiences of taste, texture, aroma, thermal quality, and visual cues. It is possible to have an intact sense of taste but impaired flavor recognition. Confusion with flavor recognition and taste is not accurately self-reported. The implications for oncology nursing practice are the following.

• Taste dysfunction is a long-term treatment side effect for head and neck cancer survivors.

• Because taste loss is upsetting and is associated with a decreased appetite and weight loss, taste changes and dysgeusia are significant nursing considerations.

• More research is needed to identify effective interventions to assist head and neck cancer survivors to adapt to these long-term complications of treatment.

ONS Research Agenda Content Areas and Priority Topics: *Cancer symptoms and side effects, late effects of cancer treatment and long-term survivorship issues, psychosocial and family issues, nursing-sensitive patient outcomes, translation science*

McLaughlin and Mahon (2014) conducted a meta-analysis of the relationship among impaired taste and treatment, treatment type, and tumor site in head and neck cancer treatment survivors (HNCTS) "to understand how taste impairment caused by head and neck cancer treatment changes over time or varies with treatment site or type" (p. E194). A literature search was conducted using the MEDLINE database to acquire reports of health-related quality of life (HRQOL) in HNCTS, which included taste function in an HRQOL instrument from 1946 to 2013. Studies deemed eligible compared taste scores from baseline to post-treatment, using two treatment types or two cancer sites. Of the 247 reports identified, 19 were found to be suitable for meta-analysis. The data were analyzed through a series of dichotomous meta-analyses using comprehensive meta-analysis software. They reported that taste scores were significantly poorer after treatment, patients treated with radiation therapy reported statistically significant worse taste function post-treatment than those who received no radiation therapy, and differences in tumor site were not a significant finding. According to McLaughlin and Mahon, taste dysfunction is a long-term complication for HNCTS, and nurses must routinely screen survivors for this sensory dysfunction.

Mucositis

ONS Research Agenda Content Areas and Priority Topics: *Cancer symptoms and side effects, late effects of cancer treatment and long-term survivorship issues, translation science*

Putwatana et al. (2009) conducted a prospective, randomized clinical trial to determine the efficacy of payayor, a Thai-prepared herbal product, as well as payayor with benzydamine in the prevention and relief of radiation-induced oral mucositis. They studied 60 patients with head and neck cancer who were randomly assigned into each treatment group. Research participants used the assigned products three times daily from the first to the last day of radiation treatment. The first group used glycerin payayor by dripping it into their mouths. The second group rinsed their mouths with benzydamine hydrochloride. The World Health Organization mucositis grading system was used to assess oral status every week during radiation treatments and every two weeks after radiation. A t-test was performed to compare the time to onset of oral mucositis, pain, severity and xerostomia; postponement of treatment; satisfaction with the solution; and subjects' body weights. The findings for the payayor group were that the average time to the onset of oral mucositis was significantly delayed, and its severity and associated discomfort scores were less than those of the benzydamine group throughout the study. Significantly higher satisfaction scores with the solution and higher body

weights at the end of the study were noted when compared to the benzydamine group. The authors concluded that payayor seemed to be more effective than benzydamine for preventing and relieving radiation-induced oral mucositis.

Nutrition

ONS Research Agenda Content Areas and Priority Topics: *Cancer symptoms and side effects, late effects of cancer treatment and long-term survivorship issues, end-of-life issues, nursing-sensitive patient outcomes, translation science*

Because home enteral nutrition (HEN) has undergone considerable development in the last 20 years and has determined economic and organizational changes in Italy, Paccagnella et al. (2008) conducted a study to evaluate the epidemiologic data of 655 patients treated in a five-year period (2001–2005) in an area of Northeast Italy. The investigation team collected and analyzed data obtained at the initiation of HEN (age, gender, pathology, Karnofsky index, type of enteral access device, presence of pressure ulcers, weight, body mass index, hematochemical tests, daily enteral intake) and then considered the length of therapy and patient survival (based on patient mortality or the patient's ability to resume oral nutrition). They found that HEN was prescribed for the following pathologies: 40.9% neurodegenerative, 26.7% neurovascular, 11.5% head and neck cancer, 9.8% abdominal cancer, 7% other pathologies, 2.6% congenital anomaly, and 1.5% head injury.

Before commencement of enteral feeding, an average weight loss of 22.9% was observed across all indications for HEN. Mean incidence of HEN was 308.7 (range 80.7–355.6) and mean prevalence was 379.8 (range 138.7–534.6). The median length of HEN was 196 days, with only 7.9% of patients resuming oral nutrition. The median survival rate was 9.1 months, which was influenced by age, gender, and the Karnofsky performance scale index. Resumption of oral nutrition was influenced by age, gender, Karnofsky index, and type of enteral access device used.

Communication—Assistive Devices

ONS Research Agenda Content Areas and Priority Topics: *Cancer symptoms and side effects, late effects of cancer treatment and long-term survivorship issues, psychosocial and family issues, nursing-sensitive patient outcomes, translation science*

In 2010, Rodriguez and Rowe reported the use of a time-series study design that tested the possibility of using a programmable speech-generating device (PSGD) in hospitalized adults with head and neck cancer who underwent treatment that left them speechless. Their sample consisted of 9 female and 12 male postoperative inpatients (mean age = 62 years) hospitalized in a tertiary care institution and who were experiencing speechlessness as a result of surgical interventions. All patients participated in a communication intervention that incorporated use of a PSGD during their hospital stay. Data regarding PSGD use, functionality, and technology-related issues were collected from the participants. The Satisfaction and Usability Instrument was used to collect and measure the variables of interest. These included satisfaction with and usability of the PSGD. The findings reported that participants confirmed significant progress in ability to use the PSGD over a four-day period for all communication functions assessed. These results also indicated that participants were "quite satisfied" with using the device and considered the technology to be "quite important" during the postoperative period. Moreover, PSGD messages generated by study participants via the hospital call system were understood by clerks. Participants admitted to intensive care units did, however, experience problems related to accessibility of the device. Specific accessibility issues reported included that the device was placed on the nightstand or at an unreachable distance when attached to the Manfrotto arm.

Rodriguez and Rowe concluded that participants demonstrated proficient and independent use of the PSGD to communicate programmed messages. Other strategies were necessary to meet their communication needs as the postoperative period progressed. The implication of these study findings and conclusions for nursing practice was that PSGDs may offer a more reliable option to facilitate communication between patients and nurses during the postoperative period. The authors also noted that technology should be tailored to meet speechless patients' unique needs as they progress through the rehabilitation process. They recommended that additional research be carried out on the technologic communication options and strategies available to tailor technology to meet the needs of speechless patients.

Pain and Anxiety

ONS Research Agenda Content Areas and Priority Topics: *Cancer symptoms and side effects, late effects of cancer treatment and long-term survivorship issues, psychosocial and family issues, translation science*

Stephenson, Swanson, Dalton, Keefe, and Engelke (2007) compared the effects of partner-delivered foot reflexology and usual care plus attention on patients' perceived pain and anxiety. They used an experimental pre- and post-test design that included 86 dyads of patients with metastatic cancer and their partners randomly assigned to an experimental (n = 42) or a control (n = 44) group. Participants represented 16 different types of cancer (23% lung cancer, followed by breast, colorectal, and head and neck cancer and lymphoma). The study setting consisted of four hospitals in the southeastern United States. The reflexology intervention included a 15–30-minute teaching session on foot reflexology delivered to the partner by a certified reflexologist, an optional 15–30-minute foot reflexology session for the partner, and

a 30-minute partner-delivered foot reflexology intervention for the patient. The control group received a 30-minute reading session from their partners.

For the treatment group, the authors found that patients experienced a significant decrease in pain intensity and anxiety following the initial partner-delivered foot reflexology. Minimal changes were seen in the control group.

The investigators concluded that the implications for nursing are that a nurse reflexologist could teach partners how to perform reflexology on patients with metastatic cancer pain in the hospital. They also suggested that hospitals could have qualified professionals offer reflexology as a complementary therapy and teach interested partners the modality.

Quality of Life

ONS Research Agenda Content Areas and Priority Topics: *Cancer symptoms and side effects, late effects of cancer treatment and long-term survivorship issues, psychosocial and family issues*

Moore, Ford, and Farah (2014) posited that head and neck cancer treatment disrupts QOL and is associated with individualized supportive care needs. Their study was designed to describe the support needs that affected the QOL of patients with head and neck cancer and to describe how patients coped with unmet support needs. They used a qualitative approach and employed semistructured interviews with eight participants who were previously treated for head and neck cancer. Participants were identified through snowball and convenience sampling methods. Content analysis was used to analyze interview data. Inductive content analysis was used to describe support needs. Directed content analysis was used according to the stress appraisal and coping model to describe coping with unmet support needs. The authors warned, however, that the conclusions from this study are limited by a small and homogenous sample. They found the following from patients.

• QOL was affected by the support received during treatment and was related to support in coping with long-term treatment side effects.
• Coping with depression and anxiety affected QOL in the first 6–12 months after treatment.
• Coping was influenced by loss of access to the hospital environment after treatment. This resulted in feelings of isolation.

From this information, they concluded that

• Patients draw support from professional and personal systems during and after treatment.
• Patients find it difficult to cope with the side effects of treatment and accessing supportive care when away from the hospital environment.
• The transactional model of stress, appraisal, and coping is useful in understanding the psychosocial outcomes of head and neck cancer.

ONS Research Agenda Content Areas and Priority Topics: *Cancer symptoms and side effects, late effects of cancer treatment and long-term survivorship issues, psychosocial and family issues, translation science*

Suzuki (2012) used a prospective, correlational, and pre- and post-test design to explore the relationship among perceived involvement in decision making, uncertainty, and QOL in patients with head and neck cancer during their pre- and post-treatment periods using Mishel's Uncertainty in Illness Theory. A convenience sample of 52 adults newly diagnosed with head and neck cancer was obtained from six outpatient clinics at urban hospitals in the northeastern United States. Study data were collected using a self-administered questionnaire containing a demographic datasheet, the Functional Assessment of Cancer Therapy–Head and Neck, Mishel's Uncertainty in Illness Scale (Adult), and the Perceived Involvement in Care Scale at pretreatment (time 1) and six weeks post-treatment (time 2). The main research variables studied were QOL, uncertainty, and perceived involvement in decision making. Suzuki found that post-treatment QOL scores were lower than pretreatment; uncertainty and employment status affected QOL at time 1 and 2; QOL scores and uncertainty during pretreatment were predictors of post-treatment QOL after adjusting for unemployment, chemoradiation, and physician; and the perception of being involved in decision making was not associated with uncertainty or QOL.

Suzuki concluded that the higher a patient's pretreatment QOL, the more likely QOL would remain stable post-treatment. Implications for nursing practice include the following.

- Financial or work-related impact needs to be taken into account when assessing QOL in patients with head and neck cancer.
- Nurses need to involve social workers and case managers early in care planning to review insurance issues, available financial resources, and synchronization of timetables to maintain employment.

The implications for nursing research include the following.

- Additional studies are needed to decrease uncertainty and to maintain employment and income.
- The antecedents of Mishel's Uncertainty in Illness Theory may need refinement for patients with head and neck cancer.

System Issues

Nursing Care Delivery Systems and Care Planning

ONS Research Agenda Content Areas and Priority Topics: *Health promotion, cancer symptoms and side effects,*

psychosocial and family issues, nursing-sensitive patient outcomes, translation science

Kagan (2009) conducted an extensive review of published research evidence pertinent to the role and influence of nursing in the management of head and neck cancer and summarized the implications for nursing practice and future research. She found that nurses can play a vital role in the management of head and neck cancer and the care of patients and their families and that the role and influence of nursing is dependent on available research evidence to support nursing's role, as well as the sociopolitical and organizational factors that shape the context for nursing and interdisciplinary practice. Nurses influence treatment for head and neck cancer through symptom management and tobacco cessation to improve QOL and patient-reported outcomes. In addition, nurses and interdisciplinary teams in the United States and Europe report successful, novel nurse-led care models that optimize their influence on management.

In summary, Kagan noted that research findings supported that nurses can influence head and neck cancer treatment through their emphasis on symptom management and tobacco and alcohol cessation and by focusing on patient and family education and care coordination. Because the research evidence for head and neck cancer nursing practice remains scant, Kagan recommended continued research, employing qualitative and quantitative approaches conducted by nursing and interdisciplinary teams to advance head and neck cancer management. Kagan also recommended that nurses optimize the influence of nursing in the patient population, suggesting that novel models for the delivery of nursing care may further improve care and patient outcomes. Evaluation of such models is required to document improvements.

ONS Research Agenda Content Areas and Priority Topics: *Cancer symptoms and side effects, psychosocial and family issues, translation science*

According to Larsson, Hedelin, and Athlin (2007), patients with head and neck cancer "have complex long-lasting physical and psychosocial needs due to illness and treatment, and studies have shown deficiencies concerning support in these respects" (p. 49). The researchers conducted a study to describe how patients with head and neck cancer with eating problems conceived the significance of a supportive nursing care clinic before, during, and after completion of radiation therapy. They carried out thematic interviews using an open-dialog strategy with 12 patients treated with radiation therapy for head and neck cancer. Their method of qualitative data analysis was phenomenology. Their findings indicated that the nurse clinic could help in meeting these patients' needs for safety and security. This was thought to be especially important before and after patients' completion of treatment when no other regular contacts in the healthcare system occurred. The significance of the nurse clinic varied depending on where patients were in their trajectory of care, what needs and problems these patients were experiencing, and how severely these needs and problems were being experienced by the individual patient. These investigators concluded that a supportive nursing care clinic could meet the patients' needs for knowledge, as well as both care and support concerning practical measures related to the disease and its treatment and emotional needs. This method of organizing care may contribute to patients' health and well-being.

ONS Research Agenda Content Areas and Priority Topics: *Late effects of cancer treatment and long-term survivorship issues, end-of-life issues, psychosocial and family issues, translation science*

Marbach and Griffie (2011) conducted an exploratory, descriptive study using an in-depth thematic and comparative analysis of four tape-recorded focus group interviews of cancer survivors to examine these patients' preferences for content and methods of delivering treatment plans, educational information, and survivorship care plans. Their research setting was an outpatient clinical cancer center in an academic medical center in the midwestern United States. Participants included 40 cancer survivors who had completed their initial treatment. Participants were grouped by disease site: prostate, genitourinary, and skin; breast and gynecologic; gastrointestinal, sarcoma, and head and neck; and brain, pancreatic, and lung. Data were grouped into four major, interconnected themes. Thematic analysis resulted in four agreed-upon categories: educational information, treatment plan, survivorship care plan, and patient support. Themes were then identified within each category.

Marbach and Griffie concluded that the number of cancer survivors continues to grow each year. Nurses should approach each cancer survivor with individualized educational information; they must assess survivors for their unique needs and intervene accordingly. An initial treatment plan, a survivorship care plan, and emotional support are all imperative.

The implications for oncology nursing practice are the following.
- Because oncology nurses assess and recognize the learning needs of each patient, they are best positioned to develop teaching content, strategies, and timing of interventions.
- The importance of written educational materials cannot be negated.
- Oncology nurses are well positioned to provide a proactive role in the development and delivery of treatment and survivorship plans of care.

Communication

ONS Research Agenda Content Areas and Priority Topics: *Translation science*

According to Liu, Mok, Wong, Xue, and Xu (2007), "Nurses have considerable needs for communication skills training in cancer care because of the general lack of education and training on oncology-specific communication skills in Mainland China" (p. 202). They undertook a study to evaluate the effectiveness of an integrated communication skills training program in which an intensive learning session was combined with practice in the clinical unit to create a supportive practice atmosphere, thus allowing nurses to practice integrated communication skills in the workplace. The investigators implemented communication skills training for 129 nurses and used a quasiexperimental research design with a nonequivalent control group. They measured basic communication skills, self-efficacy in oncology-specific communication skills, communication outcome expectancies, and self-perceived support for communication. Measures were made in the training group at pretraining evaluation, one month after training (formative evaluation), and six months after training (summative evaluation). The control group was evaluated only at the time of pretraining and six months after training (i.e., formative evaluation was not carried out in the control group). The results of this study were that continued significant improvement was noted in overall basic communication skills, self-efficacy, outcome expectancy beliefs, and perceived support in the integrated communication skills training group. In addition, no significant improvement in the control group was noted over the same period of time. The investigators concluded that nurses' communication skills can be developed and consolidated using the integrated communication skills training model. Development of effective interventions to change nurses' negative outcome expectations in communication with cancer patients requires further study.

Nurse-Managed Care

ONS Research Agenda Content Areas and Priority Topics: *Cancer symptoms and side effects, late effects of cancer treatment and long-term survivorship issues, psychosocial and family issues, nursing-sensitive patient outcomes, translation science*

To determine whether improved monitoring through close follow-up with a nurse practitioner (NP) could enhance treatment compliance and decrease frequency of hospitalizations, Mason, DeRubeis, Foster, Taylor, and Worden (2013) conducted a retrospective chart review in an academic National Cancer Institute–designated comprehensive cancer center. Their sample consisted of 151 patients aged 45–65 years old who were diagnosed with stage III or IV oropharyngeal cancer. These patients were nonrandomized into one of two groups: a pre-chemotherapy clinic group and a weekly NP-led clinic group. Descriptive statistics were examined, followed by multiple linear and logistic regression comparisons of these groups across patient outcomes. The research variables studied were hospitalization, chemotherapy dose deviations, and chemotherapy treatment completion. The findings were the following.

- The average number of visits during traditional treatment doubled after initiation of the NP-led clinic.
- The hospitalization rate was nearly cut in half from 28% in the traditional clinic group to 12% in the NP-led group.
- The rate of chemotherapy dose deviations was 48% in the traditional clinic group and decreased to 6% in the NP-led clinic group.
- Only 46% of patients in the traditional clinic group tolerated the full seven scheduled doses of chemotherapy compared to 90% of patients in the NP-led clinic group.

Mason et al. concluded that a weekly NP-led symptom management clinic reduces rates of hospitalization and chemotherapy dose deviations and increases chemotherapy completion in patients receiving intensive chemoradiotherapy for oropharyngeal cancer. The most important implication of the findings of this study for oncology nursing practice is that patients receiving chemoradiotherapy benefit from close monitoring for toxicities by NPs and may therefore successfully complete their treatment and avoid hospitalization. Further translation of this knowledge into practice indicates that early interventions to manage toxicities in patients with head and neck cancer can improve outcomes. In addition, NPs are in a key position to manage these toxicities, and costs are reduced when symptoms are controlled.

ONS Research Agenda Content Areas and Priority Topics: *Health promotion—developing or testing interventions to adopt or maintain health behaviors that reduce or prevent cancer, late effects of cancer treatment and long-term survivorship issues, psychosocial and family issues, translation science*

According to Sharp, Johansson, Fagerström, and Rutqvist (2008), "Many cancer patients continue to smoke past diagnosis and treatment, even though smoking in some cases may cause more side effects and increase the risk of treatment failure" (p. 114). These investigators developed and evaluated a nurse-led smoking cessation program with 50 patients with head and neck cancer who were undergoing radiation therapy with one-year follow-up. Their study was designed to evaluate the effectiveness of the program by evaluating the proportion of smoke-free patients. Smoking status was tested by measuring carbon monoxide in patients' expired air. Thirty-seven patients (74%) tested weekly as being smoke-free during the radiation therapy period. At the one-year follow-up visit, 28 patients (68%) tested as being smoke-free. These rates of being smoke-free are high in comparison to other reported smoking cessation studies with patients with cancer. The results indicated that even patients with head and neck cancer with a heavy smoking history and long-time nicotine dependence could quit smoking with systematic support. These investigators recommended that a more sophisticated evaluation of smoking cessation in this population be pursued, including the research strategy of obtaining larger study samples and control groups.

ONS Research Agenda Content Areas and Priority Topics: *Cancer symptoms and side effects, late effects of cancer treatment and long-term survivorship issues, psychosocial and family issues, nursing-sensitive patient outcomes, translation science*

Wells et al. (2008) evaluated a nurse-led clinic for patients undergoing radiation therapy for head and neck cancer. According to these investigators, "the side effects of radiotherapy to the head and neck are superimposed on already significant physical and psychological morbidity" (Wells et al., 2008, p. 1428). They noted that medical review clinics typically focus on treatment complications but that there is evidence that specialist nurses may provide more holistic care for patients with head and neck cancer. However, skepticism remained an issue regarding the appropriateness of a nurse-led review in this patient population. Comparisons were made regarding medical on-treatment review (phase 1) with a nurse-led clinic (phase 2) for patients undergoing radiation therapy, using a historical control group. Twenty patients with head and neck cancer were reviewed by their medical consultant and 23 by a nurse specialist, using a clinic protocol. A mixed-method approach to data collection was used. Patients completed weekly QOL questionnaires that asked about their experiences regarding support and care. General practitioners completed a questionnaire about the communication received from the clinic. Checklists assessed the content of clinic consultations. Patients valued the relationship that developed with the nurse specialist, and they had longer and more frequent consultations. In addition, they were more likely to be referred to the multidisciplinary team. The nurse specialist successfully managed 83% of consultations without referral to the medical consultant. Few significant differences in QOL were found between the groups. Oral and nutritional problems were managed more effectively in the nurse-led clinic, although emotional functioning was higher in the medical group. General medical practitioners were optimistic about the timing and content of information received by patients with head and neck cancer.

Wells et al. concluded that on-treatment review for patients with head and neck cancer can be effectively managed by nurse specialists. The implication for nursing practice is that radiation therapy nurse specialists may make important contributions to the supportive care of patients with head and neck cancer. More investment in employing these nurse specialists will be required to maximize their contribution.

Professional Patient Navigators

ONS Research Agenda Content Areas and Priority Topics: *Cancer symptoms and side effects, late effects of cancer treatment and long-term survivorship issues, translation science*

Fillion et al. (2009) discussed professional cancer navigation roles, models, implementation processes, and outcomes of patients and families dealing with head and neck cancer. After they reviewed published scientific papers, research review articles, and implementation studies, they presented and reviewed one specific research study as an illustration. In the study presented, two independent cohorts of patients with head and neck cancers were compared according to the presence of the professional navigator (exposed cohort n = 83) or not (historical cohort n = 75). The exposed cohort showed a better profile on several outcome indicators. The investigators concluded that there was a positive association between the presence of the professional navigator and continuity of care (i.e., higher satisfaction and shorter duration of hospitalization) and empowerment (i.e., fewer cancer-related problems, including body image concerns, better emotional QOL). They suggested that oncology nurses play an important role in not only continuity of care but also supportive care by helping patients to cope better with cancer treatments and issues related to recovery, cancer progression, and death issues.

ONS Research Agenda Content Areas and Priority Topics: *Cancer symptoms and side effects, late effects of cancer treatment and long-term survivorship issues, translation science*

Fillion et al. (2006) conducted a qualitative study that provides a descriptive assessment for implementing an oncology patient navigator nurse (OPN) in the head and neck oncology area of a university hospital center with a supra-regional model for oncology. They profiled the role and functions of an OPN and the preliminary phases to implementing this role within a team specializing in oncology. Three groups of stakeholders (individuals with cancer and their families, caregivers, and network partners) were interviewed before, during, and after implementation. The results indicated that the new OPN role can be integrated within a team that specializes in oncology. The investigators described the beneficial effects of this role on the process of adaptation to illness, interdisciplinary work, and continuity of care. Among their conclusions and recommendations was noting the importance of addressing the implementation process from an organizational change perspective.

Monitoring Patients With Head and Neck Cancer

ONS Research Agenda Content Areas and Priority Topics: *Cancer symptoms and side effects, late effects of cancer treatment and long-term survivorship issues, translation science*

Fox, Barrett-McNeil, Khoo, and Middleton (2011) advocated for frequent management of patients with head and neck cancer to improve the course of treatment for head and neck radiation therapy. To achieve this in a busy practice environment, they suggested the use of "streamlined" tools such as electronic toxicity scoring. They maintained that close attention using biweekly electronic toxicity scoring should improve monitoring of head and neck radiation therapy toxicities. Fox et al. studied a convenience sample of 20 patients undergoing head and neck radiation therapy

and recorded their toxicity data on a biweekly basis, including dysphagia, mucositis, skin reaction, and weight loss. They found that the efficiencies offered by an electronic medical record allowed comprehensive toxicity data to be recorded and analyzed effortlessly. The average time taken to review these patients on a biweekly basis was 6.97 minutes and contained an average of 60 words of toxicity description and action. The investigators concluded that electronic toxicity scoring offers advantages to radiation oncology nurses by increasing efficiency, thus allowing for more frequent patient interactions, which is expected to aid adherence.

Future Directions

A new ONS Research Agenda was published in 2014 that will serve as an important guide for ONS research and evidence-based practice initiatives from 2014 to 2018 (ONS, 2014). It will also guide ONS in "funding oncology nursing research, scholarships, awards, and educational programs" (ONS, 2014, p. 3). The new content areas and priority topics for oncology nursing research are symptoms, long-term/late effects of cancer treatment and survivorship care, palliative and end-of-life care, self-management, aging, family and caregivers, improving health systems, and risk reduction (ONS, 2014). The ONS 2014–2018 Research Agenda content leaders and experts also identified four innovative "cross-cutting themes": bioinformatics, biomarkers, comparative effectiveness research, and dissemination and implementation science (ONS, 2014).

Summary

In the past decade, the quantity and quality of scholarly nursing research publication regarding head and neck cancer and the care of patients with head and neck cancer and their families have increased. This chapter reviewed 25 representative studies of the more than 130 head and neck cancer–related research studies available. These research studies addressed many of the ONS Research Agenda's targeted content areas and priority topics for 2009–2013. Several gaps do, however, persist in adequately addressing the Agenda's prescriptions. For example, although numerous studies were found that addressed the assessment and management of patients' clinical signs and symptoms as well as the side effects and late effects of cancer treatment, few studies were found that directly addressed health promotion, psychosocial and family issues, and nursing-sensitive patient outcomes for the head and neck cancer population. Few studies were found that directly addressed patients' long-term survivorship issues. No relevant studies were found that could be categorized as addressing "design/methods issues" or that directly addressed end-of-life issues for patients with head and neck cancer.

There are other limitations in the extant body of nursing research literature regarding head and neck cancer. These limitations illustrate the many challenges that research investigators face in trying to address this patient population. For example, many of the published studies reviewed here are descriptive in nature when more intervention-testing and experimental studies, particularly randomized controlled clinical trials (RCTs), are needed to facilitate evidence-based practice to better benefit patients with head and neck cancer and their families. It should also be noted that many of these studies employed small sample sizes, which bring into question these studies' validity and the generalizability of their findings. The descriptive level of nursing research studies and the frequent use of small sample sizes in attempting to answer important research questions are pervasive problems in nursing research. These problems often reflect the extremely limited if not nonexistent extramural funding to support more sophisticated research designs, larger sample sizes, and multisite studies. An additional challenge in head and neck cancer research is that these patients represent a relatively small percentage of the general cancer population and may not be available in sufficient numbers for investigators with limited research funding to adequately study.

Encouraging, however, are the number of studies reviewed here that were strengthened because they were conducted by interdisciplinary research teams. These studies are in accordance with the Institute of Medicine (IOM) report, *The Future of Nursing: Leading Change, Advancing Health* (IOM, 2010). The report prescribes that collaborative teams of nurses and other healthcare professionals should identify and address the main barriers of interdisciplinary collaboration in conducting the scientific research needed to support the evidence-based practice of healthcare professional teams. In addition, teams should identify and test new and existing models of interdisciplinary teams that have the potential to add value to the healthcare system, as well as educational innovations that have the potential to increase the effectiveness of healthcare teams. These IOM prescriptions should be considered as ONS moves forward in revising and reformulating its future research agendas.

Other directions also should be considered for nursing research that is important to patients living with head and neck cancer, as well as their families and communities. No doctoral dissertation research studies directly addressing head and neck cancer were found for the past decade. Doctoral students in nursing should, therefore, be encouraged to pursue research studies regarding this patient population. More qualitative studies should be conducted, as these will assist in increasing understanding and insight regarding head and neck cancer diagnoses and their impact on those affected by this life challenge. Qualitative studies would also contribute important new knowledge useful in guiding subsequent quantitative research. Such quantitative research might address psychosocial variables not yet iden-tified as important for this patient population. More studies are needed regarding the role that nurses play in prevention and early detection of head and neck cancer. A need also exists for studies that demonstrate and document causal links between effective nursing actions/interventions and predictable positive patient outcomes. As more patients are surviving longer with the disease and the sequelae of its treatment, more longitudinal studies of head and neck cancer survivors would be helpful. Although QOL is a recurrent variable of interest in this patient population, more scientific study of human relatedness and human sexuality issues is warranted. Finally, studies addressing the emergent healthcare needs and the prevention and elimination of healthcare disparities related to head and neck cancer would be of tremendous value to this diverse and vulnerable patient population.

The authors would like to acknowledge Mary Jo Drop-kin, PhD, RN, for her contribution to this chapter that remains unchanged from the first edition of this book.

References

Deng, J., Ridner, S.H., Dietrich, M.S., Wells, N., & Murphy, B.A. (2013). Assessment of external lymphedema in patients with head and neck cancer: A comparison of four scales. *Oncology Nursing Forum, 40,* 501–506. doi:10.1188/13.ONF.501-506

Deng, J., Ridner, S.H., & Murphy, B.A. (2011). Lymphedema in patients with head and neck cancer [Online exclusive]. *Oncology Nursing Forum, 38,* E1–E10. doi:10.1188/11.ONF.E1-E10

Duffy, S.A., Scheumann, A.L., Fowler, K.E., Darling-Fisher, C., & Terrell, J.E. (2010). Perceived difficulty quitting predicts enrollment in a smoking-cessation program for patients with head and neck cancer. *Oncology Nursing Forum, 37,* 349–356. doi:10.1188/10.ONF.349-356

Fillion, L., de Serres, M., Cook, S., Goupil, R.L., Bairati, I., & Doll, R. (2009). Professional patient navigation in head and neck cancer. *Seminars in Oncology Nursing, 25,* 212–221. doi:10.1016/j.soncn.2009.05.004

Fillion, L., de Serres, M., Lapointe-Goupil, R., Bairati, I., Gagnon, P., Deschamps, M., ... Demers, G. (2006). Implementing the role of patient-navigator nurse at a university hospital centre. *Canadian Oncology Nursing Journal, 16,* 11–17. doi:10.5737/1181912x1611117

Fox, E., Barrett-McNeil, K., Khoo, L.H., & Middleton, M. (2011). Nurse led electronic toxicity scoring in head and neck radiotherapy. *European Journal of Oncology Nursing, 15,* 112–117. doi:10.1016/j.ejon.2010.06.007

Garon, B.R., Sierzant, T., & Ormiston, C. (2009). Silent aspiration: Results of 2,000 video fluoroscopic evaluations. *Journal of Neuroscience Nursing, 41,* 178–185. doi:10.1097/JNN.0b013e3181aaaade

Haisfield-Wolfe, M.E., McGuire, D.B., Soeken, K., Geiger-Brown, J., & De Forge, B.R. (2009). Prevalence and correlates of depression among patients with head and neck cancer: A systematic review of implications for research [Online exclusive]. *Oncology Nursing Forum, 36,* E107–E125. doi:10.1188/09.ONF.E107-E125

Institute of Medicine. (2010). *The future of nursing: Leading change, advancing health.* Washington, DC: National Academies Press.

Kagan, S.H. (2009). The influence of nursing in head and neck cancer management. *Current Opinion in Oncology, 21,* 248–253. doi:10.1097/CCO.0b013e328329b819

Larsson, M., Hedelin, B., & Athlin, E. (2007). A supportive nursing care clinic: Conceptions of patients with head and neck cancer. *European Journal of Oncology Nursing, 11,* 49–59. doi:10.1016/j.ejon.2006.04.033

Liu, J., Mok, E., Wong, T., Xue, L., & Xu, B. (2007). Evaluation of an integrated communication skills training program for nurses in cancer care in Beijing, China. *Nursing Research, 56*, 202–209. doi:10.1097/01.NNR.0000270030.82736.8c

Marbach, T.J., & Griffie, J. (2011). Patient preferences concerning treatment plans, survivorship care plans, education, and support services. *Oncology Nursing Forum, 38*, 335–342. doi:10.1188/11.ONF.335-342

Mason, H., DeRubeis, M.B., Foster, J.C., Taylor, J.M., & Worden, F.P. (2013). Outcomes evaluation of a weekly nurse practitioner-managed symptom management clinic for patients with head and neck cancer treated with chemoradiotherapy. *Oncology Nursing Forum, 40*, 581–586. doi:10.1188/13.ONF.40-06AP

McLaughlin, L. (2013). Taste dysfunction in head and neck cancer survivors [Online exclusive]. *Oncology Nursing Forum, 40*, E4–E13. doi:10.1188/13.ONF.E4-E13

McLaughlin, L., & Mahon, S. (2014). A meta-analysis of the relationship among impaired taste and treatment, treatment type, and tumor site in head and neck cancer treatment survivors [Online exclusive]. *Oncology Nursing Forum, 41*, E194–E202. doi:10.1188/14.ONF.E194-E202

Moore, K.A., Ford, P.J., & Farah, P.J. (2014). "I have quality of life . . . but . . .": Exploring support needs important to quality of life in head and neck cancer. *European Journal of Oncology Nursing, 18*, 192–200. doi:10.1016/j.ejon.2013.10.010

Ogama, N., & Ogama, N. (2013). Development of an oral assessment tool to evaluate appetite in patients with head and neck cancer receiving radiotherapy. *European Journal of Oncology Nursing, 17*, 474–481. doi:10.1016/j.ejon.2012.10.010

Oncology Nursing Society. (2011). Oncology Nursing Society 2009–2013 research agenda. Retrieved from https://www.ons.org/sites/default/files/research-agenda-executive-summary-2009-2013.pdf

Oncology Nursing Society. (2014). Oncology Nursing Society 2014–2018 research agenda. Retrieved from https://www.ons.org/sites/default/files/2014-2018%20ONS%20Research%20Agenda.pdf

Paccagnella, A., Baruffi, C., Pizzolato, D., Favaro, V., Marcon, M.L., Morello, M., ... Foscolo, G. (2008). Home enteral nutrition in adults: A five-year (2001–2005) epidemiological analysis. *Clinical Nutrition, 27*, 378–385. doi:10.1016/j.clnu.2008.03.005

Putwatana, P., Sanmanowong, P., Oonprasertpong, L., Junda, T., Pitiporn, S., & Narkwong, L. (2009). Relief of radiation-induced oral mucositis in head and neck cancer. *Cancer Nursing, 32*, 82–87. doi:10.1097/01.NCC.0000343362.68129.ed

Rodriguez, C., & Rowe, M. (2010). Use of a speech-generating device for hospitalized postoperative patients with head and neck cancer experiencing speechlessness. *Oncology Nursing Forum, 37*, 199–205. doi:10.1188/10.ONF.199-205

Sharp, L., Johansson, H., Fagerström, K., & Rutqvist, L. (2008). Smoking cessation among patients with head and neck cancer: Cancer as a "teachable moment." *European Journal of Cancer Care, 17*, 114–119. doi:10.1111/j.1365-2354.2007.00815.x

Stephenson, N.L., Swanson, M., Dalton, J., Keefe, F.J., & Engelke, M. (2007). Partner-delivered reflexology: Effects on cancer pain and anxiety. *Oncology Nursing Forum, 34*, 127–132. doi:10.1188/07.ONF.127-132

Suzuki, M. (2012). Quality of life, uncertainty, and perceived involvement in decision making in patients with head and neck cancer. *Oncology Nursing Forum, 39*, 541–548. doi:10.1188/12.ONF.541-548

Wells, M., Donnan, P.T., Sharp, L., Ackland, C., Fletcher, J., & Dewar, J.A. (2008). A study to evaluate nurse-led on-treatment review for patients undergoing radiotherapy for head and neck cancer. *Journal of Clinical Nursing, 17*, 1428–1439. doi:10.1111/j.1365-2702.2007.01976.x

Williams, P.D., Piamjariyakul, U., Ducey, K., Badura, J., Boltz, K.D., Olberding, K., ... Williams, A.R. (2006). Cancer treatment, symptom monitoring, and self-care in adults: Pilot study. *Cancer Nursing, 29*, 347–355. doi:10.1097/00002820-200609000-00001

Index

The letter f after a page number indicates that relevant content appears in a figure; the letter t, in a table.